BLASTOCYST IMPLANTATION

Koji Yoshinaga

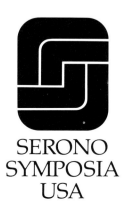

SERONO SYMPOSIA USA

Published by:
Adams Publishing Group, Ltd., 1989
Box 263   Prudential Center
Boston, MA 02199
ISBN 0-944903-04-5

Copyright by:
Serono Symposia, USA

Preface

An International Symposium on Blastocyst Implantation was scheduled to be held in December of 1988, but it did not come to pass... Because great expenditure had been made in terms of effort and planning, and since a meeting of such international scale had not been held in over a decade, we decided it would be important nonetheless to record the current status of blastocyst implantation research.

This volume, containing 30 papers contributed by the principal participants-to-be of the International Symposium, represents our current understanding of blastocyst implantation. The excellent list of the contributors to this volume is the outcome of the teamwork of the committee members: Drs. Allen C. Enders, Michael J.K. Harper, Alexandre Psychoyos, and R. Michael Roberts. As you read through this volume, you will find these papers to be of top quality in each aspect of implantation research, and I hope you will be able to grasp the trends and directions of this difficult area. The research on implantation is not easy, first, because it is impossible to carry out for human implantation. Second, even in laboratory animals the research is difficult because the phenomenon of implantation takes place in a minute area of the uterus to which one has only limited access and the amount of samples obtainable is extremely small. Finally, there is a wide range of species variation in the mode of implantation. Despite these difficulties, the researchers have been trying very hard to understand human implantation by extrapolating from the information available in different species of animals.

The recent advancements in endocrinology, cell biology, immunology, and other disciplines have revealed the importance of paracrine/autocrine mechanisms in modulating hormone action at target tissues and in intercellular communication. Because the implantation phenomenon consists of a series of successive interactions between trophoblast cells and uterine cells and/or extracellular matrix components, the studies of the paracrine/autocrine mechanisms are extremely important. Establishment of good *in vitro* model systems for implantation research is eagerly awaited because they will help to clarify these stage-specific cellular interactions. Increasing availability of extracellular matrix reagents for culture system development; of growth regulating peptide molecules and their antibodies; and of advanced cellular and molecular biological techniques is expected to advance our knowledge on implantation. We hope that this volume will be a milestone in implantation research and serve as a foundation upon which new findings and development will flourish. I would like to express my profound gratitude to all of the contributors to this book for their thoughtful commitment and dedication despite their busy schedules.

My sincere thanks go to Professor Roy O. Greep who made a special contribution to this volume. His views on science make one think about where implantation researchers are positioned within the world of science and about the significance of their contributions within the mainstream of scientific progress.

I would like to express my gratitude to Serono Symposia, USA for providing me the opportunity and pleasure of compiling the fruits of the recent progress in implantation research in this volume. The tireless assistance provided by Drs. James T. Posillico and L. Lisa Kern and their support of "the implantation project" is much appreciated. The extraordinary effort of Mr. Joseph Adams, Adams Publishing Group, Ltd., in the production of this book of an impressive quality with a marvelous speed and efficiency, deserves a special commendation.

Koji Yoshinaga

Contents

Preface iii
    Koji Yoshinaga

SPECIAL CONTRIBUTION

A Biologist Looks at Life and the Universe 1
    R.O. Greep

SECTION I: PROGRAMMING FOR IMPLANTATION

The Expansion of the Mouse Blastocyst 11
    M.H. Johnson, T.P. Fleming

The Role of Embryonic Signals in the Control of Blastocyst Implantation 17
    S. Fleming, C. O'Neill, M. Collier, N.R. Spinks, J.P. Ryan, A.J. Ammit

Embryonic Mediators of Maternal Recognition of Pregnancy 25
    R.M. Roberts, C.E. Farin, K. Imakawa

Protein and mRNA Synthesis in the Pre-implantation Rat Endometrium 31
    J. Mulholland, F. Leroy

Energy Metabolism of the Blastocyst and Uterus at Implantation 39
    H.J. Leese

SECTION II: SPECIES VARIATION. IN VITRO MODEL SYSTEMS

Species Variation, Location and Attachment of Blastocysts 47
    C.A. Finn

Comparisons of the Ability of Cells from Rat and Mouse Blastocysts and Rat Uterus to Alter Complex Extracellular Matrix In Vitro 55
    A.O. Welsh, A.C. Enders

Isolated Endometrial Cells as In Vitro Models to Study the Establishment of Pregnancy ... 75
    J.K. Findlay, L.A. Salamonsen, R.A. Cherny

Implantation: In Vitro Models Utilizing Human Tissues 83
    H.J. Kliman, C. Coutifaris, R.F. Feinberg, J.F. Strauss III, J.E. Haimowitz

SECTION III: ENDOMETRIAL INVASION

Is Trophoblastic Invasion Hemotropic in the Rabbit? 95
    L.H. Hoffman, V.P. Winfrey

Epithelial Cell Death During Rodent Embryo Implantation 105
    E.L. Parr, M.B. Parr

Fetomaternal Cell Fusion at Ruminant Implantation 117
    F.B.P. Wooding, G. Morgan

SECTION IV: DECIDUALIZATION. IMMUNOLOGICAL CONSIDERATIONS

Morphology of the Decidua 127
    P.A. Abrahamsohn

Mediators Involved in Decidualization 135
    T.G. Kennedy, P.M. Squires, G.M. Yee

Expression of mRNAs and Synthesis of Proteins by Rat Antimesometrial and Mesometrial Decidua 145
    P.G. Jayatilak, T.K. Puryear, Z. Herz, A. Fazleabas, G. Gibori

Comparative Aspects of Secretory Proteins of the Endometrium and Decidua in the Human and Non-human Primates 151
    S.C. Bell, A.T. Fazleabas, H.G. Verhage

The Barrier Role of the Primary Decidual Zone 163
    M.B. Parr, E.L. Parr

Determinants of Embryo Survival in the Peri- and Post-implantation Period 171
    D.A. Clark, G. Chaouat

Hormonal Dependence of the Metrial Gland 179
    D. Martel, M.N. Monier, V.J. De Feo, A. Psychoyos

A Possible Immunological Action Mechanism of Ovine Trophoblast Protein-1 (oTP-1) 185
    K. Yoshinaga

SECTION V: MAINTENANCE OF PREGNANCY

Role of the Mammalian Corpus Luteum in the Maintenance of Early Pregnancy 189
    R.A. Mead

Hormonal Requirement for the Establishment of Pregnancy in Primates 195
    N. Ravindranath, N.R. Moudgal

Pregnancy Deferred: An Unusual Role for Prolactin in a Marsupial 201
    L.A. Hinds

Control of the Endocrine Function of the Human Placenta by cyclic AMP 209
    G.E. Ringler, L.-C. Kao, A. Ulloa-Aguirre, J.F. Strauss III

SECTION VI: IMPLANTATION WINDOW

Biomolecular Markers for the Window of Uterine Receptivity 219
    T.L. Anderson

Scanning Electron Microscopy of the Uterine Luminal Epithelium as a Marker of the Implantation Window 225
    D. Martel, R. Frydman, L. Sarantis, D. Roche, A. Psychoyos

Uterine Receptivity for Implantation: Human Studies 231
    P.A.W. Rogers, C.R. Murphy

The Luteal Phase and Nidation in Relation to In Vitro Fertilization Treatment 239
    B. Lejeune, F. Leroy

SPECIAL CONTRIBUTION

A BIOLOGIST LOOKS AT LIFE AND THE UNIVERSE
From Inception to the Modern Era and Beyond

Roy O. Greep

Professor Emeritus
Harvard University
Cambridge, Massachusetts 02138   USA

PRIOR to retirement, I was generally asked to contribute on some specific topic within my special field of interest. Now that I am long removed from the mainstream of science and research, I am simply asked to cogitate or ruminate. This clearly signifies recognition that the days when I could claim some expertise are long gone. I am, as they say, "Over the hill," but not so far gone as to risk a commentary on implantation in concert with the world's leading authorities.

Throughout my professional career my energies were predominantly consumed by research on problems in endocrinology along with numerous editorial and administrative duties. My outlook on the physical world in which we live and the broad issues of human society were inevitably constricted. This is the price most of us pay for trying to remain competitive in one's own field of expertise. For me, that all came to an end with mandatory retirement twelve years ago. That was admittedly a wrenching experience. The way of life that I had known for forty-six years collapsed overnight. I learned that the command which was once at my beck and call belonged to the position held and not to the occupant.

It was not long before compensating opportunities for personal development and fulfillment began filling the void. It was a golden opportunity for me to learn more about the world in which we all live, including matters such as the origin of the universe, the creation of life, and man's place in nature. Questions such as these titillate the mind. After a long professional career of exploring the unknown with much satisfaction, I have been paddling about in my later years in the vast sea of the known, where learning has its own rewards. Blastocyst implantation, one of an orderly series of stages in the growth and differentiation of an individual organism, stems from a background of biological evolution extending for 3½ billion years. I shall provide some perspective on this event by a kaleidoscopic scan of prior developments in the physical world that made possible a hospitable home for living things that have multiplied in kind and quantity. Among them there ultimately appeared a unique primate *Homo sapiens* that acquired conscious behavior and cognitive ability. This multitudinous species has become king of all predators, inheritor of the earth, and spoiler of the land, sea and air. Being the only species ever able to determine its own destiny, question exists as to what the future holds. There is reason for hope and cause for concern. On all these matters I am simply an interested observer, not an authority.

From the dawn of *Homo sapiens* as conscious beings, the universe has been viewed with wonderment, mystique, and superstition. These early concepts were based on fabrications of the imagination too bizarre to merit comment here. Even the claims of Aristotle in the fourth century B.C. and of Ptolemy in the second century A.D. that the earth is stationary and at the center of the universe, though totally unfounded, were unchallenged for more than a millenium. We credit the Greeks for claiming that the earth is round not flat for the simple observation that sails on ships passing over the horizon were last to disappear.

The well-known observations of Nicholas Copernicus, Johannes Kepler, and Galileo Galilei in the 16th and 17th century yielded the first firm knowledge of the arrangement and movement of heavenly bodies visible to the naked eye or with an early telescope as in the hands of Galileo. They visualized the makeup and operation of the solar system and perceived the sun as the center of the universe. Later evidence has, of course, shown that neither the sun nor even the solar system is at the center of the universe as we now know it.

In the modern era it is the origin of the universe that is at the center of attention. It has been proposed that the universe originated 12 to 20 billion years ago as the result of an explosion of incomprehensible magnitude termed the *Big Bang*. This revolutionary concept came about as the consequence of some ground breaking observations in astronomy that need to be reviewed briefly.

In 1687, Sir Isaac Newton, one of the great intellects of all time, developed mathematical equations for the forces of gravity that control the movement of celestial bodies and explain the reason for their elliptical orbits. He firmly held that the universe is static; that it has always existed in its present state and would thus remain forever. His view dominated thinking for the next 300 years and well into the twentieth century. The Newton era came to an end with the advent of Albert Einstein, a man of equal intellectual genius whose name is synonymous with the theory of relativity. I think it is not widely understood that this theory was put forth in two parts. In 1905, Einstein, then a clerk in the patent office in Bern, Switzerland, published his theory of *restricted* or *special relativity* which dealt with the fact that nothing could ever exceed the speed of light. This had some seemingly absurd implications. For example, if an object measuring one meter were to approach the speed of light, it would shorten and eventually reach zero. A clock in a similar situation would slow to a stop at the ultimate speed and time would stand still. This was received with considerable skepticism by his German colleagues. Twelve years later Einstein (1917) published his theory of *general relativity*, the impact of which has increased our understanding of the microcosm as well as the macrocosm immeasurably. The heart of his theory is stated in that most famous equation ever devised, $E = MC^2$, where E is for energy, M is for mass, and C^2 is for the speed of light squared. In this equation, Einstein combined two separate and longstanding axioms or laws, (1) the conservation of energy and (2) the conservation of mass, by showing that they are equivalent and interchangeable. The consequences of Einstein's equation made possible his letter to President Roosevelt in 1939 urging the development of an atom bomb, an undertaking that has altered history in a manner that cannot yet be fully assessed.

Getting back to the origin of the universe, Einstein, a rather devout man, was distressed to learn that a Dutch physicist, Villem de Sitter, had used the mathematics behind his theory to predict that the universe was not static but expanding. Einstein called this "senseless," but de Sitter's predictions which were at first ignored were later to be substantiated. Indeed, in 1913 an American astronmer, Vesto Slipher, established by direct observation on a dozen galaxies that they were moving away from the observer and from each other at speeds ranging up to 2 million miles per hour. This was the first hint that the universe is expanding.

In the mid-twenties Edwin Hubble, a former champion boxer and later lawyer turned astronomer, working at the Mt. Wilson Observatory, persuaded Milton Humason, a former mule driver and self-taught astronomer, to join him in a detailed study of the expanding universe. Hubble measured the distance to many receding galaxies and Humason measured their speed of recession which ranged up to 200 million miles per hour. Both determinations were made by means of the so-called red shift. The details of that important methodology are explained briefly in the legend to Figure 1. Hubble then plotted distance against speed and demonstrated that the farther away a galaxy is the faster it moves. This discovery known as Hubble's law had far-reaching implications. An expanding universe meant that if the record of cosmological history were played backward, the universe would shrink and reach a point where the expansion began. Hubble's observations were in agreement with de Sitter's earlier predictions based on Einstein's theory of general relativity. Thus, with both observation and theory pointing to the same conclusion, astronomers everywhere began to accept the idea that the universe is expanding and did indeed have a beginning, the Big Bang. Even so, this revolutionary idea remained in need of supporting evidence.

Pursuit of this intriguing problem during the 1940's led George Gamow, Ralph Alpher, and Robert Herman to predict that the explosion of the cosmic fireball would have produced microwave radiation of a specific wave length. With this cue, Robert Dicke and James Peebles of Princeton University proposed that remanents of that radiation should still be hanging around, perhaps detectable. In 1965, Arno Penzias and Robert Wilson of Bell Telephone Laboratories, using a horn-shaped antenna in their search for a radio signal from the *Milky Way*, were troubled by a noise that came from whatever direction the

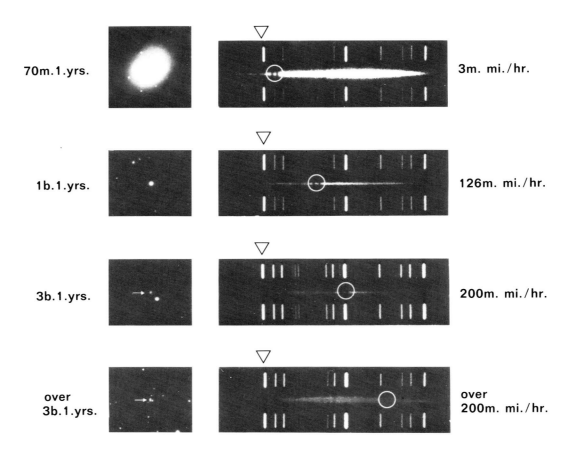

Figure 1. *This photograph shows the relationship between the red shift, distance to light source, and speed of galaxy recession. The second column from the left shows five different galaxies. Their distance in light years is at the left. The tapering bands of light in the third column show the spectrum for each galaxy. The triangles point to the superimposed markers for light from a nonmoving source. The white circles each enclose a pair of bands that stem from calcium in the light source. The position of these bands measures the red shift. The distance that these bands move to the right corresponds to the speed of recession of the light source and is proportional to its distance.*

The red shift is the result of a Doppler phenomenon that applies to light waves in the same manner as it does to sound waves. With a receding light source, the wave lengths of light increase (toward the red end of the spectrum). When the light source is moving toward the observer, the wave length decreases and shifts to the blue end of the spectrum.

As modified from Robert Jastrow, God and the Astronomers, *p. 89, W.W. Norton Company, Inc. 1978.*

receiving antenna was pointed. It also remained constant through day and night and during all seasons. Some of you will remember the account of their suspicion that pigeons nesting in the antenna might be the source of this strange reception. As you will already have deduced, the problem was not solved by doing away with the pigeons and their residue.

Indeed, it was remanents of the radiation produced at the time of the Big Bang that Penzias and Wilson were receiving and for which they were awarded the Nobel Prize in 1978. They were alerted to the probable solution to their problem by hearing about the prior work of Dicke and Peebles who received several lesser awards. That is par for the course in science, where he or she who makes the crowning achievement stands on the shoulders of those whose work helped make that achievement possible. Awards aside, the discovery of this radiation provided proof of the Big Bang origin of the universe and stands as one of the greatest discoveries of the century. Now with proof of the Big Bang in hand comes the question: When did this Big Bang occur? In other words, what is the age of the universe? Most estimates range from 15 to 20 billion years. What is more certain is that the minimum age is 12 billion years because that is the time necessary for light from the most distant galaxy observable to reach the earth. A recent newspaper account reports the discovery of an even more distant galaxy that would place the minimum age at 13 billion years, and an article in the August 19, 1988 issue of *Science* would extend that minimum to 15 billion years. It is unlikely that the exact age will ever be known, nor will the precise size and nature of the fireball just prior to the explosion. One thing certain is that the fireball was unimaginably hot and of infinite density. Victor Weisskopf, speaking last May at the American Academy of Arts and Sciences on "The Origin of the Universe," estimated the temperature at one millionth of a second after the *Primal Bang* (as he prefers to call it) to be 10,000 billion degrees Farenheit. Steven Weinberg, author of a small book entitled, *The First Three Minutes*, estimated that the temperature which is proportional to density would have registered 100 trillion degrees Kelvin at 1/100th of a second and within three minutes would have dropped to a mere one billion degrees K. Weinberg has also calculated that at 1/100th of a second, the density would have been 4000 million times that of water and others have estimated the density in grams per cubic inch at 10^{50}. These figures are literally and figuratively astronomical and beyond comprehension. On a more mundane level, they are mindful of the number of hamburgers sold each year by a certain fast-food chain, leaving aside the profit in dollars per square mile of these standard morsels. It may also help to note that of the nearly six billion inhabitants of the earth, one billion persons smoked five trillion cigarettes last year. With the tremendous temperatures existing at the time of the Big Bang, and for many thousands of years thereafter, all matter would remain in the form of nuclear particles, i.e., electrons, protons, neutrons, photons, and many others including the three quarks in each proton and neutron. Altogether there may be a hundred or more nuclear particles, some having so short an existence as a billionth of a second. Moreover, for every particle of matter there is a corresponding piece of antimatter. The actual number of nuclear particles existing at the time of the Big Bang may never be known because these conditions cannot be duplicated. Temperature is equatable with energy, and the energy needed to keep nuclear particles apart is measured in electron volts. At the time of the Big Bang, energy in the form of electron volts was of such colossal magnitude that it may never be achieved by any man-made particle accelerator and collider.

After about 300,000 years, the universe cooled to the point of permitting electrons to orbit nuclei, forming atoms of heavy hydrogen and later helium. With further cooling over a couple billion years the universe was filled with 90% hydrogen and 10% helium. Local condensations of these gases under the influence of gravity gave rise to 100 billion or more galaxies, each with a similar number of stars.

Newly forming stars soon start generating thermonuclear reactions due to fusion of hydrogen and helium and become factories for the production of different chemical elements like iron, copper, gold, silver, etc. When stars run out of hydrogen fuel they often explode, scattering their ionized chemical elements into space for incorporation into succeeding generations of stars. Most stars are comprised of 93% hydrogen, 6% helium, and 1% matter. It is the latter that is of prime importance to the human race.

There you have it. Our present universe is expanding at the rate of 5 to 10% every thousand million years and is likely to continue doing so indefinitely. The universe has cooled down to a temperature of -454° F, which is just short of absolute zero, and it is undergoing constant decompression. Should these trends ever be reversed, it can be assumed that the universe would collapse back into another fireball and complete a cycle. Should that happen, it is said that the earth would be reduced to the size of a golf ball. It is, of course, possible to speculate that the fireball for our universe came from the collapse of a previous universe. No one will ever know.

It was a result of this generation of chemicals out of the raw material of hydrogen that set the stage on the planet earth for the most fantastic happening of all time, the creation of living matter. By a most incredible happenstance, every chemical element that was needed for the creation of life was in place in the form of a chemical soup containing newly formed carbon and nitrogen-containing macromolecules. That all of these were present is evident from the fact that they are recoverable from the rocks of that period.

The earth came into existence as a molten sphere 4.6 billion years ago. By its first billionth birthday it, too, had cooled to form a surface crust that would later develop cracks forming a few large tectonic plates that literally float on the molten magma beneath. Obviously, no one knows what triggered the initiation of life, but much effort is being expended trying to duplicate that first step, and with enough progress via synthetic steps induced by electrical discharges to suggest that the goal is possible.

The earth's original atmosphere was totally lacking in oxygen and this might seem a handicap to the generation of life, but it was in fact a favoring circumstance. Oxygen without the enzymes needed for its metabolism would have been a poison. Whatever the nature of this earliest living substance may have been, it was not a complete cell but it had to have a replicating mechanism. This suggests that linear polymers of nucleic acid were present at the beginning and led to the evolution of anerobic microbes that are now a part of the fossil record. Oxygen began appearing in the atmosphere as early as two billion years ago but did not reach its present level of 20% until 400 million years ago. Since our solar system came into being 5 billion years ago the flow of energy from the sun, which is the sole support of all living things, was available at the initiation of life. Life has existed for 3.5 billion years but microbes held sole dominion over the earth for the first 2 billion years. The appearance of primitive multicellular organisms was delayed to a mere 670 million years ago. A late but crucial advance. What has happened in the meantime is so remarkable that it would be unbelievable were it not a fact that during this tick of the geologic clock millions upon millions of different species of plants and animals have evolved. It is said that 99% of all the species that ever lived have perished along the way. Among the estimated 5 million species that exist today, only 1½ million have been catalogued.

Among the intellectual triumphs that have shaped our view of the natural world, none has had a greater impact than Charles Darwin's theory on the origin of the species through evolution based on genetic variability, natural selection, and survival of the fittest. This view of life and of human origin rocked the world of thoughtful people and challenged the biblical concept of divine creation. It is strange that the idea of evolution took so long to be realized when the evidence based on comparative anatomy, embryology, and the orderly sequence of fossils found in the geologic record all pointed to that conclusion.

Evolution is now a fact of nature and reference to it as theory is a misrepresentation of the evidence now overwhelmingly compelling. Biological evolution is a one-way street on which there is no turning back. Every new species represents a positive advantage in the struggle to adapt and survive. Evolution is the sole basis of order among all plants and animals, living or extinct. The course of evolution is not predictable. The creation of humankind was not the ultimate goal of the evolutionary process. We did not arrive here by design or direction but by chance genetic mutations that favored survival among our earlier kin.

Modern students of evolution are in disagreement over the pace of the evolutionary process. Darwin contended that evolution proceeds at a fairly steady pace as the result of competition for survival among individuals of the same species. This mechanism termed "phylogenetic gradualism" or "incrementalism" still has many supporters. Over the past two decades, the field has been jolted by a new theory put forward by Stephen J. Gould and associates of Harvard University under the banner of neoDarwinism and termed "punctuated equilibrium." They propose that evolution has occurred in sudden bursts of speciation and involves entire species or groups of species rather than individuals. They hold that waves of extinction caused by harsh changes in climate or other harmful conditions left environmental voids that were soon filled by new species better able to cope. The proliferation of new species of mammals following extinction of the dinosaurs is a case in point. In an operational sense neoDarwinism is basically Darwinian evolution.

My particular interest in evolution centers on the origin of our own species. Despite much disagreement among the experts on this matter, all agree that we share a common heritage with other members of the animal kingdom. To put it simply, we are a part of, and not apart from, the natural world as many would have it. This fact, humbling to some and shocking to others, has completely altered our view of ourselves and our place in the world.

Contrary to an earlier popular notion, we did not descend from monkeys. Our closest living relatives in terms of comparative anatomy, immunology, fossil evidence, and molecular genetics are the great apes, and among them we relate most closely to the chimpanzees. In fact, we share with them 98% of our DNA. We did not, however, descend from the apes but we share with them a common ancestor that lived some 7 to 10 million years ago. Although fossil evidence for this particular ancestor has not yet been found few doubt that it will be. There are disputed claims that such an ancestral fossil may have already been found in Egypt.

The supposition is that our earliest ancestors known as hominids were in transition from tree dwelling to knuckle walking on the savannas. There are many conflicting theories as to how and why our ancestors became bipedal. All agree that this was clearly an early adaption to land dwelling with emphasis on food and feeding habits. The finding by Mary Leakey of normal appearing human footprints in volcanic ash laid down in Africa 3.6 million years ago is clear evidence that our ancestors were walking upright that long ago. By great good fortune the earliest prehuman fossil found to date is the fairly complete skeleton of a bipedal female who lived 3.5 million years ago.

She was 3 feet, 8 inches in height and is enshrined in the literature as "Lucy" for the odd reason that the Beatles' song "Lucy in the Sky with Diamonds" was playing on a nearby radio at the time of the find. Because Lucy had extra long arms for her height, reduced brain capacity and a somewhat pointed mandible, she was not classed with the genus *Homo* by her discoverer, Donald Johansen, but she was on the way. He classed her as *Australopithecus afarensis* after the region in Ethiopia, Afar, where she was found. Evidence for the presence of about half a dozen other species of this genus has been found. They were a bit ape-like in facial features.

While the focus of attention currently centers on those rare fossils of greatest age in the human lineage, fossils of more recent origin are available in abundance. Obviously, many new species came into existence and vanished leaving no successors. Thus, the human family tree is better defined as a bush than a tree. It is only the major branches that are of concern here.

The earliest specimen of the genus *Homo* found in Africa by Richard Leakey and named *Homo gracilis* dates back only 1.8 million years. As the name suggests, they were short and slender with small canines and moderate brain volume. They roamed Africa for about 200,000 years before being succeeded by *Homo erectus* believed to be the direct ancestor of *Homo sapiens*. *Erectus* was tall, muscular, skilled in making stone tools, lived in groups, and used fire. Over a period of 2 million years *Homo erectus* spread to the far corners of the earth before being succeeded by *Homo sapiens* just 100,000 years ago. It must be obvious that evolutionary progress among the early hominids had been proceeding at a very slow pace but phenomenal acceleration lay ahead. With the appearance of *Homo sapiens*, having a well-developed frontal cortex and increased evidence of cognitive ability, their human potential began to express itself. By 30,000 years ago *Homo sapiens* had taken over the European continent and met up with two other hominids of uncertain origin, the Cro-Magnons of the Levant and the Neanderthals of Germany. They were both cave dwellers and obviously considerably advanced as shown by their beautiful cave paintings. Curiously, both groups vanished with the influx of *Homo sapiens*. The Cro-Magnons were of modern build and are classified by some authors as *Homo sapiens*. The Neanderthals were, by contrast, of the muscular type and very strong. They had heavy brow ridges, walked on the outer edge of their feet, and their big toes were well apart from the others. Their extinction is regrettable in that they would have found lucrative service as linesmen in professional football. Their replacement by *Homo sapiens* possibly either by disease, combat, or hybridization coincides with the beginning of accelerating human development and the exercise of conscious behavior as signified by symbolic language inscribed on the shoulder blades of prey and on cave walls. These early *sapiens* sought shelter in caves and organized themselves into communal groups for hunting and gathering. They were rapidly becoming more human than animal. They learned to domesticate plants and animals long before the beginning of recorded history 7 or 8 thousand years ago. Once they were able to transmit information from one generation to the next by means other than genetic inheritance, they were off to the races. As Erwin Laszlo states in his new book *Evolution, the Grand Synthesis*, knowledge of human evolution is no longer genetic it is sociocultural, and cultural evolution is far more rapid than biological evolution. The critical point here is that we became the only species ever to be able to direct its own evolutionary destiny.

The engine that has been driving the evolution of human society from the beginning is technology, equitable with know-how and problem-solving. Just learning to fashion a sharp-pointed spear revolutionized the yield of food from large mammals such as the mammoth and elephant. Technology predated science by many millenia but it is now the handmaiden of science.

Today we live in an era of science and technology that has raised the standard of living by quantum leaps over the past half century. We fly through the air at close to or beyond the speed of sound. We transmit sight and sound instantaneously to any point on the globe. We enjoy the benefits of greatly improved medical care and our life expectancy has been nearly doubled in the span of a single lifetime.

These benefits have been distributed unevenly among members of the human race. The world is now divided between a small group of highly industrialized and wealthy states with low birth rates that stand in sharp contrast with a much larger number of underdeveloped nations that are adding to their distress by excessive population growth. No satisfactory means of solving this unhappy and dangerous situation wherein poverty breeds discontent has yet been found.

Members of human society are also divided on the basis of race and religion. Groups differing in skin color, language, or religious faiths all want to preserve their own cultural heritage and their sovereign status. These ethnic and religious differences have led to brutal and bloody strife throughout recorded history. I need only mention the Persian Gulf and Northern Ireland to make the point.

Threats to modern society arise from many quarters and

are of grave concern. We are depleting the earth's non-renewable resources with harmful chemicals of man-made origin. The greenhouse phenomenon has already made an appearance and loss of protection from the sun's carcinogenic radiation through damage to an overhead layer of ozone has become a looming reality. Our forests, streams, and lakes are being ravaged by acid rain, and even our oceans are being seriously threatened by ill-advised dumping therein of sewerage and all manner of hazardous wastes. Earlier I referred to man as the king of all predators. The heartless extinction of wildlife by loss of habitat and wanton killing is a sad commentary on the only species ever to acquire a conscience or appreciate the importance of balance of nature. All of these circumstances are consequences of extreme population pressure, a problem that all world leaders choose to ignore even though the threat to human welfare is second only to that of a nuclear holocaust.

Human society is obviously undergoing rapid cultural changes, the consequences of which remain in doubt. These changes include a decline in the nuclear family, cohabitation, a 50% divorce rate (till death do us part has taken on a hollow ritualistic ring), single parent families, mothers in the work place, crime in the street, millions on drugs (30 million in the U.S. alone), declining educational test scores, unruly classroom behavior, a shortage of qualified teachers, and boob tube interference with proper study habits.

Reflecting on the lessons of history, scores of other advanced cultures now reduced to buried ruins are known to have fallen by the wayside. What of our own destiny? Are we falling victim to our own excesses, wasteful habits, environmental tampering, lowering standards of moral and ethical conduct in business and in science, and yes, evangelism as well? Clearly, we are in no danger on a short-term basis, but trends are in motion that need serious attention. Surely, a better understanding of how we got here will provide some valuable insight into our future.

An old aphorism states that those who ignore history are bound to repeat it. Lessons from the history of biological evolution are not repeatable but they can reveal a lot about human nature. Lessons from sociocultural evolution are repeatable whether beneficial or otherwise. We can, therefore, return to the exercise of high moral standards in all aspects of business, science, and religion. We can stem the epidemic of procreation among the poor and the ignorant. We can stop the production of acid rain. We can stop using the ocean as a dumping place for harmful wastes. We can replant our forests. We can stop the killing of whales and other forms of wildlife. We can stop war as the means of resolving international disputes. We can control or at least reduce the use of harmful drugs. Yes, we can do all of these things, and as I stated earlier, *Homo sapiens* is the only species ever to have control of its destiny. At this point in history we can take encouragement from the fact that small gains are being made or are under serious consideration on all of these matters.

Louis Leakey, former head of the great Leakey dynasty in paleoanthropology, speaking to an audience on the desecration of the land, sea and air proclaimed that "we must save man from himself," but concluded that "time is growing dangerously short." I am neither an optimist nor a pessimist but a realist and I share that view. Laszlo is of the same opinion, "*Homo* is still alive and dominant. But he now lives within sociocultural systems that he no longer knows how to control. His future will be decided by...his ability to steer the course of their evolution."

Finally, this account would not be complete without mention of God whom many regard as creator of the firmament and of all living things. The formation of the universe and its continuing expansion based on sound physical principles seems difficult to reconcile with the biblical account whereby God created the Heavens and earth out of nothing. Another seeming discrepancy that can be accounted for by flexible interpretation involves the creation of light. On Day one God said "Let there be light" but then creation of the sun was delayed to Day four. Similarly, the Big Bang created light immediately but it was several billion years before the solar system came into existence. The Book of Genesis also reveals God's creation of man in his own image but this is so out of keeping with scientific evidence as to be incredulous and not worthy of comment before an audience of informed and intelligent people. I emphasize the distinction between intelligent and informed because there are millions of intelligent but poorly informed people who accept the word of God as the literal truth and are respected for their views. The crucial point is that religious beliefs are founded on faith whereas science is founded on verifiable factual evidence.

Science and religion have each both ennobled and endangered human life. Religious faiths of all denominations foster admirable human qualities such as goodness, compassion, and integrity. On the opposite side of that coin lies the long history of religious wars. The Bible itself contains a litany of slayings on massive scales. Then there is the Inquisition decreed by the Catholic orthodoxy against heretics. It started in the fourth century A.D., spread throughout Europe and lasted for nearly 1300 years reaching the height of unspeakable horror with the Spanish Inquisition supported by Ferdinand and Isabella. The church-appointed Inquisitors were prosecutor, judge and jury. The accused were subjected to unmerciful torture including use of the head crusher, or more often, burning at the stake. In England, the Inquisition ended in 1696 with the hanging of an eighteen-year-old medical student in Edinburgh.

That science has been of enormous benefit to human welfare is patently obvious. That it has also endangered all humankind is starkly evident by the array of intercontinental missiles capable of extinguishing life now 3½ billion years in the making.

Newton believed in God but there were serious flaws in his character. He used his elevated status to deny Gottfried Leibniz, his contemporary codeveloper of integral calculus, the right to publish. He also sought unsuccessfully to preempt and publish data provided by a competing astronomer. He castigated everyone who disagreed with his ideas and later, as Warden of the Royal Mint, he sent counterfeiters to the gallows.

When Einstein was asked if he believed in God, he said, "I believe in Spinoza's God who reveals himself in the orderly harmony of what exists, not in a God who concerns himself with the fate and actions of human beings." Einstein opposed the idea of an expanding universe until he saw Hubble's plates in 1932 and then agreed somewhat grudgingly that the universe is not static. He also opposed the idea of the Big Bang until just before his death in 1955. Believing in Spinoza's God is revealing as to Einstein's views on the Bible.

Benedictus De Spinoza, a contemporary of Sir Isaac Newton, was an independent thinker and late renaissance philosopher of great renown. He is best known for his classic work, *Ethics*. He held that the Bible "cannot prevent us from holding that to be true which our reason prompts us to believe." He also wrote, "The Bible is in parts imperfect, corrupt, erroneous, and inconsistent with itself." Spinoza was scorned for a century but the intelligent world gradually came round to his views and agreed that true religion is not something written in books but "Inscribed on the heart and mind of Man." To Spinoza, God and nature were identical. Spinoza's father, I might note, fled Portugal with his family to escape the Inquisition and took up residence in Amsterdam where Spinoza spent most of his life alone except for contact with other scholars of his time such as Descartes, Newton, and Galileo. He made a meager living grinding lenses for eyeglasses and telescopes and died at 44 due to dust inhalation from grinding lenses.

Last we have the view of Stephen Hawking, a British physicist judged to be of the same extraordinary intellectual caliber as Newton and Einstein. In his new book, *A Brief History of Time*, Hawking states that he is simply trying to "read the mind of God." For me, that is a rather tangential answer, perhaps purposely so, to a question of monumental concern to the Christian world.

As a final note, it may be well to remind ourselves that physics does not provide all the answers. Last May, Victor Weisskopf, Professor Emeritus of nuclear physics at MIT and former member of the Manhattan Project, speaking on *The Origin of the Universe*, took most of his audience by surprise in stating that to the shame of all astronomers and physicists, 90% of the universe is comprised of something called dark matter. It is invisible and its substance is unknown, but proof of its existence is beyond question.

By way of summary, I have tried to describe for you what, to me, is the drama of the unfolding history of the world, how we got here as conscious beings, and where we appear to be headed in terms of the evolution of our complex society and, therefore, of civilization itself.

SECTION I: PROGRAMMING FOR IMPLANTATION

THE EXPANSION OF THE MOUSE BLASTOCYST

Martin H. Johnson and Tom P. Fleming*

Department of Anatomy
Cambridge University
Downing Street
Cambridge CB2 3DY, United Kingdom

*Present address:
Department of Biology
Medical and Biological Sciences Building
University of Southampton
Bassett Crescent East
Southampton SO9 3TU, United Kingdom

THE formation of a fluid-filled blastocoel is an early and invariant feature of mammalian development. The process of blastocyst formation involves a rapid increase in embryonic volume without the requirement for an increase in mass; the resulting increase in size may facilitate the transfer of the embryo along the genital tract as well as the process of implantation. The process of blastocyst formation also converts a three-dimensional structure into a set of two-dimensional cell monolayers within and between which occur the critical interactions that lead to the early generation of cellular heterogeneity.

The formation of a blastocoel requires two complementary types of biological process. First, there is a requirement for the vectorial transport of fluid, which itself depends upon the development and coordinated activity of polarized cell function. Second, there must be a mechanism for preventing paracellular leakage of the transported fluid; this is provided by the development of a *zonular occludens* (tight) junction between the polarized cells and is supported by desmosomal and adherens junctions with their associated cytoskeletal elements. Both the development of polarized cell function and the development of tight junctions commence during the 8-cell stage, but neither process reaches maturity until over two cell cycles later at the late 32- to early 64-cell stage when the nascent blastocoel forms. During the intervening period, individual cells within the morula mature asynchronously, so that some achieve a full transport capacity and a tight junctional seal with their neighbors before others. The precise timing and pattern of nascent blastocoel formation will therefore vary between different embryos depending upon the degree of heterogeneity of cells within each, and this variation may influence the establishment of axes within the embryo. In this paper, we review first and briefly the evidence relating to the establishment of polarized cell function, second and more extensively the evidence relating to the establishment of a junctional seal, and third the data relating the effects of cell heterogeneity to the pattern and timing of nascent blastocyst formation.

POLARIZED CELL FUNCTION

The process by which cells first polarize and subsequently elaborate their polar features to form a mature epithelium has been the subject of two recent and detailed reviews.[1,2] Here we summarize the principal features of this process.

The earliest evidence of polarized cell organization that marks the beginning of trophectoderm formation is found at the 8-cell stage during compaction. At this stage, cell interaction, mediated at least in part by the activity of the Ca^{2+}-sensitive cell-cell adhesion molecule E-cadherin (also uvomorulin or L-CAM), leads to the setting up of a stable polar organization within each cell that is manifested primarily in the organization of the cytocortex. This cytocortical asymmetry determines secondarily the organization of the cytoskeleton, which in turn leads to a polarized organization of cytoplasmic contents. This process of polarization is regulated entirely at a post-translational level[3] and may involve the mediation of the IP_3 second messenger system.[4] Functionally, polarized 8-cells show preferential endocytotic activity apically[5] and a polarized ion flux along the long axis of each cell.[6]

During the subsequent division of each polarized 8-cell blastomere to yield a couplet of 16-cells, the axis of cytocortical polarity is retained, which gives the possibility, depending upon the orientation of the cleavage plane in relation to the axis of polarity, of either a differentiative division, in which one daughter cell is polar and the other nonpolar, or a conservative division in which both offspring are polar.[7] The different adhesive properties of the polar and nonpolar daughter cells ensure that the former enclose the latter, so that the cells differ in both inherited phenotype and relative position. During the 16-cell stage a further maturation of the polar phenotype of the outer cells occurs, involving the maturation of endocytotic trafficking and processing systems and the elaboration of a more complex cytoskeletal organization.[2] However, at this stage there is no decisive evidence to favor a major and stable heterogeneity of molecular determinants within the surface membrane of each cell, in particular, the activity of Na^+-K^+-ATPase is not restricted to the basolateral domain of the cells. Only after division to the 32-cell stage does such an activity appear in a stabilized basolateral distribution pattern, at about the same time that blastocoel formation becomes evident.[8] It seems that the process of epithelialization occurs serially and progressively, elaborating the mature phenotype over two to three developmental cell cycles.[2,9]

JUNCTION FORMATION

The earliest ultrastructural evidence of tight junction formation is the occasional focal junction at the 8-cell stage.[10,11] In succeeding cell cycles, focal junctions are detected more frequently and become organized increasingly in a linear pattern as visualized in freeze fracture, until by the blastocyst stage a complete and multi-layered zonular junction appears to be present. The recent development of molecular probes for the tight junctional proteins ZO-1[12-14] and cingulin[15] has made it possible to examine the details of junction formation more closely using biochemical and immunocytochemical approaches. We review here recent studies[16] on the process of junction formation *de novo* using monoclonal antibodies to the molecular marker ZO-1, a monomeric phospho-protein of M_r 215-225 kDa associated with the cytoplasmic face of the tight junction possibly via a short intramembranous tail.

Although immunoblotting studies show trace levels of ZO-1 protein at the 4-cell stage, immunocytochemical techniques demonstrate that surface assembly of ZO-1 initiates at the 8-cell stage, at around the time that junction formation can first be detected ultrastructurally. Studies on pairs of 8-cell blastomeres, formed by division of experimentally isolated 4-cell blastomeres, and cultured as quasi-synchronous cohorts for varying times during the 10-12 hrs of the 8-cell stage before examination, reveal few cells positive for ZO-1 prior to 6 hrs into the cell cycle, with a steep rise in the incidence of positive cells thereafter. In most cell couplets, the ZO-1 localizes in discrete spots to the contact boundary between cells (Fig. 1A), but in a few the ZO-1 is scattered apparently randomly over the whole surface of the cells. This latter pattern is seen invariably either if newly formed 8-cells are isolated and cultured singly rather than in pairs or if pairs are cultured in the absence of calcium, thereby preventing the development of more extensive intercellular contacts (Fig. 1B). The appearance of the ZO-1 is blocked almost completely if protein synthesis is inhibited. This result distinguishes ZO-1 regulation from that of most other developing contemporary features relating to cell polarization and intercellular flattening which are resistant to the effects of protein synthesis inhibition.

Taken together these observations suggest that ZO-1 production occurs contemporaneously with, and thus could be limiting for, tight junction assembly, and that cellular interactions influence strikingly the spatial patterns of junctional protein assembly *de novo*. The results of further experiments suggest that there is specificity to these cell interactions. Thus, if an 8-cell blastomere synthesizing ZO-1 is aggregated with, and flattens upon, a 4-cell blastomere lacking ZO-1, then the ZO-1 in the 8-cell is distributed randomly and is not focused to the boundary of intercellular contact with the 4-cell. If, in contrast, two 8-cell blastomeres are aggregated with, and flatten on, a 4-cell blastomere, the ZO-1 in each of the 8-cells is focused to the boundary of contact between 8-cells but is excluded from the boundary each makes with the 4-cell. This result indicates that intercellular flattening, although necessary, is not sufficient for focusing junctional proteins. Complementary competence is also required; whether of ZO-1 expression or of some other intramembranous linker molecule is the subject of investigation. It will be of interest to see whether a similar examination of cingulin distribution and regulation now under way leads to similar conclusions, or if the relative roles of each junctional protein in the assembly process are different.

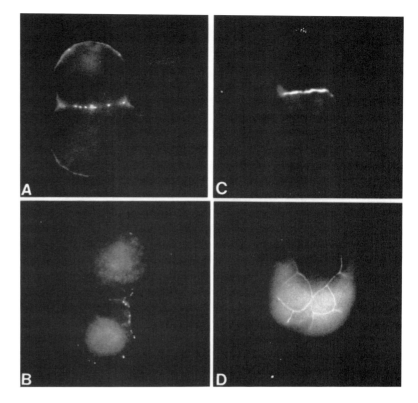

Figure 1. Cells of the early mouse embryo stained for the distribution of the tight junction associated protein ZO-1. (A) A pair of 8-cell blastomeres approximately halfway through the 8-cell stage; note that foci of ZO-1 stain only at the boundary of the interface between cells. (B) A pair of late 8-cell blastomeres that had been cultured in medium low in calcium to prevent intercellular contact; note that ZO-1 foci are not restricted to the region between the cells. (C) A pair of late 8-cell blastomeres in which the distribution of ZO-1 has become more extensive in the intercellular region. (D) A blastocyst in which contacts between adjacent trophoblast cells are stained continuously for ZO-1 (see ref. 16 for details).

Analysis of cell clusters or whole embryos at stages of development progressively later than the 8-cell stage reveals that the initially punctate distribution pattern of ZO-1 localized to the contact boundary region becomes increasingly linear (Fig. 1A,B), until by the blastocyst stage a more or less continuous linear array of ZO-1 is present between trophectoderm cells (Fig. 1C,D). It is this linear array, equivalent to the tight junctional strands,[13] that presumably gives to the trophectoderm of the blastocyst its fluid-retaining properties. It may also be the appearance of a continuous junctional array that allows the clearly delineated segregation of Na^+-K^+-ATPase to the basolateral membrane domain and thereby leads to the efficient vectorial transport of fluid into the developing blastocoelic cavity. Thus, tight junctional maturity may be the limiting component not only for the seal but also for the pump. Early in blastocyst formation, the tight junction may not perform these tasks very reliably, since there is evidence for its sporadic leakiness, with loss of blastocoelic fluid and collapse of the blastocoel.[17] Only with greater maturity does collapse become a rare event. It is likely that the efficiency with which the tight junction performs is determined by the state of development of an ancillary set of junctions, namely, the desmosomes and the adherens junctions, which may have the more mechanical function of holding firmly together trophectodermal cells under tension from the accumulating fluid.

The *adherens* junction of the early mouse blastocyst does indeed seem relatively underdeveloped. It is associated with a concentration of E-cadherin, but the details of its time of appearance and the way in which this is regulated are not well documented.[18] In contrast, a little more is known about desmosome formation, where there is evidence of structural[19] and molecular (unpublished data) immaturity during the early stages of blastocyst formation. Thus, whilst desmosomes are first evident at the 32-cell stage when the blastocoel forms,[10,11] an analysis of their molecular composition using a panel of antibodies against different desmosomal proteins and glycoproteins reveals that even by the time that blastocyst expansion has occurred the desmosomes lack the full complement of glycoprotein components. Since the glycoproteins are believed to be important for the strong adhesive properties of desmosomes, these immature desmosomes may indeed be less effective. It is also clear that, despite the rapid elaboration of a complex network of cytokeratin filaments during the 16- and 32-cell stage of development,[20] it is only after blastocyst expansion has occurred that most trophectodermal cells have well-defined patterns of cytokeratin fibers associated with the lateral boundaries between cells, again suggesting a contributory cause to the inefficiency of tight junctional function early in blastocyst expansion.

TIMING AND SITE OF BLASTOCOEL FORMATION

A number of studies have indicated that the time of blastocyst formation is related to the number of developmental cell cycles traversed, tending to occur when cells are in their sixth developmental cell cycle.[21] However, as pointed out earlier, cells within an embryo do not develop synchronously. It has been proposed that this asynchrony may be an important determinant of the site of the nascent blastocoel. This proposal has a wider developmental significance, since the site of the nascent blastocoel may mark the abembryonic pole of the embryonic:abembryonic axis[22] and so cell asynchrony might determine the spatial arrangement within the developing conceptus.

Two models have been put forward to explain how cell asynchrony might influence the site of the abembryonic pole, but one makes directly opposite assumptions to the other. Surani and Barton[22] have suggested that during the transition from 16 to 32 cells those outer cells that are relatively delayed in their progress through the cell cycles of early development will tend to become stretched by the accumulation of cells internally. Stretched cells, it is argued, will be less likely to undergo cytokinesis and are therefore more likely to become polynucleate. Since the cells at the abembryonic pole are known to be polyploid, it is suggested that the appearance of the polynucleate cells indicates premature terminal differentiation into trophectoderm and therefore identifies the first cells capable of forming and retaining blastocoelic fluid (see also Ref. 23). In contrast, an alternative model suggests that the competence to form and retain fluid is dependent simply on maturity and that this maturity will be acquired first by the most advanced cells, which will therefore mark the site of the nascent blastocoel and the abembryonic pole. Thus, both models assume that temporal heterogeneity among cells contributes to the generation of spatial heterogeneity, but each makes quite contradictory predictions.

The two models have been tested experimentally by marking the most advanced or most delayed cells within an embryo and following their fate. The results of these studies show that there is indeed a positive correlation between the position of the *earliest* dividing cells and the position of the nascent blastocoel; the notion that the delayed cells might mark this site is therefore not sustained.[24] However, the positive correlation is not absolute and invariant, a finding that need not surprise us, since, as outlined above, the processes whereby fluid is vectorially transported and retained are complex. Thus, the retention of fluid will depend upon a whole cluster of adjacent cells being competent to form a junctional seal not just on the more advanced cells that happen to have been marked. These studies have also shown that the position of the nascent blastocoel is positively correlated with the position of the abembryonic pole. However, again the correlation is not 100%, in many expanded blastocysts the site of the nascent blastocoel being adjacent to, rather than opposite, the ICM. In these embryos, it is possible that the nascent ICM is particularly firmly anchored to the overlying trophectoderm such that the blastocoel spreads around it from its initial site of formation. The reasons why this might occur are discussed in more detail by Garbutt and her colleagues.[24]

CONCLUSION

The expansion of the blastocoel marks a critical transition in the development of the conceptus. The initiation of blastocoel formation coincides with some of the earliest maturational events of the relatively atypical cleaving blastomeres. The fact that the junctional complexes and cytoplasmic organization of the early blastomeres are primitive and mature progressively over several cell cycles[2] means that the development of a capacity to form and sustain a blastocoel is correspondingly protracted. The leisurely pace of development allows temporal differences between cells to impose on the developing blastocyst spatial heterogeneities among cells.

Acknowledgment

We wish to acknowledge the financial support of the Medical Research Council and the Cancer Research Campaign.

References

1. Johnson MH, Maro B. Time and space in the early mouse embryo: a cell biological approach to cell diversification. In: Rossant J, Pedersen RA, eds. *Experimental approaches to mammalian embryonic development.* New York: Cambridge University Press, 1986:35-66.
2. Fleming TP, Johnson MH. From egg to epithelium. *An Rev Cell Biol* 1988; 4:459-485.

3. Levy JB, Johnson MH, Goodall H, Maro B. Control of timing of compaction: a major transition in mouse early development. *J Embryol Exp Morph* 1986; 95:213-237.
4. Bloom T. The effects of phorbol ester on mouse blastomeres; a role for protein kinase C in compaction? *Development* 1989; in press.
5. Fleming TP, Pickering SJ. Maturation and polarisation of the endocytotic system in outside blastomeres during mouse preimplantation development. *J Embryol Exp Morph* 1985; 89:175-208.
6. Nuccitelli R, Wiley L. Polarity of isolated blastomeres from mouse morulae: detection of transcellular ion currents. *Dev Biol* 1985; 109:452-463.
7. Johnson MH, Pickering SJ, Dhiman A, Radcliffe GS, Maro B. Cytocortical organisation during natural and prolonged mitosis of mouse 8-cell blastomeres. *Development* 1988; 102:143-158.
8. Watson AJ, Kidder CM. Immunofluorescent assessment of the timing of appearance and cellular distribution of Na/K-ATPase during mouse embryogenesis. *Dev Biol* 1988; 126:80-90.
9. Batten BE, Albertini DF, Ducibella T. Patterns of organelle distribution in mouse embryos during preimplantation development. *Am J Anat* 1987; 178:204-213.
10. Ducibella T, Albertini DF, Anderson E, Biggers JD. The preimplantation mammalian embryo: characterization of intercellular junctions and their appearance during development. *Dev Biol* 1975; 45:231-250.
11. Magnuson T, Demsey A, Stackpole CW. Characterization of intercellular junctions in the preimplantation mouse embryo by freeze fracture and thin section electron microscopy. *Dev Biol* 1978; 76:214-224.
12. Anderson JM, Stevenson BR, Jesaitis LA, Goodenough DA, Moosekar MS. Characterization of ZO-1, a protein component of the tight junction from mouse liver and Madin-Darby canine kidney cells. *J Cell Biol* 1987; 106:1141-1149.
13. Stevenson BR, Anderson JM, Bullivant S. The epithelial tight junction: structure, function and preliminary characterization. *Molec Cell Biochem* 1989; in press.
14. Stevenson BR, Siliciano JD, Moosekar MS, Goodenough DA. Identification of ZO-1: a high molecular weight polypeptide associated with the tight junction (zonula occludens) in a variety of epithelia. *J Cell Biol* 1986; 103:755-766.
15. Citi S, Sabanay H, Jakes R, Geiger B, Kendrick-Jones J. Cingulin, a new peripheral component of tight junctions. *Nature* 1988; 333:272-276.
16. Fleming TP, McConnell J, Johnson MH, Stevenson BR. Development of tight junctions de novo in the mouse early embryo: the control of assembly of the tight junction-specific protein, ZO-1. *J Cell Biol* 1989; 108:1407-1418.
17. Smith R, McLaren A. Functional test of tight junctions in the mouse blastocyst. *Nature* 1977; 267:351-352.
18. Vestweber D, Gossler A, Boller K, Kemler R. Expression and distribution of cell adhesion molecule uvomorulin in mouse preimplantation embryos. *Dev Biol* 1987; 124:451-456.
19. Jackson BW, Grund C, Schmid E, Burki K, Franke MW, Illmensee K. Formation of cytoskeletal elements during mouse embryogenesis. *Differentiation* 1980; 17:161-179.
20. Chisholm JC, Houliston E. Cytokeratin filament assembly in the preimplantation mouse embryo. *Development* 1987; 101:565-582.
21. Smith R. McLaren A. Factors affecting the time of formation of the mouse blastocoele. *J Embryol Exp Morph* 1977; 41:79-92.
22. Surani MAH, Barton SC. Spatial distribution of blastomeres is dependent on cell division order and interactions in mouse morulae. *Dev Biol* 1984; 102:335-343.
23. Soltynska MS, Balakier H, Witkowska A, Karaslewicz J. Binucleate cells in mouse morulae. *Wilhelm Roux' Arch Dev Biol* 1985; 194:173-177.
24. Garbutt CL, Chisholm JC, Johnson MH. The establishment of the embryonic-abembryonic axis in the mouse embryo. *Development* 1987; 100:125-134.

THE ROLE OF EMBRYONIC SIGNALS IN THE CONTROL OF BLASTOCYST IMPLANTATION

S. Fleming, C. O'Neill, M. Collier, N.R. Spinks, J.P. Ryan, A.J. Ammit

Human Reproduction Unit
Royal North Shore Hospital of Sydney
St. Leonards
New South Wales 2065, Australia

IMPLANTATION may be considered as a sequence of biochemical and physical interactions between the embryo and the uterus. It is an inherently complex process and involves communication between the embryo and uterus, as well as transduction of information between epithelial and stromal tissues of the endometrium. It has been most widely studied in rodents and species of agricultural importance, such as sheep. Fundamental differences in the biology of implantation exist between these two groups of animals, however. The rodents, in particular mice and rats, share broad similarities with implantation in man, although there are specific differences. The preimplantation embryo is a free-floating organism with obvious limitations for presenting physical signals to the mother. Accordingly, research has concentrated on identifying soluble factors produced by the embryo. Whilst it is now generally accepted that the embryo produces soluble luteotrophins and/or anti-luteolysins,[1-7] this review will concentrate on putative embryonic signals that influence implantation in the mouse.

In rodents, the 'rescue' of the corpus luteum occurs sometime after implantation is established, which suggests a likely differentiation between embryonic signals specific to these events. The first observed responses of the endometrium to implantation are increased capillary permeability and decidualization of stromal cells adjacent to blastocysts.[8,9] This occurs during attachment of the blastocyst and is preceded by interdigitation of microvilli and cell membrane apposition between blastocyst trophectoderm and uterine epithelium.[10,11] A decidual cell response can be elicited by a variety of agents, however, including Arachis oil and air bubbles.[11,12] This is not a nonspecific phenomenon though, since cleavage stage embryos are unable to induce decidualization.[11] Neither can a blastocyst induce this response within a uterus which is not appropriately primed hormonally.[13]

During pregnancy in mice the uterus becomes primed by pre-ovulatory estrogen and luteal progesterone. Luteal or nidatory estradiol, however, is necessary to sensitize the stromal cells to a decidual stimulus from the blastocyst. This provides a narrow 'window' for implantation, of 12-18 hours duration, after which the uterus becomes refractory and is unable to undergo decidualization.[9] Experimentally, the dose of nidatory estradiol that can be given has a critical upper limit, above which results in a totally refractive uterus.[9] Nidatory estradiol is believed to either stimulate endometrial synthesis of factors that induce blastocyst implantation,[14] or inhibit the synthesis of factors that prevent implantation.[15,16] Most recent data suggest that a combination of these mechanisms exists.[17,18] Monoclonal antibodies to progesterone block endometrial responses to deciduogenic stimuli and inhibit implantation.[19,20] Hence, both progesterone and estradiol are obligatory for implantation to occur.

EMBRYONIC SIGNALS

A number of hormones and proteins have been forwarded for consideration as embryonic signals. Criteria that may characterize a factor as an embryonic signal include synthesis and release from the preimplantation embryo, and blockade of implantation through the use of specific antagonists or antibodies to these factors. Disagreement persists, however, as to the relative importance of the various signals proposed.

Steroids

Hydroxysteroid dehydrogenases, key enzymes of steroid biosynthesis, have been detected within preimplantation embryos by histochemistry.[21,22] On this basis, it has been suggested that embryos synthesize steroids necessary for implantation. Others, however, have been unable to demonstrate the synthesis of steroids in preimplantation embryos.[23] Also, the presence of an enzyme does not necessarily mean that it is active in vivo. Nevertheless, culture of blastocysts in the presence of an anti-estrogen reduces their implantation rate on transfer to pseudopregnant hosts.[24] Recently, blastocysts have also been shown to metabolize progesterone in vitro.[25] Consequently, a role for steroids of blastocyst origin in implantation may exist, perhaps through modulation of pro-inflammatory agents at the adjacent endometrium.

Histamine

The role of histamine in implantation has been mostly studied in the rabbit and the rat. In the mouse, Dey and Johnson have proposed that blastocysts synthesize histamine through their ability to convert histidine to histamine.[26] As a working hypothesis, they suggest that embryonic histamine could stimulate endometrial prostaglandin production, so initiating implantation. In support of this, a competitive antagonist of histidine decarboxylase, DL-methylhistidine dihydrochloride, inhibits embryogenesis and implantation in the rabbit, this being reversible with concomitant administration of histidine.[27,28] Contrary to their hypothesis, decidualization in mice[29] and rabbits[30] has been found not to occur in response to histamine. Also, the trauma-induced decidual cell response in mice is merely progesterone-dependent[12] whereas estradiol is obligatory for histamine to initiate implantation in the rat.[31]

Histaminergic H-2 receptors have recently been demonstrated to activate ornithine decarboxylase in neonatal rat brain.[32] Therefore, histamine may influence implantation through the stimulation of polyamine synthesis. Consistent with this hypothesis, inhibition of ornithine decarboxylase has been shown to prevent blastocyst outgrowth in vitro whereas it may be promoted using mixed polyamines.[33] Hence, histamine may also prove to be an embryonic autacoid, yet its role in implantation remains unclear.

Prostaglandins

It has been proposed that murine blastocysts synthesize prostaglandins and, indeed, there is evidence to support this view.[4] On the other hand, Racowsky and Biggers were unable to demonstrate the synthesis of prostaglandins by mouse blastocysts.[34] Recent studies, however, using antisera to prostaglandin E_2 with immunofluorescence, have localized prostaglandin E_2 within the cytoplasm of ova through to blastocysts, both in vitro and in vivo.[35] The most intense fluorescence was observed in 8-cell and morula stages. Furthermore, this fluorescence was markedly diminished with indomethacin, an inhibitor of prostaglandin synthesis. Of interest, prostaglandin E_2 has been reported to play a major role in the hatching of blastocysts[36] and in the initiation of implantation,[37] these events being inhibited by indomethacin and other prostaglandin antagonists. Many of these studies, however, have been conducted without inhibition of uterine prostaglandins believed to participate in changes in endometrial capillary permeability. Nevertheless, prostaglandins are considered obligatory for implantation in the mouse.[4]

Stage-Specific Proteins

In mice, a high molecular weight glycoprotein was found to be synthesized and released by blastocysts prior to implantation.[38] And recently, using two-dimensional polyacrylamide gel electrophoresis, qualitative and quantitative changes in the synthesis and secretion of embryonic proteins have been identified.[39] Compared with day 4 embryos, 22 extra proteins were isolated from the conditioned medium of day 5 embryos. These were shown to be mostly glycosylated proteins and they were not detectable within the embryos, indicating their synthesis for secretion alone. Of significance was the close temporal correlation between the appearance of these proteins and subsequent changes in the synthesis of uterine proteins, consistent with their having both inhibitory and stimulatory effects. Two-dimensional gels are notoriously difficult to interpret, however, and glycosylation or phosphorylation of proteins can alter their mobility in a misleading manner.[40] Some of these proteins may be growth factors. For example, peri-implantation mouse embryos have been suggested to release transforming growth factors.[41]

Ovum Factor

An embryo-dependent immunomodulation by low molecular weight immunosuppressive proteins of ovarian and oviductal origin has been ascribed to a substance termed *early pregnancy factor* (EPF).[42,43] It is first observed within hours of fertilization and is dependent upon the continued production of a so-called *ovum factor*. Its physiological role and the validity of the rosette inhibition test,[44] by which EPF is measured, have been questioned.[45] Mice injected with conditioned medium from fertilized eggs express serum EPF activity, and it is suggested that an ovum factor induces activation of an inactive precursor.[46] An assay for ovum factor itself would help resolve the issue, and consequently, a role for ovum factor or EPF in implantation remains to be shown.

Embryo-Derived Platelet-Activating Factor

Platelet-activating factor (PAF), 1-o-alkyl-2-acetyl-sn-glyceryl-3-phosphocholine, is one of the most potent members in a family of biologically active phospholipids.[47,48] As such, it modulates increases in vascular permeability and initiates many events associated with inflammation.[49,50] Indeed, a variety of cells involved in the inflammatory response, including platelets and leucocytes, release and/or are activated by PAF.[51]

Embryo-derived PAF was first shown to be released by preimplantation mouse embryo by O'Neill in 1985.[52] Subsequently, embryo-derived PAF of both human and mouse origin was demonstrated to share structural and biochemical homology with synthetic PAF.[53,54] Preimplantation embryos of both species produce PAF within hours of fertilization and this was correlated with their ability to implant.[52,55] Furthermore, a maternal thrombocytopenia which is embryo-dependent and inducible with PAF suggests that embryo-derived PAF mediates the *maternal recognition of pregnancy*.[56] It has since become apparent that PAF of embryonic origin probably plays a crucial role in the establishment of pregnancy. These findings have been reviewed in the literature.[55,57,58]

EVIDENCE FOR THE INVOLVEMENT OF PAF IN IMPLANTATION

Autocrine Actions

There is evidence to suggest that PAF is an embryonic autacoid.[57,58] The addition of synthetic PAF to culture medium for three days was found to augment the metabolic rate of 2-cell through to blastocyst stage preimplantation embryos by 30%, with a concomitant increase in cell number.[59-61] Expanded blastocysts, cultured in this manner, were transferred to pseudopregnant recipients, control and PAF-treated embryos being placed in separate uterine horns. The implantation rate and fetal viability of embryos cultured in the presence of PAF was significantly greater than that of controls. Of interest, the embryos did not appear to undergo desensitization to the continued presence of PAF in the culture medium, and yet, higher doses of PAF proved inhibitory. This may be explained by a toxic action of PAF on the embryo at higher doses.

The mechanisms by which embryo-derived PAF exerts its actions are largely unknown. In other systems, however, PAF is known to stimulate phospholipase C, which initiates the catabolism of phosphatidylinositol with the formation of phosphatidic acid and inositol triphosphate.[62] This leads to calcium mobilization and the phosphorylation of proteins.

Paracrine Actions

Blastocyst outgrowth, considered by some to be the *in vitro* correlate of implantation[63,64] has been shown to be supported by whole serum but not by serum derived from platelet-depleted plasma.[65] This phenomenon probably reflects a requirement for platelet-derived growth factors and/or attachment factors. Indeed, a recent study demonstrates that platelet factor IV supports embryo attachment and outgrowth,[66] similar to the other heparin/heparan sulphate-binding proteins, laminin and fibronectin. Whereas laminin and fibronectin have not been observed at the apical surfaces of murine uterine epithelia,[67,68] PAF-induced platelet activation would result in the extravasation of serum and platelet-derived proteins *in vivo*. It is also conceivable that embryo-derived PAF may induce the expression of attachment factors and/or growth factors by the preimplantation embryo itself.

Actions Upon Maternal Physiology

A significant reduction in maternal platelet count from days 1-7 of pregnancy and following transfer of fertilized eggs to pseudopregnant recipients has been demonstrated in mice.[56] The latter finding was correlated with the number of viable embryos within the uterus. Parthenogenetically activated ova were also found to cause a maternal thrombocytopenia.[56] Furthermore, injection of culture medium, conditioned by embryos, was shown to induce a dose-dependent thrombocytopenia in splenectomized mice.[52] An embryo-derived PAF was identified as the factor responsible for these effects.[52,54]

Alprazolam, Iloprost, and SRI 63-441, inhibitors of platelet activation, have been shown to block PAF-induced thrombocytopenia in splenectomized mice.[69] Iloprost and SRI 63-441 also blocked implantation in pregnant mice, simultaneous administration of synthetic PAF reestablishing pregnancy rates to those of controls. In these studies, however, a poor correlation was found between the ability of these inhibitors to inhibit PAF-induced thrombocytopenia and implantation. This observation infers that PAF does not affect implantation via platelet activation alone. Circulating levels of progesterone were unaffected by these antagonists and their inhibitory effects could not be overcome with administration of estradiol, suggesting an effect other than the disruption of these nidatory steroids. Contrary to this finding, the production of progesterone by human granulosa cells *in vitro* has been found to be enhanced by the presence of PAF in the culture medium.[55] This apparent discrepancy may be due to differences between *in vivo* and *in vitro* studies.

Consistent with the effects of embryo-derived PAF in pregnancy, injection of mice with anti-platelet antiserum on days 4 and 7 of pregnancy has been found to cause thrombocytopenia and a 50% reduction in implantation rate.[70] It was also recently demonstrated that synthetic PAF injected into mature mice during diestrus, pro-estrus, or estrus induced the expression of EPF, which implies that ovum factor could be embryo-derived PAF.[71] Studies in the rat, using the specific PAF antagonist BN 52021, have also shown a dose-dependent inhibition of the implantation rate.[72]

CONCLUSIONS

In spite of the range of substances thought to act as embryonic signals for the establishment of pregnancy in the mouse, a unified concept is beginning to emerge. Implantation in this species is, in many respects, analogous to the inflammatory response and, in all likelihood, requires the participation of a number of metabolites in the arachidonic acid cascade. For example, Kennedy and Armstrong have proposed that increased endometrial vascular permeability requires two mediators;[73] prostaglandins of the E or I series to induce vasodilation, and histamine to increase vascular permeability. It would not be surprising if embryo-derived PAF were to initiate these changes in endometrial physiology. Indeed, recent studies using dispersed glandular endometrial cells removed in the secretory phase of the menstrual cycle, have demonstrated that synthetic PAF stimulates the synthesis of prostaglandin E_2 whilst slightly reducing the release of prostaglandin $F_2\alpha$.[74]

An autocrine action of embryo-derived PAF seems likely from the evidence to date. It is tempting to speculate that the production of preimplantation embryonic factors, such as stage-specific proteins, is modulated by PAF. Similarly, PAF may play a part in the activation of blastocysts prior to implantation, perhaps through the stimulation of maternal platelets to cause the release of platelet-derived growth factors. Endometrial PAF, detected in the rat and the rabbit,[75,76] may be more important in this respect. Compared to non-pregnant animals in estrus, endometrial PAF concentrations were found to rise dramatically during pregnancy, reaching maximal levels prior to implantation on day 5 and returning to control levels by day 7.[76] Of note, these levels were significantly decreased in regions apposed to the implanting embryo.

Embryo-derived PAF appears to hold a central role in the initiation of implantation as an embryonic signal of early pregnancy. It would seem likely that PAF is important at both the embryonic and the uterine level and, as such, probably modulates the activity of various other factors. Therefore, the importance of other agents reported to initiate blastocyst implantation should not be underestimated.

References

1. Heap RB, Rider V, Wooding FBP, Flint AP. Molecular and cellular signalling and embryo survival. In: *Current topics in veterinary medicine and animal science.* 1986:46-73.
2. Hearn JP. The embryo-maternal dialogue during early pregnancy in primates. *J Reprod Fert* 1986; 76:809-819.
3. Bazer FW, Vallet JL, Roberts RM, Sharp DC, Thatcher WW. Role of conceptus secretory products in establishment of pregnancy. *J Reprod Fert* 1986; 76:841-850.
4. Kennedy TG. Embryonic signals and the initiation of blastocyst implantation. *Aust J Biol Sci* 1983; 36:531-543.
5. Heap RB, Flint APF, Gadsby JE. Role of embryonic signals in the establishment of pregnancy. *Br Med Bull* 1979; 35:129-135.
6. Dey SK, Johnson DC. Embryonic signals in pregnancy. *Ann NY Acad Sci* 1986; 476:49-62.
7. Heap RB, Flint APF, Gadsby JE. Embryonic signals and maternal recognition. In: Glasser SR, Bullock DW, eds. *Cellular and molecular aspects of implantation.* New York: Plenum Press, 1981:311-326.
8. Finn CA. The biology of decidual cells. *Adv Reprod Physiol* 1972; 5:1-26.

9. Psychoyos A. Hormonal control of ovoimplantation. *Vitams Horm* 1973; 31:201-256.
10. Enders AC, Schlafke S. Comparative aspects of blastocyst-endometrial interactions at implantation. *Ciba Found Symp* 1979; 64:3-32.
11. Sherman MI, Wudl LR. The implanting mouse blastocyst. In: Poste G, Nicolson GL, eds. *The cell surface in animal embryogenesis and development.* Amsterdam: Elsevier/North Holland, 1976:81-125.
12. Finn CA, Hinchliffe JR. Reaction of the mouse uterus during implantation and deciduoma formation as demonstrated by changes in the distribution of alkaline phosphatase. *J Reprod Fert* 1964; 8:331-338.
13. Cowell TP. Implantation and development of mouse eggs transferred to the uteri of non-progestational mice. *J Reprod Fert* 1969; 19:239-245.
14. Heald PJ. Biochemical aspects of implantation. *J Reprod Fert* Suppl 1976; 25:29-52.
15. Finn CA. The induction of implantation in mice by actinomycin D. *J Endocrinol* 1974; 60:199-200.
16. O'Neill C, Quinn P. Inhibitory influence of uterine secretions on mouse blastocysts decreases at the time of blastocyst activation. *J Reprod Fert* 1983; 68:269-274.
17. Lejeune B, Dehou MF, Leroy F. Tentative extrapolation of animal data to human implantation. *Ann NY Acad Sci* 1986; 476:63-74.
18. Nieder GL, Macon GR. Uterine and oviducal protein secretion during early pregnancy in the mouse. *J Reprod Fert* 1987; 81:287-294.
19. Wright LJ, Feinstein A, Heap RB, Saunders JC, Bennett RC, Wany M-Y. Progesterone monoclonal antibody blocks implantation in mice. *Nature* 1982; 295:415-417.
20. Rider V, McRae A, Heap RB, Feinstein A. Passive immunization against progesterone inhibits endometrial sensitization in pseudopregnant mice and has antifertility effects in pregnant mice which are reversible by steroid treatment. *J Endocrinol* 1985; 104:153-158.
21. Dickmann Z, Dey SK, Gupta JS. A new concept: control of early pregnancy by steroid hormones originating in the preimplantation embryo. *Vitams Horm* 1976; 34:215-242.
22. Wu J-T, Lin GM. The presence of 17β-hydroxysteroid dehydrogenase activity in preimplantation rat and mouse blastocysts. *J Exp Zool* 1982; 220:121-124.
23. Sherman MI, Atienza SB. Production and metabolism of progesterone and androstenedione by cultured mouse blastocysts. *Biol Reprod* 1977; 16:190-199.
24. Sengupta J, Roy SK, Manchanda SK. Effect of an antiestrogen on implantation of mouse blastocysts. *J Reprod Fert* 1981; 62:433-436.
25. Wu J-T. Metabolism of progesterone by preimplantation mouse blastocysts in culture. *Biol Reprod* 1987; 36:549-556.
26. Dey SK, Johnson DC. Histamine formation by mouse preimplantation embryos. *J Reprod Fert* 1980; 60:457-460.
27. Dey SK, Johnson DC, Santos JG. Is histamine production by the blastocyst required for implantation in the rabbit? *Biol Reprod* 1979; 21:1169-1173.
28. Dey SK. Role of histamine in implantation: inhibition of histidine decarboxylase induces delayed implantation in the rabbit. *Biol Reprod* 1981; 24:867-869.
29. Humphrey KW, Martin L. Attempted induction of deciduomata in mice with mast-cell, capillary permeability and tissue inflammatory factors. *J Endocrinol* 1968; 42:129-141.
30. Hoffman LH, Strong GB, Davenport GR, Frolich JC. Deciduogenic effect of prostaglandins in the pseudopregnant rabbit. *J Reprod Fert* 1977; 50:231-237.
31. Johnson DC, Dey SK. Role of histamine in implantation: dexamethasone inhibits estradiol-induced implantation in the rat. *Biol Reprod* 1980; 22:1136-1141.
32. Rodriguez J, Toledo A, Brandner R, Rodriguez R, Sabria J, Blanco I. Histamine H_2-receptor mediated activation of neonatal rat brain ornithine decarboxylase in vivo. *Biochem Pharmacol* 1988; 37:551-4.
33. Van Winkle LJ, Campione AL. Effect of inhibitors of polyamine synthesis on activation of diapausing mouse blastocysts in vitro. *J Reprod Fert* 1983; 68:437-444.
34. Racowsky C, Biggers JD. Are blastocyst prostaglandins produced endogenously? *Biol Reprod* 1983; 29:379-388.
35. Niimura S, Ishida K. Immunohistochemical demonstration of prostaglandin E_2 in preimplantation mouse embryos. *J Reprod Fert* 1987; 80:505-508.
36. Baskar JF, Torchiana DF, Biggers JD, Corey EJ, Andersen NH, Subramanian N. Inhibition of hatching of mouse blastocysts in vitro by various prostaglandin antagonists. *J Reprod Fert* 1981; 63:359-363.
37. Holmes PV, Gordashko BJ. Evidence of prostaglandin involvement in blastocyst implantation. *J Embryol Exp Morph* 1980; 55:109-122.
38. Fishel SB, Surani MAH. Evidence for the synthesis and release of a glycoprotein by mouse blastocysts. *J Reprod Fert* 1980; 59:181-185.
39. Nieder GL, Weitlauf HM, Suda-Hartman M. Synthesis and secretion of stage-specific proteins by peri-implantation mouse embryos. *Biol Reprod* 1987; 36:687-699.
40. Cullen BR, Emigholz K, Monahan JJ. Protein patterns of early mouse embryos during development. *Differentiation* 1980; 17:151-160.

41. Rizzino A. Early mouse embryos produce and release factors with transforming growth factor activity. *In Vitro Cell Dev Biol* 1985; 21:531-536.
42. Morton H, Rolfe BE, NcNiell L, Clarke FM, Clunie GJA. Early pregnancy factor: tissues involved in its production in the mouse. *J Reprod Immunol* 1980; 2:73-82.
43. Cavanagh AC. Production in vitro of mouse early pregnancy factor and purification to homogeneity. *J Reprod Fert* 1984; 71:581-592.
44. Morton H, Hegh V, Clunie GJA. Studies of the rosette inhibition test in pregnant mice: evidence of immunosuppression? *Proc R Soc B* 1976; 193:413-419.
45. Whyte A, Heap RB. Early pregnancy factor. *Nature* 1983; 304:121-122.
46. Morton H. Early pregnancy factor (EPF): a link between fertilization and immunomodulation. *Aust J Biol Sci* 1984; 37:393-407.
47. Hanahan DJ, Kumar R. Platelet activating factor; chemical and biochemical characteristics. *Prog Lipid Res* 1987; 25:1-28.
48. Braquet P, Touqui L, Shen TY, Vargaftig BB. Perspectives in platelet-activating factor research. *Pharmacol Rev* 1987; 39:97-145.
49. Vargaftig BB, Braquet PG. PAF-acether today — Relevance for acute experimental anaphylaxis. *Br Med Bull* 1987; 43:312-335.
50. McManus LM. Pathobiology of platelet-activating factors. *Pathol Immunopathol Res* 1986; 5:104-117.
51. Braquet P, Rola-Pleszczynski M. Platelet-activating factor and cellular immune responses. *Immunol Today* 1987; 8:345-352.
52. O'Neill C. Examination of the causes of early pregnancy associated thrombocytopenia in mice. *J Reprod Fert* 1985; 73:578-585.
53. O'Neill C. Partial characterization of the embryo-derived platelet-activating factor in mice. *J Reprod Fert* 1985; 75:375-380.
54. Collier M, O'Neill C, Ammit AJ, Saunders DM. Biochemical and pharmacological characterization of human embryo-derived platelet activating factor. *Human Reprod* 1988; 3:993-998.
55. O'Neill C. Embryo-derived platelet-activating factor: a preimplantation embryo mediator of maternal recognition of pregnancy. *Dom Anim Endocrinol* 1987; 4:69-86.
56. O'Neill C. Thrombocytopenia is an initial maternal response to fertilization in mice. *J Reprod Fert* 1985; 73:559-566.
57. O'Neill C, Collier M, Ryan JP, Spinks NR. Embryo-derived platelet-activating factor. *J Reprod Fert* Suppl 1989; 37:19-27.
58. O'Neill C, Spinks NR, Ryan JP, et al. The role of platelet activating factor in early pregnancy. In: Handley DA, Saunders RN, Houlihan, Tomesch JC, eds. *Platelet activating factor in endotoxin and immune diseases.* New York: Marcel Dekker Inc., 1989; in press.
59. Ryan JP, Wiegand MH, O'Neill C, Wales RG. In vitro development and metabolism of lactate by mouse embryos in the presence of platelet activating factor (PAF) (Abstract). *Proc Austr Soc Reprod Biol* 1987; 19:47.
60. Ryan JP, Spinks NR, O'Neill C, Saunders DM, Wales RG. Enhanced rates of implantation and increased metabolism of mouse embryos cultured in the presence of platelet activating factor (Abstract). *Proc Fert Soc Austr* 1987; 6:47.
61. Ryan JP, Spinks NR, O'Neill C, Wales RG. Implantation potential and fetal viability of embryos cultured in the presence of platelet activating factor (Abstract). *Proc Austr Soc Reprod Biol* 1988; 20:47.
62. Berridge MJ, Heslop JP, Irvine RF, Brown KD. Inositol triphosphate formation and calcium mobilization in Swiss 3T3 cells in response to platelet-derived growth factors. *Biochem J* 1984; 222:195-201.
63. Bryson DL. Development of mouse eggs in diffusion chambers. *Science* 1964; 144:1351-1352.
64. Gwatkin RBL. Amino acid requirements for attachment and outgrowth of the mouse blastocyst in vitro. *J Cell Physiol* 1966; 68:335-344.
65. O'Neill C. The role of blood platelets in the establishment of pregnancy. In: Hau J, ed. *Pregnancy proteins in animals.* Berlin: Walter de Gruyter, 1986:225-233.
66. Farach MC, Tang JP, Decker GL, Carson DD. Heparin/Heparan sulfate is involved in attachment and spreading of mouse embryos in vitro. *Dev Biol* 1987; 123:401-410.
67. Wartiovaara J, Leivo I, Vaheri A. Expression of the cell surface-associated glycoprotein, fibronectin, in the early mouse embryo. *Dev Biol* 1979; 69:247-257.
68. Leivo I, Vaheri A, Timpl R, Wartiovaara J. Appearance and distribution of collagens and laminins in the early mouse embryo. *Dev Biol* 1980; 76:100-114.
69. Spinks NR, O'Neill C. Antagonists of embryo-derived platelet-activating factor prevent implantation of mouse embryos. *J Reprod Fert* 1988; 84:89-98.
70. Gasic GJ, Gasic TB. Total suppression of pregnancy in mice by post-coital administration of neuraminidase. *Proc Natl Acad Sci* 1970; 67:793-798.
71. Orozco C, Perkins T, Clarke FM. Platelet-activating factor induces the expression of early pregnancy factor activity in female mice. *J Reprod Fert* 1986; 78:549-555.
72. Acker G, Hecquet F, Etienne A, Braquet P, Mencia-Huerta JM. Role of platelet-activating factor (PAF) in the ovo-implantation in the rat: effect of the specific PAF-acether

antagonist, BN52021. *Prostaglandins* 1988; 35:233-241.
73. Kennedy TG, Armstrong DT. The role of prostaglandins in endometrial vascular changes at implantation. In: Glasser SR, Bullock DW, eds. *Cellular and molecular aspects of implantation.* New York: Plenum Press, 1981:349-363.
74. Smith SK, Kelly RW. Effect of platelet-activating factor on the release of $PGF_2\alpha$ and PGE_2 by separated cells of human endometrium. *J Reprod Fert* 1988; 82:271-276.
75. Yasuda K, Satouchi K, Saito K. Platelet-activating factor in normal rat uterus. *Biochem Biophys Res Commun* 1986; 138:1231-1236.
76. Angle MJ, Jones MA, McManus LM, Pinckard RN, Harper MJK. Platelet-activating factor in the rabbit uterus during early pregnancy. *J Reprod Fert* 1988; 83:711-722.

EMBRYONIC MEDIATORS OF MATERNAL RECOGNITION OF PREGNANCY

R. Michael Roberts, Charlotte E. Farin, Kazuhiko Imakawa

Departments of Animal Sciences and Biochemistry
University of Missouri-Columbia
Columbia, Missouri 65211 USA

PHYSIOLOGICAL recognition of the presence of an embryo by the mother occurs as a result of the production of biochemical mediators by the embryo.[1] In most mammalian species this phenomenon may provide for extended luteal function either by prevention of luteolysis, as is seen in domestic ruminants such as sheep and cattle, and/or by direct luteotropic support, as is found in the primate species where luteal function is supplemented by the production of chorionic gonadotropin. In addition to alteration of maternal ovarian function, embryonic mediators are also necessary to prepare the uterus for implantation or decidualization. Finally, since the embryo is not congenic with maternal tissues, it has been proposed that embryonic mediators must also act locally in some manner to retard maternal immune defenses. In this short paper we focus on two proteins produced by the sheep and cow conceptus respectively during the period that coincides with blastocyst expansion and initial attachment and that immediately precedes implantation. It is within this period that the corpus luteum must be "rescued" if the pregnancy is to survive.

CONCEPTUS-DERIVED PROTEINS: ROLE IN MATERNAL RECOGNITION OF PREGNANCY IN CATTLE AND SHEEP

The most commonly recognized change in maternal physiology associated with pregnancy is the extension of the functional lifespan of the corpus luteum. In sheep, the timing of the release of the embryonic signal(s) critical for luteal extension is quite specific, and first occurs between days 12 and 13 post-mating.[2,3] This phenomenon of conceptus-maternal signaling resulting in the extension of luteal function has been classically designated *maternal recognition of pregnancy*. Intrauterine infusions of conceptus homogenates or conceptus secretory proteins and intrauterine transfer of trophoblastic vesicles have been used to demonstrate that conceptus secretions are responsible for extending luteal function and that the signal(s) originates from the trophoblast layer of the developing embryo.[4-7]

In cattle, maternal recognition of pregnancy occurs between days 16 and 17 of gestation.[8,9] Similar studies to those in sheep have been used to demonstrate that embryo-derived products are responsible for extended luteal function in cattle.[9-11]

OVINE AND BOVINE TROPHOBLAST PROTEIN-1

Based on analysis of proteins secreted by cultured ovine conceptuses of different age, a protein postulated to be a primary component responsible for maternal recognition of pregnancy in the sheep has been identified.[5,7,12] Originally designated as an ill-defined factor, trophoblastin, by Martal et al.[5] and later purified and named ovine trophoblast protein-1 by Godkin et al.,[12] this protein is first produced at about day 13 of gestation and is the major

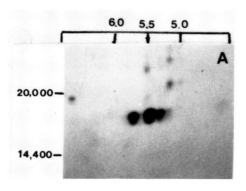
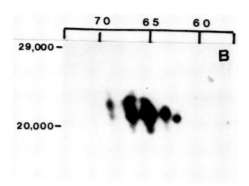

Figure 1. *Fluorographs of portions of two-dimensional polyacrylamide gels used for analysis of the polypeptides secreted by day 17 sheep conceptuses (A) or day 19 bovine conceptuses (B). The main product released by the ovine conceptus is oTP-1, shown here as a group of 3-4 isoforms. In the bovine, bTP-1 is evident as a cluster of several polypeptides (Data from Ref. 14).*

secretory product of conceptuses between day 13-21 of pregnancy[7] (Fig. 1A). It has a molecular weight of ~17,000 and consists of 3 to 4 isoelectric variants with pI's in the range 5.3 to 5.7 (Fig. 1A).

In addition, oTP-1 is the dominant translation product of mRNA isolated from ovine conceptuses on day 16 of pregnancy.[13,14] The isoforms of oTP-1 are probably derived from transcription of a set of unique oTP-1 genes and are not products of post-transcriptional modification.[15-17]

Bovine embryos also secrete a characteristic early product, designated bovine trophoblast protein-1 (bTP-1), which is immunologically cross-reactive with oTP-1 antibody.[18] BTP-1 is produced between days 16 and 33 of gestation[18,19] and shows approximately 80% predicted amino acid identity with oTP-1 based on analysis of cloned bTP-1 cDNA's.[20] Unlike oTP-1, however, bTP-1 is a glycoprotein whose seven to nine isomers (pI 6.0-6.7) are divided between two size classes of either 22,000 or 24,000 relative molecular mass (Fig. 1B).[14,21] These differences in molecular weight probably arise from differences either in the number of N-linked carbohydrate chains or in the relative degree of processing of these chains from high mannose to complex types.[14]

CLONING OF cDNA'S FOR oTP-1 AND bTP-1

Analyses of the sequence of cloned oTP-1 DNA led to the novel observation that oTP-1 may be a member of the α-interferon family of peptides.[15] Similar conclusions have been reported based on analysis of N-terminal amino acid sequences for purified oTP-1.[16,17] Based on their predicted amino acid sequences, both oTP-1 and bTP-1 are 172 amino acid polypeptides and have predicted molecular weight of approximately 19,000 Da.[15] This value does not take into account the carbohydrate on bTP-1. Ovine TP-1 and bTP-1 both show approximately 70% sequence identity with bovine α_{II}-interferon and 40-55% identity with mouse, rat, pig, bovine, and human IFN-α_I.[15,20] The α_{II} subfamily, to which oTP-1 and bTP-1 seem to belong, is a recent addition to the large alpha interferon family of proteins.[22] Its existence has been inferred only from screening human and bovine genomic DNA. In the bovine, at least a dozen α_{II} genes exist, although many may be non-functional. Unlike the IFN-α_I's, which are 166 amino acids in length, members of the α_{II} subfamily are 172 amino acids long, with a 23-residue long signal sequence. The positions of the cysteines at positions 1, 29, 99 and 139 are conserved, as is a cluster of amino acids at positions 139-146. The remainder of the primary structures of the α_{II}IFN's show about 60 to 65% identity with their α_I homologs, but the differences are scattered widely throughout the molecules and are not confined to any particular region.[22]

The nucleotide sequences of the oTP-1, bTP-1 and bovine IFN-α_I and IFN-α_{II} genes are compared diagrammatically in Fig. 2. It may be significant that oTP-1 and bTP-1 resemble each other in both amino acid sequence and in the nucleotide sequence of their genes more than bTP-1 resembles boIFN-α_{II}. Finally, the 3'-nontranslated region of bTP-1 mRNA is very different from that inferred for boIFN-α_{II} mRNA.[20] It is, therefore, possible that bTP-1 (and by inference oTP-1) form another subgroup within

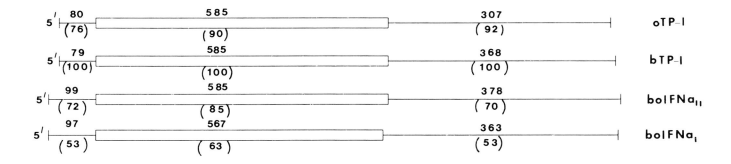

Figure 2. *Diagrammatic representation of the mRNA's for oTP-1, bTP-1, a bovine IFN-α_{II} and a bovine IFN-α_I. The numbers of nucleotides in the 5'-untranslated region (single line) within the open reading frame (boxed) and in the 3'-untranslated region are shown above each structure. Numbers in parentheses below each structure are percent identities in nucleotide sequence. The data are from Imakawa et al.*[15,20] *and Capon et al.*[22] *Note that there are several distinct mRNA's for each of the above interferons.*

the IFN gene family. Whether the large number of boIFN-α_{II} genes from the bovine genomic library recognized by Capon et al.[22] include the bTP-1 genes is unclear since their Southern analyses employed conditions that were highly stringent.

ARE oTP-1 AND bTP-1 ACTING AS FUNCTIONAL IFN'S?

The fact that oTP-1 and bTP-1 appear to belong to a subfamily of IFN's that have not been recognized as major products induced in leukocytes in response to a virus challenge has suggested they may have a specialized function. Alternatively, they may possess the normal range of biological activities of an IFN-α but be expressed only under very specialized conditions.

Recently, a considerable amount of evidence has accumulated to suggest that oTP-1 and bTP-1 have the properties of functional IFN-α's. For example, (1) intrauterine infusion of large doses of recombinant bovine interferon (IFN) α_I into ewes or heifers during the mid and late luteal phase extends the estrous cycle in a manner comparable to that following treatment with ovine or bovine conceptus secretory proteins;[23,24] (2) oTP-1 inhibits virally-induced destruction of cultured bovine kidney cells [25,26] and ³H-thymidine incorporation by Concanavalin A or phytohemagglutinin-stimulated lymphocytes *in vitro*;[26] (3) IFN-α can mimic the effects of oTP-1 protein secretion by cultured endometrial cells[28] and endometrial explants;[29] (4) recombinant bovine IFN-α will displace oTP-1 specific binding from endometrial tissue;[16,23,27] (5) IFN and oTP-1 reduce the production of PGF$_2\alpha$ and PGE by ovine endometrial cells in a comparable manner.[28] Together these results suggest that oTP-1 and bTP-1 act on the endometrium as IFN-α's. What appears to be unusual is the magnitude of their synthesis and the fact that production occurs in absence of a known viral stimulus. However, it cannot be ruled out at this stage that these trophoblast interferons have some specialized function not mediated, for example, through usual IFN-α receptors.

LOCALIZATION AND TIME OF oTP-1 AND bTP-1 SYNTHESIS

Based on biosynthetic studies[7] and Northern analysis of total cellular RNA obtained from ovine conceptuses between days 12 and 22 of gestation,[30] it appears that oTP-1 messenger RNA is present in embryonic tissues between days 13 and 18 of gestation, with highest levels present on Day 14. Detection of oTP-1 mRNA by utilizing the more sensitive technique of *in situ* hybridization leads to the conclusion that oTP-1 mRNAs are detectable at least as early as day 11 of gestation but that their levels are extremely low (C. Farin and R.M. Roberts, unpublished results). Levels of mRNA per cell appear maximal at around Day 13 and then decline to very low levels after Day 21 of pregnancy. In agreement with previous immunocytochemical studies of oTP-1 localization,[12] mRNA for oTP-1 is present in the trophectodermal layer of the conceptus. In contrast, oTP-1 mRNA is not found in underlying extraembryonic endoderm or in cells associated with the embryonic disc.

EMBRYONIC IFN'S ARE ANTILUTEOLYTIC SUBSTANCES

The action of both the ovine and bovine conceptus in initiating luteal rescue associated with maternal recognition of pregnancy appears to be primarily anti-luteolytic in nature. Luteolysis in these species results from the action of prostaglandin (PG) $F_2\alpha$ on the corpus luteum, with production of $PGF_2\alpha$ possibly occurring in response to binding of uterine receptors by oxytocin.[31] In both cattle and sheep, pregnancy is associated with a decrease in the number and frequency of luteolytic pulses of $PGF_2\alpha$ and a decrease in responsiveness of the uterine endometrium to estradiol or oxytocin-stimulated PGF production (see Ref. 1). Similarly, intrauterine infusion of secretory proteins from day 14 ovine conceptuses, which are known to contain primarily oTP-1,[7] resulted in reduced endometrial $PGF_2\alpha$ production in response to estradiol or oxytocin treatment.[33] Intrauterine infusion in cattle of secretory proteins from day 17-18 bovine conceptuses also results in suppression of uterine $PGF_2\alpha$ production in response to a luteolytic challenge by estradiol.[34] Thus, the anti-luteolytic action of conceptus signals at the time of maternal recognition of pregnancy involve a reduction in the ability of the endometrium to produce $PGF_2\alpha$.

The site of the action of oTP-1 appears to be primarily intrauterine, although specific binding of oTP-1 to luteal tissues has been reported.[12] Ovine TP-1 specifically binds to the uterine endometrium and superficial portions of the uterine glands and does not appear to be transported from the uterus.[12] Associated with its uterine binding activity, oTP-1 induces the production of specific secreted proteins by the uterine endometrium,[12,28,29,35] and reduces $PGF_2\alpha$ and PGE production by ovine epithelial cells. Interferons have been reported by others to inhibit the synthesis of prostaglandin in some mammalian cells.[36-38] Whatever the basis of the regulation of $PGF_2\alpha$ production in the uterus, it may represent a means whereby IFN-α's in general can be employed pharmacologically to delay the onset of luteolysis in sheep and cattle.

oTP-1 AND bTP-1 AS IMMUNOMODULATORS

IFN-α's are potent cellular regulatory molecules.[39] They inhibit the proliferation of a variety of cells in culture and the incorporation of [^{3}H]-thymidine into T-lymphocytes activated by mitogens or antigen. They can, in addition, enhance the differentiation of certain cells of the immune system yet inhibit the differentiation of others. Of particular interest in relation to pregnancy is their ability to delay rejection of grafts. The IFN's seem to play a complex role within the network of reactions constituting the immune response. Since the conceptus is not rejected by the maternal immune system during pregnancy yet is known to generate an immune reaction in the mother, these embryonic IFN's could play a pivotal role in controlling cell-cell interactions at the interface between maternal and conceptus tissue.

SUMMARY

Two proteins, ovine trophoblast protein-1 (oTP-1) and bovine trophoblast protein-1 (bTP-1), secreted by the trophoblast of sheep and cow conceptuses, respectively, during the period of maternal recognition of pregnancy have been implicated in reducing the synthesis or release of the uterine luteolysin prostaglandin $F_2\alpha$. Molecular cloning studies have revealed that these two products are closely related to alpha interferons (IFN-α's) and specifically to a little studied α_{II} subfamily whose members are 172 amino acids in length (in contrast to the 166 residue long IFN-α_I's). Both oTP-1 and bTP-1 possess many of the biological properties, including the antiviral activity, of IFN-α's and some of the physiological effects of oTP-1, can be mimicked by recombinant bovine IFN-α_I. It is not known how the expression of the oTP-1 genes are controlled, although they are expressed for only a limited time in early pregnancy. Their mRNA is confined entirely to cells of the trophectoderm. In addition to a role in maternal recognition of pregnancy, oTP-1 and bTP-1, because they are IFN's, may play a role in immunoregulation at the conceptus-maternal interface.

Acknowledgment

The authors thank Dr. Thomas Hansen, Dr. Mohammad Kazemi, Dr. Russell Anthony, Dr. Jay Cross and Ms. Harriet Francis for their contributions to this study, and Gail Foristal for typing the manuscript. The research was supported by NIH grant HD21896.

References

1. Bazer FW, Vallet JL, Roberts RM, Sharp DC, Thatcher WW. Role of conceptus secretory products in establishment of pregnancy. *J Reprod Fert* 1986; 76:841-850.
2. Moor RM, Rowson LEA. The corpus luteum of the sheep: Functional relationships between the embryo and the corpus luteum. *J Endocrinol* 1966; 34:233-239.
3. Moor RM, Rowson LEA. The corpus luteum of the sheep: Effect of the removal of embryos on luteal function. *J Endocrinol* 1966; 34:497-502.

4. Rowson LEA, Moor RM. The influence of embryonic tissue homogenate infused into the uterus, on the lifespan of the corpus luteum in sheep. *J Reprod Fert* 1967; 13:511-516.
5. Martal J, Lacroix MC, Loudes C, Saunier M, Wintenberger-Torres S. Trophoblastin, an antiluteolytic protein present in early pregnancy in sheep. *J Reprod Fert* 1979; 56:63-73.
6. Ellinwood WE, Nett TM, Niswender GD. Maintenance of the corpus luteum of early pregnancy in the ewe. I. Luteotropic properties of embryonic homogenates. *Biol Reprod* 1979; 212:281-288.
7. Godkin JD, Bazer FW, Moffatt J, Sessions F, Roberts RM. Purification and properties of a major, low molecular weight protein released by the trophoblast of sheep blastocysts on day 13-21. *J Reprod Fert* 1982; 65:141-150.
8. Betteridge KJ, Eaglesome ND, Randall GCB, Mitchell D, Lugden EA. Maternal progesterone levels as evidence of luteotrophic or antiluteolytic effects on embryos transferred to heifers 12-17 days after estrus. *Theriogenology* 1978; 9:86-93.
9. Northey DL, French LR. The effect of embryo removal and intrauterine infusion of embryonic homogenates on the lifespan of the bovine corpus luteum. *J Anim Sci* 1980; 50:298-302.
10. Heyman Y, Camous S, Fevre J, Mezious W, Martal J. Maintenance of the corpus luteum after uterine transfer of trophoblastic vesicles to cyclic cows and ewes. *J Reprod Fert* 1984; 70:533-540.
11. Knickerbocker JJ, Thatcher WW, Bazer FW, Drost M, Barron DH, Fincher KB, Roberts RM. Proteins secreted by day-16 to -18 bovine conceptuses extend corpus luteum function in cows. *J Reprod Fert* 1986; 77:381-391.
12. Godkin JD, Bazer FW, Roberts RM. Ovine trophoblast protein-1, an early secreted blastocyst protein, binds specifically to uterine endometrium and affects protein synthesis. *Endocrinology* 1984; 114:120-130.
13. Hanson PJ, Anthony RV, Bazer FW, Baumbach GA, Roberts RM. In vitro synthesis and secretion of ovine trophoblast protein-1 during the period of maternal recognition of pregnancy. *Endocrinology* 1985; 117:1424-1430.
14. Anthony RV, Helmer SD, Sharif SF, Roberts RM, Hansen PJ, Thatcher WW, Bazer FW. *Endocrinology* 1988; 123: 1274-1280.
15. Imakawa K, Anthony RV, Kazemi M, Marotti KR, Polites HG, Roberts RM. Interferon-like sequence of ovine trophoblast protein secreted by embryonic trophectoderm. *Nature* 1987; 330:377-379.
16. Stewart HJ, McCann SHE, Barker PJ, Lee KE, Lamming GE, Flint APF. Interferon sequence homology and receptor binding activity of ovine trophoblast antiluteolytic protein. *J Endocr* 1987; 115:R13-R15.
17. Charpigny G, Reinaud P, Huet J-C, Guillomot M, Charlier M, Pernollet J-C, Martal J. High homology between a trophoblast protein (trophoblastin) isolated from ovine embryo and α-interferons. *FEBS Lett* 1988; 228:12-16.
18. Helmer SD, Hansen PJ, Anthony RV, Thatcher WW, Bazer FW, Roberts RM. Identification of bovine trophoblast protein-1, a secretory protein immunologically related to ovine trophoblast protein-1. *J Reprod Fert* 1987; 79:83-91.
19. Godkin JD, Lifsey BJ Jr., Gillespie BE. Characterization of bovine conceptus proteins produced during the peri- and postattachment periods of early pregnancy. *Biol Reprod* 1988; 38:703-711.
20. Imakawa K, Hansen TR, Malathy PV, Anthony RV, Polites HG, Marotti KR, Roberts RM. Molecular cloning and characterization of cDNA's corresponding to bovine trophoblast protein-1. A comparison with ovine trophoblast protein-1 and bovine interferon-α_{II}. *Molec Endocr* 1989; 3:127-139.
21. Bartol FF, Roberts RM, Bazer FW, Lewis GS, Godkin JD, Thatcher WW. Characterization of proteins produced in vitro by periattachment bovine conceptuses. *Biol Reprod* 1985; 32:681-693.
22. Capon DJ, Shepard HM, Goeddel DV. Two distinct families of human and bovine interferon-α genes are coordinately expressed and encode functional polypeptides. *Molec Cell Biol* 1985; 5:768-779.
23. Stewart HJ, McCann SHE, Lamming GE, Flint APF. Evidence for a role for interferon in the maternal recognition of pregnancy. *J Reprod Fert* 1988; (Suppl 1), in press.
24. Thatcher WW, Hansen PJ, Gross TS, Helmer SD, Plante C, Bazer FW. Antiluteolytic effects of bovine trophoblast protein-one. *J Reprod Fert* 1988; (Suppl 1), in press.
25. Pontzer CH, Torres BA, Valet JL, Bazer FW, Johnson HM. Antiviral activity of the pregnancy recognition hormone ovine trophoblast protein-1. *Biochem Biophys Res Commun* 1988; 152:801-807.
26. Roberts RM, Imakawa K, Niwano Y, Kazemi M, Malathy PV, Hansen TR, Glass AA, Kronenberg LH. Interferon production by the preimplantation sheep embryo. *J Interferon Res* 1989; 19:175-187.
27. Hansen TR, Kazemi M, Keisler DH, Malathy PV, Imakawa K, Roberts RM. Complex binding of the embryonic interferon ovine trophoblast protein-1 to endometrial receptors. *J Interferon Res*, 1989; 9:215-225.
28. Salamonsen LA, Stuchbery SJ, O'Grady CH, Godkin JD, Findlay JK. Interferon-α mimics effects of ovine trophoblast protein 1 on prostaglandin and protein secretion by ovine endometrial cells in vitro. *J Endocr* 1988; 117:R1-R4.
29. Silcox RW, Francis H, Roberts RM. The effects of ovine

29. trophoblast protein-1 (oTP-1) on ovine endometrial protein synthesis are mimicked by human alpha-1 interferon. *J Anim Sci* 1988; 66(Suppl. 1):153-154.
30. Hansen TR, Imakawa K, Polites HG, Marotti KR, Anthony RV, Roberts RM. Interferon RNA of embryonic origin is expressed transiently during early pregnancy in the ewe. *J Biol Chem* 1988; 263:12801-12804.
31. McCracken JA, Schramm W, Okulicz WC. Hormone receptor control of pulsatile secretion of $PGF_2\alpha$ from the ovine uterus during luteolysis and its abrogation in early pregnancy. *Anim Reprod Sci* 1984; 7:31-55.
32. Barcikowski B, Carlson JC, Wilson L, McCracken JA. The effect of endogenous and exogenous estradiol 17β on the release of prostaglandin $F_2\alpha$ from the ovine uterus. *Endocrinology* 1974; 95:1340-1349.
33. Fincher KB, Bazer FW, Hansen PJ, Thatcher WW, Roberts RM. Proteins secreted by the sheep conceptus suppress induction of uterine prostaglandin $F_2\alpha$ release by estradiol and oxytocin. *J Reprod Fert* 1986; 76:425-433.
34. Knickerbocker JJ, Thatcher WW, Bazer FW, Barron DH, Roberts RM. Inhibition of uterine prostaglandin-$F_2\alpha$ production by bovine conceptus secretory proteins. *Prostaglandins* 1986; 31:777-793.
35. Sharif S, Harris HG, Keisler DH, Roberts RM. Correlation between release of oTP-1 by the conceptus and the production of an acidic polypeptide by the maternal endometrium (Abstract). *Biol Reprod* 1987; 36(Suppl. 1):68.
36. Dore-Duffy P, Perry W, Kuo HH. Interferon-mediated inhibition of prostaglandin synthesis in human mononuclear leukocytes. *Cellul Immunol* 1983; 79:232-239.
37. Boraschi D, Cinsini S, Bartalini M, Tagliabue A. Regulation of arachidonic acid metabolism in macrophages by immune and nonimmune interferons. *J Immunol* 1985; 135:502-505.
38. Browning JL, Ribolini A. Interferon blocks interleukin-1 prostaglandin release from human peripheral monocytes. *J Immunol* 1987; 138:2857-2863.
39. Lengyel P. Biochemistry of interferons and their actions. *Ann Rev Biochem* 1982; 51:251-282.

PROTEIN AND mRNA SYNTHESIS IN THE PERI-IMPLANTATION RAT ENDOMETRIUM

Joy Mulholland*† and Fernand Leroy†

*Department of Cell Biology
Baylor College of Medicine
Houston, TX 77030 USA

†Human Reproduction Research Unit
St. Pierre University Hospital
B-1000 Brussels, Belgium

ATTACHMENT of the blastocyst to the uterine endometrium, which initiates implantation and establishes pregnancy, can occur only during a restricted period of the reproductive cycle. The hormonal regimen necessary to prepare a non-receptive uterus to receive embryos and permit implantation was defined in studies with the ovariectomized rat.[1] This has provided a useful experimental model for studying the regulation of implantation in other mammalian species. In the rat model, a minimum of 48 hrs treatment with progesterone is required to develop a "prereceptive" uterus which will accommodate the presence of embryos. The prereceptive rat uterus is also sensitive to decidual stimuli but does not permit embryo attachment. This condition is maintained by continued daily progesterone treatment. If a single minimal dose of estradiol is administered to prereceptive rats, the uterus enters a brief receptive period, extending from 12-36 hrs after estradiol injection, during which time it is receptive to attachment of the blastocyst. Embryo attachment can now take place and luminal epithelial cells respond to this first step in implantation by transducing some signal which initiates differentiation of the cells in the subjacent stromal compartment into decidual cells. This estradiol treatment has historically been referred to as "nidatory" estradiol since it stimulates those changes in epithelial and stromal cells which characterize the receptive status of the endometrium. Receptivity is transient and nidatory estradiol apparently also regulates the transformation of a receptive endometrium to the subsequent refractory status during which embryo attachment can no longer occur. The refractory endometrium differs from the prereceptive endometrium in that embryos cannot be maintained in the lumen of refractory uteri and the tissues no longer respond to decidual stimuli. Although nidatory estradiol is apparently responsible for initiating refractoriness, this condition is maintained by continued daily progesterone treatment. Withdrawal of progesterone for 48 hrs returns the refractory uterus to a neutral condition which can again be made prereceptive with resumed progesterone treatment.[2]

While the hormonal regulation of these phases of uterine development has been established, their biochemical mechanism of action has yet to be defined at a cellular or molecular level. Currently, a receptive endometrium is defined as one which permits implantation and decidualization, a refractory endometrium as one which does not. Changes that occur in luminal epithelial cells that permit them to respond to blastocyst signals and transduce these signals to the stroma and those that prepare a stromal cell to acknowledge these signals and begin to differentiate into a decidual cell remain undisclosed. The molecular levels at which nidatory estradiol acts in epithelial or stromal cells to initiate these changes and the ways in which these disparate cell types communicate with each other to effect peri-implantation uterine development also have yet to be established.

Differences in the proteins synthesized in response to progesterone or estradiol have been implicated in mediating uterine development by several kinds of analysis. In studies that addressed the effects of nidatory estradiol on the development of the refractory state it was shown that this condition could be delayed by administration of cycloheximide within 12-16 hours of estradiol injection.[3] These results suggest that proteins synthesized within this period are involved in establishing the refractory phase. Indirect evidence that some change in the profile of proteins present is involved in initiating receptivity and refractoriness has also been provided by the investigation of RNA transcription. Treatment of ovariectomized rats with progesterone for 48 hours increased the number of RNA initiation sites in uterine chromatin five-fold. Subsequent treatment of these prereceptive animals with a nidatory dose of estradiol caused the number of transcriptional sites to drop to control levels within 4 hours of treatment.[4] Estrogen can apparently restrict progesterone-induced transcription, implying that the course of RNA, and subsequently, protein synthesis has been altered. An analysis of the effects of priming estradiol, progesterone, and nidatory estradiol on proteins synthesized by luminal epithelial and stromal cells in ovariectomized rats was previously conducted using two-dimensional gel electrophoresis to map the proteins.[5] Estrogen priming stimulated synthesis of several proteins, but production of these proteins was subsequently blocked by three days of progesterone treatment. Synthesis of a different group of proteins was induced by progesterone in both luminal epithelial and stromal cells. At 16 hrs after nidatory estradiol treatment, production of several induced proteins was repressed in both the epithelium and stroma, and this effect was more pronounced in epithelial cells. The repression of progesterone-induced proteins was accompanied by the synthesis of some of the proteins which were characteristic of the estrogen-primed uterus. But nidatory estradiol treatment failed to induce synthesis of new species of proteins at this time point. These results support the idea that nidatory estradiol acts by interfering with the progesterone-maintained pattern of protein synthesis.

Increasing effort has been directed towards the analysis of proteins in order to identify specific macromolecules which characterize the stages of hormonally directed uterine development. Most of these studies have focused on either the pre-implantation or the pregnant uterus.[6] Effectively, no studies have sought to analyze the proteins of the refractory uterus. The experiments discussed below extend previous observations to earlier and later time points which encompass the receptive period and include the early refractory phase. Because luminal epithelium and stroma differ in several responses to progesterone and estradiol,[5,7-10] the proteins synthesized by each of these endometrial compartments were again examined. The aim of these studies was to identify proteins which might distinguish prereceptive, receptive, or refractory uterine cells by examining cytosolic proteins synthesized by luminal epithelial and stromal cells during these three developmental stages and to examine the role of nidatory estradiol in the regulation of protein synthesis.

EXPERIMENTS

Mature (150 g) Wistar rats that had been ovariectomized for at least 2 weeks were treated as follows:

Day	1	2	3	4	5	6	7	8	9
Prereceptive phase	E	E	-	-	P	P	P	K	
Receptive phase	E	E	-	-	P	P	Pe	K	
Refractory phase	E	E	-	-	P	P	Pe	P	K

E is 1 μg estradiol, P is 5 mg progesterone, e is 50 ng estradiol (nidatory), K is killed.

Timing of receptive and refractory periods was determined by subjecting one group of rats at each time point to an artificial decidual stimulus and measuring the change in uterine weights after 4 days. Animals sacrificed after three injections of progesterone (day 8) and at 6 hrs after nidatory estradiol injection were considered to be prereceptive. Animals killed 12, 16, 24, and 36 hrs after nidatory estradiol provided receptive phase cells and those at 40 and 64 hrs refractory cells. Epithelial cells were isolated by the method of Bitton-Casimiri et al.[11] and stromal cells were scraped away from the myometrium with a scalpel blade. Following a 4 hour incubation in minimal essential medium containing 100 μCi/ml ^{35}S-methionine, cells were collected by centrifugation and processed for two-dimensional gel electrophoresis as described by O'Farrell.[12] Only cytosol proteins were examined in this study. Gel samples consisted of equal numbers of precipitable ^{35}S counts. Following fluorography[13] films of radiolabeled proteins were compared visually. Three to five films from different groups of animals were examined for each time point.

Proteins Synthesized During the Receptive and Refractory Periods

The two-dimensional protein patterns for luminal epithelial cells are shown in Figure 1, A-C and for stromal cells in Figure 1, D-F. Table I presents a chronology of the appearance of these proteins in luminal epithelial and stromal cells.

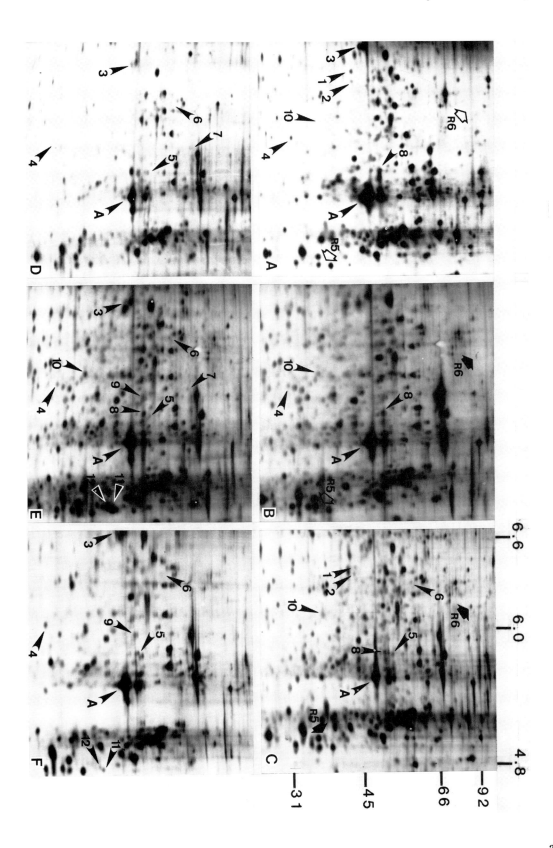

Figure 1. Profiles of proteins synthesized by epithelial (A-C) and stromal (D-F) cells during the prereceptive (A,D), receptive (B,E), and refractory (C,F) periods. The thick arrows denote the presence (dark arrows) or absence (clear arrows) of proteins R5 and R6. Molecular weight markers are noted in kDa, and the pH gradient is marked at the top of C. Protein "A" is actin.

Table I. *Proteins synthesized by uterine epithelium (UE) and stroma (US) during uterine development.*

Spot	MW*	Prereceptive UE	Prereceptive US	Receptive UE	Receptive US	Refractory UE	Refractory US
1	40.7	+	−	−	−	+	−
2	40.7	+	−	−	−	+	−
3	43.5	+	+	−	+	−	+
4	27.3	+	+	+	+	−	+
5	50.7	−	+	−	+	+	+
6	58.1	−	+	−	+	+	+
7	65.4	−	+	−	+	−	−
8	49.4	+	−	+	+	+	−
9	50.0	−	−	−	+	−	+
10	33.5	+	−	+	+	+	−
11	38.7	−	−	−	+	−	+
12	40.0	−	−	−	+	−	+

*MW is apparent molecular weight in kilodaltons.

Compared with prereceptive luminal epithelial cells, nidatory estradiol treatment resulted in the loss of three proteins (nos. 1,2,3) during the receptive period. No labeled proteins were detected which were not also present in prereceptive epithelial cells. In stromal tissue, however, all the proteins present in prereceptive cells were maintained in receptive stromal cells and, in addition, nidatory estradiol treatment induced synthesis of five proteins not labeled in prereceptive stroma (nos. 8,9,10,11,12). Thus, in the receptive period, nidatory estradiol appeared to repress synthesis of particular proteins in the luminal epithelium while inducing synthesis of new protein species in the stromal compartment.

By 40 hrs after nidatory estradiol treatment, luminal epithelial cells of the refractory uterus begin to synthesize two proteins not previously seen (nos. 5,6). Furthermore, two proteins whose synthesis was repressed during the receptive period (nos. 1,2) reappear. One protein which was synthesized throughout the prereceptive and receptive periods (no. 4) was no longer produced. In the stromal compartment, three proteins synthesized during the prereceptive and/or receptive intervals no longer appear in the gel profiles or refractory cells (nos. 7,8,10) and three of the five proteins induced during the receptive period (nos. 9,11,12) continue to be labeled in stromal cells 40 to 64 hrs after injection of nidatory estradiol. Unlike the luminal epithelium, no proteins were found in stromal cells which were synthesized only during the refractory period.

Comparison of gels of luminal epithelial and stromal proteins revealed a striking similarity between the protein patterns. Although stromal cells were rarely found in epithelial cell samples examined by electron microscopy, stromal tissue samples did contain glandular epithelium. There are relatively few glands in the rat uterus, but it is possible that these cells do contribute to the stromal cell protein pattern and may account for the similarity between stromal and epithelial cell protein profiles. This issue remains to be clarified. Analysis of stromal proteins is further complicated by the melange of cells which comprise this tissue.[14] Changes in the protein pattern undoubtedly reflect the number of each cell type present in the stromal compartment at each developmental period. Nonetheless, proteins specific to luminal epithelial or stromal cell samples were observed (Table I, nos. 1,2,7,9,11,12). One of the most notable observations from these experiments is that nidatory estradiol can affect synthesis of the same protein differentially in luminal epithelial and stromal cells. Proteins 5 and 6, for example, are only synthesized in the luminal epithelium during the refractory period, but these proteins are constitutively synthesized in stroma. Similarly, protein 8 is always synthesized by luminal epithelial cells, but is only labeled in stromal cells during the receptive period.

Effects of Nidatory Estradiol on mRNA Synthesis in Epithelial Cells

To assess the effect of nidatory estradiol on transcription, RNA was extracted from luminal epithelial cells before and after nidatory estradiol treatment and translated *in vitro* in a rabbit reticulocyte lysate system using ^{35}S-

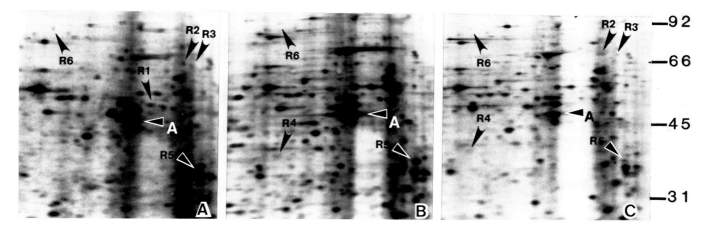

Figure 2. Profiles of proteins translated in vitro from RNA isolated from prereceptive (A), receptive (B), and refractory (C) epithelial cells. Protein "A" is actin.

methionine to label proteins.[15,16] Translation products were then separated by two-dimensional gel electrophoresis. Animals were treated as described above and sacrificed after three progesterone injections or 6, 12, 24, or 40 hrs after nidatory estradiol. The profiles of proteins synthesized in vitro from isolated mRNA transcripts are shown in Figure 2.

Messenger RNA for one protein (R1, 52.5 kDa) was present only in prereceptive epithelial cells. Two other proteins, R2 (68.8 kDa) and R3 (67.6 kDa), were synthesized from transcripts present during the prereceptive and refractory phases, but not during the receptive period. These results are again consonant with estradiol-induced repression of progesterone action, this time at the transcriptional level. Estradiol also appeared to induce synthesis of mRNA for one protein (R4, 33.2 kDa) beginning 24 hrs after treatment and continuing in refractory cells.

We attempted to test for the presence of untranslated messages by comparing the patterns of in vitro translated proteins with those of cell-synthesized proteins from the same time points. It was difficult to match minor spots on the paired gels and the analysis was further complicated by the lack of post-translational protein modifications in in vitro translated samples. However, in the case of at least two proteins, in vitro translation of isolated mRNA demonstrates that the transcripts for these proteins are present in luminal epithelial cells at times when they are not being actively synthesized. Messenger RNA for protein R5 (MW 33.8 kDa) was found in prereceptive, receptive, and refractory phase epithelial cells. In isolated luminal epithelial cells, however, this protein was only synthesized during the refractory period. Protein R6 (MW 85.0 kDa) was never found in labeled proteins of prereceptive cells, but mRNA for this protein was present in these cells.

DISCUSSION

These results support the implication that receptivity in epithelial cells is effected by estrogenic repression of progesterone-directed gene expression and subsequent loss of certain proteins rather than the stimulated synthesis of new proteins. De novo synthesis of cytosol proteins was not observed in luminal epithelial cells of the receptive uterus, but antithetically, other proteins synthesized by prereceptive cells were no longer produced during this period. Epithelial plasma membrane or secreted proteins, which would not be present in cytosol extracts, may have been induced during this period, however. Early analyses of uterine luminal proteins during gestation and in hormonally treated animals also demonstrated that progesterone and estradiol could each antagonize the other's effect on the proteins present in the lumen, but these experiments could not identify the cellular origins of the affected proteins.[17-19] Recent studies of hormonal effects of progesterone and estradiol on uterine protein secretion are attempting to define whether these hormones act at the level of transcription, translation, or post-translational modification and which cell types are being affected.[20,21] Taken together the results of many investigations of hormonal action on RNA transcription, protein synthesis, and secretion in the rat uterus emphasize that it is the interaction between progesterone and estradiol which regulates these processes in both epithelial and stromal cells as well as the interactions between these cell types which are responsible for regulating development of the peri-implantation uterus.

Nidatory estradiol appears to induce synthesis of several stromal proteins expressed during the receptive period. Since the uterine stroma of rats treated with progesterone alone is sensitive to deciduogenic stimuli,[22] the role of these proteins in overreceptivity is unclear. They may be involved in the initial stages of decidualization or initiate changes which contribute to refractoriness. It is not known if nidatory estradiol causes stromal cells *per se* to become refractory or to produce factors which render epithelial cells refractory to attachment. Protein synthesis occurring within 16 hrs of nidatory estradiol has been shown to play a role in initiating the refractory phase.[3] The proteins involved have not been identified, but our results suggest that they are of stromal origin.

Since the changes that render the epithelial cell refractory may occur at a number of levels, i.e., changes in protein synthesis, loss of apical attachment sites, changes in luminal secretions, the definition of refractoriness is complex. Currently it is defined by the inability of blastocysts to attach to the apical surface of luminal epithelial cells and the failure of the epithelium to transduce a deciduogenic stimulus to stromal cells. Blastocyst attachment also fails to occur during the prereceptive period, but since the luminal secretions of the refractory uterus are detrimental to blastocysts,[23] refractoriness is not just a return to the prereceptive state. We have not analyzed the apical membrane proteins of luminal epithelial cells or the profiles of secreted proteins, but we have demonstrated the presence of two proteins in epithelial cytosol which are produced only during the refractory period. These proteins are attractive candidates for cell-specific markers of the refractory uterus.

Defining epithelial cell refractoriness solely in terms of stromal decidualization can be misleading since several possibilities exist as to why stromal cells fail to differentiate. These include: (1) the epithelium is not transducing a signal, (2) the signal is not being acknowledged by the stromal cells, (3) the stromal cells fail to respond to the signal. Only the first possibility represents refractoriness in epithelial cells. In each of these cases, however, the epithelium is responsible for controlling stromal responses elicited via a transduced signal. This leads to the hypotheses that both receptivity and refractoriness may initially be controlled by the luminal epithelium and that both might arise from the direct action of nidatory estradiol on the epithelium. The demonstration that receptive phase stromal cells fail to respond to decidual stimuli in the absence of the luminal epithelium provides compelling evidence that the presence of the luminal epithelium is requisite to decidualization of the stroma.[24]

The possibility that these developmental phases are regulated independently in the luminal epithelium and stroma by nidatory estradiol and progesterone should also be considered. While decidualization may be induced in prereceptive stromal cells,[22] epithelial receptivity requires exposure to nidatory estradiol.[1] Thus stromal responsiveness precedes that of the epithelium. While the transition from receptivity to refractoriness is integrated in the uterine epithelium and stroma, this development need not occur concomitantly in both compartments. Estrogen induction of selective protein synthesis is receptor-mediated. The increase in stromal estrogen receptors in progesterone-treated animals[10] may facilitate their response to nidatory estradiol. During the pre-implantation period in pregnant rats, the number of epithelial estrogen receptors falls as progesterone titers rise.[25] Nevertheless, progesterone-dominated (prereceptive) epithelial cells exhibit a response to nidatory estradiol in the repression of protein synthesis.

Our analysis of *in vitro* translated proteins demonstrated that only a small percentage of the isolated epithelial cell RNA appeared to have been affected by nidatory estradiol. Similarly, quantitative but not qualitative differences were found in *in vitro* translated proteins from RNA extracted from rats treated with estrogen, progesterone, or a combination of these hormones.[26] These observations may result from the loss or degradation of RNA during isolation, differential rates of translation of messages in the reticulocyte lysate system, or low abundance of the affected mRNA. The similarity of *in vitro* translated protein patterns from RNA extracted before and after nidatory estradiol could also be accounted for if translation, as well as transcription, is being regulated by this hormonal treatment. A model which applies this hypothesis to the rat uterus has been proposed which suggests the presence of masked mRNA in prereceptive cells.[27] We have now found two proteins which support the idea that estrogen can act at the translational level to regulate uterine protein synthesis. This concept raises the possibility that transcription of mRNA for a particular protein can be induced by one hormone (i.e., progesterone) and its translation by another (i.e., estradiol).

To understand how the uterus is prepared for blastocyst attachment it will be necessary to define the cellular and molecular mechanisms through which the individual endometrial cell types develop from prereceptivity through to their refractory condition. These experiments have contributed two proteins which may serve as markers of refractoriness in luminal epithelial cells. In addition they demonstrate that epithelial and stromal cell protein synthesis can be independently regulated by progesterone and estradiol and that these hormones can affect protein syntheis at both the transcriptional and translational levels. Development of *in vitro* models for uterine epithelial cell differentiation and stromal decidualization and the analysis of cDNA libraries from prereceptive, receptive, and refractory epithelial and stromal cells should help to resolve questions addressing the inductive and repressive effects of steroid hormones on individual cell types and the regulation of the epithelial-stromal interactions which permit embryo attachment and the subsequent steps of implantation.

Acknowledgment

The proficient technical assistance of Mme. Jeannine Van Hoeck and critical review of the manuscript of Dr. Stanley Glasser are gratefully acknowledged. This research was generously funded by the Lalor Foundation and the Belgian FRSM.

References

1. Psychoyos A. Hormonal control of ovoimplantation. *Vitam Horm* 1973; 31:201-256.
2. Meyers KP. Hormonal requirements for the maintenance of estradiol-induced inhibition of uterine sensitivity in the ovariectomized rat. *J Endocr* 1970; 46:341-346.
3. Leroy F, Van Hoeck J, Lejeune B. Effects of cycloheximide on the uterine refractory state induced by nidatory estrogen in rats. *J Reprod Fert* 1979; 56:187-191.
4. Glasser SR, McCormack SA. Estrogen-mediated uterine gene transcription in relation to decidualization. *Endocrinology* 1979; 104:1112-1118.
5. Lejeune B, Lecocq R, Lamy R, Deschacht J, Leroy F. Patterns of protein synthesis in endometrial tissues from ovariectomized rats treated with estradiol and progesterone. *J Reprod Fert* 1985; 73:223-228.
6. Bell SC. Comparative aspects of decidualization in rodents and humans; cell types, secreted products and associated function. In: Edwards RG, Purdy JM, Steptoe PC, eds. *Implantation of the human embryo*. London: Academic Press, 1985:71-122.
7. Tachi C, Tachi S, Lindner HR. Modification by progesterone of estradiol-induced cell proliferation, RNA synthesis and estradiol distribution in the rat uterus. *J Reprod Fert* 1972; 31:59-76.
8. McCormack SA, Glasser SR. Differential response of individual uterine cell types from immature rats treated with estradiol. *Endocrinology* 1980; 106:1634-1649.
9. Markaverich BM, Upchurch S, McCormack SA, Glasser SR, Clark JH. Differential stimulation of uterine cells by nafoxidine and clomiphene: relationship between nuclear estrogen receptors and type II estrogen binding sites and cellular growth. *Biol Reprod* 1981; 24:171-181.
10. Martel D, Psychoyos A. Different responses of rat endometrial epithelium and stroma to induction of estradiol binding sites by progesterone. *J Reprod Fert* 1982; 64:387-389.
11. Bitton-Casimiri V, Rath NC, Psychoyos A. A simple method for separation and culture of rat uterine epithelial cells. *J Endocr* 1977; 73:537-538.
12. O'Farrell PH. High resolution two-dimensional electrophoresis of proteins. *J. Biol Chem* 1975; 250:4007-4021.
13. Laskey RA, Mills AD. Quantitative film detection of ^{3}H and ^{14}C in polyacrylamide gels by fluorography. *Eur J Bioch* 1975; 56:335-341.
14. Padykula HA. Shifts in uterine stromal cell populations during pregnancy and regression. In: Glasser SR, Bullock DW, eds. *Cellular and molecular aspects of implantation*. New York: Plenum Press, 1981:197-216.
15. Chirgwin JM, Pryzbyla AE, MacDonald RJ, Rutter WJ. Isolation of biologically active ribonucleic acid from sources enriched in ribonuclease. *Biochemistry* 1979; 18:5294-5299.
16. Pelham HRB, Jackson RJ. An efficient mRNA-dependent translation system from reticulocyte lysates. *Eur J Biochem* 1976; 67:247-256.
17. Surani MAH. Cellular and molecular approaches to blastocyst uterine interactions at implantation. In: Johnson MH, ed. *Development in mammals*. Vol. I. Amsterdam: North Holland Publ. Co., 1977:245-305.
18. Jacobs MH, Lyttle CR. Uterine media proteins in the rat during gestation. *Biol Reprod* 1987; 36:157-165.
19. Wheeler C, Komm BS, Lyttle CR. Estrogen regulation of protein synthesis in the immature rat uterus: the effects of progesterone on proteins released into the medium during *in vitro* incubations. *Endocrinology* 1987; 120:919-923.
20. Takeda A. Identification and characterization of an estrogen-inducible glycoprotein (uterine secretory protein-1) synthesized and secreted by rat uterine epithelial cells. *Endocrinology* 1988; 122:105-113.
21. Takeda A. Progesterone and antiprogesterone (RU 38486) modulation of estrogen-inducible glycoprotein (USP-1) syn-

thesis and secretion in rat uterine epithelial cells. *Endocrinology* 1988; 122:1559-1564.
22. Glasser SR, Clark JH. A determinant role for progesterone in the development of uterine sensitivity to decidualization and ovo-implantation. In: *Proceedings of the thirty-third symposium of the Society for Developmental Biology.* New York: Academic Press, 1975:311-345.
23. Psychoyos A, Casimiri V. Uterine blastotoxic factors. In: Glasser SR, Bullock DW, eds. *Cellular and molecular aspects of implantation.* New York: Plenum, 1981:327-334.
24. Lejeune B, Leroy F. Role of the uterine epithelium in inducing the decidual cell reaction. *Prog Reprod Biol* 1981; 7:92-101.
25. Glasser SR, McCormack SA. Analysis of hormonal responses of the rat endometrium by the use of separated uterine cell types. In: Kimball FA, ed. *The endometrium.* New York: Spectrum Publ. 1980:173-192.
26. Komm BS, Lyttle CR. Steroidal regulation of rat uterine *in vitro* mRNA translation products. *J Steroid Biochem* 1984; 21:571-577.
27. Leroy F, Schetgen G, Camus M. Initiation of implantation at the subcellular level. *Prog Reprod Biol* 1980; 7:200-215.

ENERGY METABOLISM OF THE BLASTOCYST AND UTERUS AT IMPLANTATION

Henry J. Leese

Department of Biology
University of York
Heslington, York, YO1 5DD
United Kingdom

THIS review focuses on the role of the uterus in the energy metabolism of the blastocyst at implantation. The emphasis will be on the rodent; specifically the rat uterus and mouse embryo.

UTERINE FLUID

Long and Evans[1] first described the accumulation of a fluid which distended the uterine lumen of rats at proestrus, was discharged at late estrus, and was absent in diestrus. Subsequent work showed that uterine fluid accumulation could be mimicked by estrogen treatment of ovariectomized rats and prevented by the concomitant administration of progesterone.[2-4]

Following mating or pseudopregnancy, the volume of the uterine lumen dramatically declines so that by day 5 of pregnancy in the rat, it is reduced to a narrow slit which closes around and clasps the blastocysts.[5] Uterine fluid volumes at this stage have to be estimated indirectly following flushing of the lumen with inert markers, and are of the order of 1-3 μl.[6]

It is surprising that little is known about the ionic basis of uterine fluid secretion. In a pioneering paper, Levin and Edwards,[7] showed that proestrus fluid was a secretion rather than a simple transudate of serum, and that the epithelial cells of the endometrium were most likely involved in its formation. The potential difference between the lumen and the serosal surface of an isolated preparation of the uterus at proestrus was 4.3 ± 0.9 mV. A similar value of 4.41 ± 0.54 mV has been recorded in my laboratory[10] using a vascular perfusion preparation based on that applied to the rabbit oviduct.[8] On days 4 and 5 of pregnancy, the potential difference falls to 2.64 and 1.23 mV, respectively.[9] This suggests that the uterine epithelium is more permeable to ions and possibly nonelectrolytes at this time. On the basis of an analysis of uterine fluid at proestrus, Levin and Edwards[7] considered that potassium and chloride ions were actively secreted into the lumen, while sodium ions were reabsorbed. To the best of my knowledge, these observations have never been followed up to provide a comprehensive picture of the ion fluxes across the uterine wall.

The organic composition of uterine secretions, particularly at proestrus, has been described for a number of species.[10-13] Glucose is the major free sugar in uterine fluid of the rat, rabbit, cow, ewe, pig, and human. It is present in rat proestrus uterine fluid at a concentration of 0.92 mM.[9] Fructose has been detected in uterine flushings from pigs during estrus, in uterine flushings from pregnant roe deer during blastocyst elongation and implantation,[14] and in rabbits, cows, and the woman.[15] Intriguingly, Zavy and colleagues[16] found that the porcine conceptus could itself produce fructose between days 14 and 18 of pregnancy, which they speculated might be channeled into the pentose phosphate pathway to provide nucleic acid precursors and NADPH for fatty acid biosynthesis. Fructose originating from seminal plasma is, of course, present in the uterine lumen of rodents immedi-

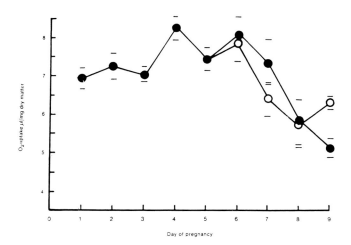

Figure 1. *Oxygen consumption per unit dry weight of uterine tissue from the pregnant rat during early pregnancy. After day 5, the tissue was divided into implanted and non-implanted areas. Each point represents the mean from 4-6 animals. Horizontal lines indicate standard errors of the mean.*
● *whole uterine tissue to day 5 and implanted areas thereafter.*
○ *non-implanted tissue.*
Reprinted by permission from: Surani MAH and Heald PJ. Acta Endocrinologica, 66, 19 (1971).

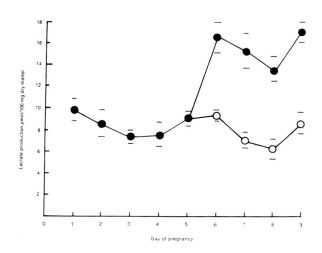

Figure 2. *Lactic acid production per unit dry matter, of the uterus of pregnant rats. Details as described in Fig. 1.*
● *whole uterine tissue to day 5 and implantation sites thereafter.*
○ *non-implanted tissue.*
Reproduced by permission from: Surani MAH and Heald PJ. Acta Endocrinologica 66, 22 (1971).

ately following mating, though it is consumed by spermatozoa at a lower rate than glucose.[17]

UTERINE METABOLISM

The oxygen uptake and glucose utilization of uterine tissue from the pregnant rat has been widely studied.[18] Of particular interest is the paper by Surani and Heald[19] who compared the oxygen consumption and lactic acid production of implanted and non-implanted areas of the rat uterus from days 1-9 of pregnancy. The results are shown in Figures 1 and 2.

The oxygen uptake was constant on days 1-3 before increasing slightly on day 4. There was a pronounced decrease in the QO_2 of both implanted and non-implanted sites from day 6 onward.

In contrast, lactic acid production from glucose by the implanted sites was markedly elevated above that of non-implanted sites on days 6-9. While studies of this type may be criticized for failing to distinguish between myometrial and endometrial metabolism, they do suggest that the oxygen supply to the decidual tissue may be reduced at these early stages. It may be significant, as first described by Krehbiel,[20] that glycogen, which could act as a substrate for lactate production, appears transiently in the primary decidual zone during the early implantation stages.

EMBRYO METABOLISM

During their early preimplantation stages, the embryos of the mouse, rabbit, and human oxidize pyruvic acid in preference to glucose.[21-23] In the mouse, glucose as sole energy source is unable to support development until the 8-cell stage. My colleague David Gardner has measured the uptake of glucose and the formation of lactic acid by single mouse embryos using an ultramicrofluorometric technique.[24] The results are shown in Figures 3 and 4.

The proportions of glucose uptake accounted for by lactate formation at the 2-cell, 8-cell, and blastocyst stages were 25% and 40%, respectively.[25] Nieder and Weitlauf[26] reported a figure of 80% of glucose converted to lactate for delayed and reactivated mouse blastocysts.

Lactate production by post-implantation mouse embryos aged 6-9 days post-coitum was investigated by Clough and Whittingham.[27] The embryos were removed from the

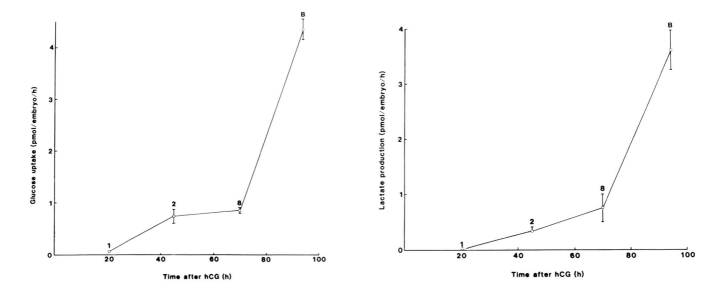

Figures 3 and 4. The uptake of 1 mM glucose (Fig. 3, left) and the formation of lactic acid (Fig. 4, right) by 1-cell (1), 2-cell (2), 8-cell (8) embryos and blastocysts (B) from the mouse. Values are mean ± standard errors of the mean of six embryos. Redrawn from DK Gardner and JH Leese, Development (in press). Reproduced with permission. Company of Biologists Ltd., Cambridge, UK.

uterus and cultured individually for 1 hour in the presence of 5 mM glucose. At each stage, more than 90% of the glucose catabolized was converted to lactate even though the embryos were cultured in medium gassed with 20% oxygen. Ellington[28] has recently shown that the energy metabolism of the rat embryo between 9.5 and 10.5 days is also characterized by high rates of glycolysis with 100% of the glucose taken up accounted for by lactate formation.

Figure 5, taken from Clough,[29] summarizes the profile of energy metabolism in early rodent embryos.

The question arises as to whether these *in vitro* studies are indicative of embryo metabolism during the peri-implantation period *in vivo*. In order to answer this question, it is necessary to consider the microvasculature of the rodent uterus at implantation.

Uterine Microvasculature

The earliest response to deciduogenic stimuli is an increase in the permeability of the endometrial capillaries. This phenomenon may be visualized as the distinct blue spots following the intravascular injection of Evans' or Ponta-mine blue dye. Evans' blue binds strongly to serum albumin, and the blue areas are indicative of local edema as macromolecules, such as albumin, leak into the surrounding tissue. The reaction may first be elicited in the rat on the evening of day 5 post-coitus.[30] It is, however, 20 hrs later that the first decidual cells appear. Local edema will increase the distance between capillaries and might therefore limit the diffusion of oxygen, predisposing the embryo to the typically anerobic metabolism observed *in vitro*.

Further evidence for the *in vitro* pattern of metabolism being a reflection of that *in vivo* lies in the work of Rogers and co-workers on the microvascular anatomy of the rat uterus at implantation.[31-33] Using the technique of microvascular corrosion casting, they were able to produce a 3-dimensional replica of the vasculature immediately surrounding the implanting rat blastocyst on day 6 of pregnancy.

In addition to the increased permeability of the endometrium in the vicinity of the implanting blastocysts, it was found that the center of the sites were characterized by the *absence* of patent capillaries in an area approximately 420 μ long by 210 μ in diameter. The size and location of this space corresponded to the primary decidual zone seen in light microscope sections taken on day 6 of pregnancy. The phenomena had previously been observed in 1937 by Krehbiel[20] who noted that:

"the primary decidual zone is comparatively free of prominent capillaries. . .".

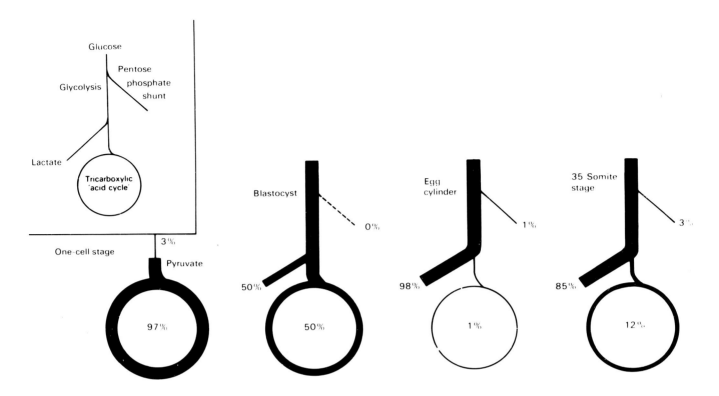

Figure 5. *Diagrammatic summary of energy metabolism in rodent embryos. The relative amounts of the major substrate metabolized via different pathways, shown in the inset, are indicated by the thickness of the lines. Reprinted by permission from:* Biochemical Society Transactions *13, 78 Copyright © (1985). The Biochemical Society, London.*

Krehbiel's observation has, however, tended to be ignored.

If the implanting blastocyst is surrounded by a region largely devoid of capillaries, it would readily explain the dependence of the embryo on the conversion of glucose to lactate in order to obtain its supply of ATP.

Furthermore, Rogers and co-workers speculate that:

"[Firstly]... it is possible that the degeneration and sloughing of the uterine epithelium in the region of the blastocyst on the morning of Day 7 or the subsequent breaching of the basement membrane and the invasion of the stromal tissue by the trophoblast are due, in part at least, to an initial local reduction in blood supply. Secondly, it may be that a reduced blood supply at implantation is involved in the process whereby the implanting blastocyst gains an early immunological privilege from the mother."[33]

Whether or not the implanting blastocyst converts glucose to lactate in response to a hypoxic environment, a high rate of glycolysis *in vitro* is characteristic of other normal and transformed cells, especially those which divide rapidly;[34] indeed, Warburg[35] proposed that the basis of malignancy was the large increase in glycolysis seen in many tumor cells.

It is also worth emphasizing that glucose is a precursor of many, particularly macromolecular, cell constituents, e.g., ribose moieties for nucleic acid biosynthesis; glycerol phosphate for the formation of phospholipids; complex sugars in mucoproteins and mucopolysaccharides; carbon moieties for glycogen.

IMPLICATIONS FOR THE OUTCOME OF IMPLANTATION

Is the ability of an embryo to implant in the uterus a function of its metabolic capacity? This question was pursued with particular reference to glucose metabolism by my colleague David Gardner[36] who measured the glucose uptake of 50 single mouse blastocysts non-invasively prior to transferring them into the uterus of pseudopregnant foster mothers. Thirty-eight of the blastocysts gave rise to live offspring; 12 embryos failed to develop. The mean glucose uptake of these 12 embryos was significantly below that of those which developed successfully, suggesting that metabolic capacity does play a part in determining the ability of an embryo to implant. The extent to which the metabolism of the uterus contributes to the success or otherwise of implantation remains to be seen.

Acknowledgment

The author's studies reported in this paper were supported by grants from the U.K. Science and Engineering Research Council and The Wellcome Trust. I thank Dr. Peter Rogers for helpful comments on the manuscript.

References

1. Long JA, Evans HM. The oestrous cycle in the rat and its associated phenomena. *Mem Univ Calif* 1922; 6:1-148.
2. Armstrong DT. Hormonal control of uterine lumen fluid retention in the rat. *Am J Physiol* 1968; 214:764-771.
3. Tantayaporn P, Mallikarjuneswara VR, De Carlo SJ, Clemetson CAB. The effects of estrogen and progesterone on the volume and electrolyte content of the uterine luminal fluid of the rat. *Endocrinology* 1974; 95:1034-1045.
4. Clemetson CAB, Verma UL, DeCarlo SJ. *J Reprod Fert* 1977; 49:183-187.
5. Enders AC, Schlafke S. A morphological analysis of the early implantation stages in the rat. *Am J Anat* 1967; 120:185-226.
6. Hoversland RC, Weitlauf HM. The volume of uterine fluid in 'implanting' and 'delayed' implanting mice. *J Reprod Fert* 1981; 60:105-109.
7. Levin RJ, Edwards F. The transuterine endometrial potential difference, its variation during the oestrous cycle and its relation to uterine secretion. *Life Sci* 1968; 7:1019-1036.
8. Leese HJ, Gray SM. Vascular perfusion: a novel means of studying oviduct function. *Am J Physiol* 1985; 248:E624-E632.
9. Gray SM, James AF, Leese HJ (unpublished).
10. Shih HE, Kennedy J, Huggins C. Chemical composition of uterine secretions. *Am J Physiol* 1940; 130:287-291.
11. Heap RB. Some chemical constituents of uterine washings: a method of analysis with results from various species. *J Endocr* 1962; 24:367-378.
12. McRae AC. The blood-uterine barrier and its possible significance in early embryo development. In: Clarke JC ed. *Oxford reviews in reproductive biology.* Oxford University Press 1984;6:129-173.
13. Beier HM. Oviduct and uterine fluids. *J Reprod Fert* 1974; 37:221-237.
14. Aitken RJ. Uterine secretion of fructose in the roe deer. *J Reprod Fert* 1976; 46:439-440.
15. Douglas CP, Garrow JS, Pugh EW. Investigation into the sugar content of endometrial secretion. *J Obstet Gynaecol Brit Commonw* 1970; 77:891-894.
16. Zavy MT, Clark WR, Sharp DC, Roberts RM, Bazer FW. Comparison of glucose, fructose, ascorbic acid and glucosephosphate isomerase enzymatic activity in uterine flushings from nonpregnant and pregnant gilts and pony mares. *Biol Reprod* 1982; 27:1147-1158.
17. Leese JH, Astley NR, Lambert D. Glucose and fructose utilization by rat spermatozoa within the uterine lumen. *J Reprod Fert* 1981; 61:435-537.
18. Yochim JM. Development of the progestational uterus: metabolic aspects. *Biol Reprod* 1975; 12:106-133.
19. Surani MAH, Heald PJ. The metabolism of glucose by rat uterus tissue in early pregnancy. *Acta Endocrinologica* 1971; 42:16-24.
20. Krehbiel RH. Cytological studies of the decidual reaction in the rat during early pregnancy and in the production of deciduoma. *Physiol Zool* 1937; 10:212-234.
21. Leese HJ, Barton AM. Pyruvate and glucose uptake by mouse ova and preimplantation embryos. *J Reprod Fert* 1984; 72:9-13.
22. Brinster RL. Nutrition and metabolism of the ovum, zygote and blastocyst. In: Greep RO, Astwood EB, eds. *Handbook of physiology.* Am Physiol Soc Washington DC 1973; Section 7, Vol II, Part 2:165-185.
23. Hardy K, Hooper MAK, Handyside AH, Rutherford AJ, Winston RML, Leese HJ. Non-invasive measurement of glucose and pyruvate uptake by individual human oocytes and preimplantation embryos. *Hum Reprod* 1989; 4:188-191.
24. Leese HJ, Biggers JD, Mroz EA, Lechene C. Nucleotides in a single mammalian ovum or preimplantation embryo. *Anal Biochem* 1984; 140:443-448.
25. Gardner DK, Leese HJ. The role of glucose and pyruvate transport in regulating nutrient utilization by preimplantation mouse embryos. *Development* 1988; 104:423-429.
26. Nieder GL, Weitlauf HM. Regulation of glycolysis in the mouse blastocyst during delayed implantation. *J Exp Zool* 1984; 231:121-129.
27. Clough JR, Whittingham DG. Metabolism of ^{14}C glucose by postimplantation mouse embryos in vitro. *J Embryol Exp Morph* 1983; 74:133-142.
28. Ellington GL, Weitlauf HM. In vitro analysis of glucose metabolism and embryonic growth in post-implantation rat embryo. *Development* 1987; 100:431-439.

29. Clough JR. Energy metabolism during mammalian embryogenesis. *Biochem Soc Trans* 1985; 13:77-79.
30. Psychoyos A. Endocrine control of egg implantation. In: Greep RO, Astwood EB, Geiger SR, eds. *Handbook of physiology.* Am Physiol Soc Washington, DC. 1973 Section 7 Vol II part 2:187-215.
31. Rogers PAW, Gannon BJ. The vascular and microvascular anatomy of the rat uterus during the estrous cycle. *Aust J Exp Biol Med Sci* 1981; 59:667-679.
32. Rogers PAW, Murphy CR, Gannon BJ. Changes in the spatial organization of the uterine vasculature during implantation in the rat. *J Reprod Fert* 1982; 65:211-214.
33. Rogers PAW, Murphy CR, Rogers AW, Gannon BJ. Capillary patency and permeability in the endometrium surrounding the implanting rat blastocyst. *Int J Microcirc Clin Exp* 1983; 2:241-249.
34. Mandel LJ. Energy metabolism of cellular activation, growth and transformation. *Current Topics Membranes and Transport* 1986; 27:261-291.
35. Warburg O. *Uber den Stoffwechsel der Tumoren.* 1926. Berlin: Springer-Verlag.
36. Gardner DK, Leese HJ. Assessment of embryo viability prior to transfer by the noninvasive measurement of glucose uptake. *J Exp Zool* 1987; 242:103-105.

SECTION II: SPECIES VARIATION, *IN VITRO* MODEL SYSTEMS

SPECIES VARIATION, LOCATION AND ATTACHMENT OF BLASTOCYSTS

C.A. Finn

Department of Veterinary Preclinical Sciences
University of Liverpool
Liverpool, United Kingdom

IN the previous section the authors have discussed some of the processes taking place in the ovum as it is transported from the ovary to the uterus. We now come to the crucial stage in which the blastocyst becomes fixed to the wall of the uterus. This is the first attachment an individual makes with another animal and is the most important. If it does not take place satisfactorily the animal will not survive.

The changes which take place in the ovum during the development of the embryo came very early in evolution and similar changes can be found in many species. Attachment and implantation of the ovum into the wall of the uterus, however, is a much more recent event in evolution. Although primitive forms of viviparity can be found in many orders of animals,[1] attachment of the young to the uterus with placenta formation has reached its peak in the eutherian and marsupial mammals.

Probably as a consequence of its late appearance in evolution, the mechanisms developed to bring about implantation of the ovum vary somewhat from species to species. Although only a minority of mammalian species has been studied in detail, it is possible from the information we have to discern a line of increasing complexity from simple attachment of the trophoblast to the luminal membrane of the uterine epithelial cells to deep embedding of the blastocyst into the wall of the uterus. Along the way, however, one finds some cellular adaptations which seem to be unique to a few species. Obviously, one has to be very careful about giving a generalized picture of implantation applicable to all species.

Before discussing the attachment of the ovum to the uterus, therefore, it will be useful to briefly survey the way in which species vary in the mechanisms of implantation. Strictly speaking, the term implantation should only be applied to cases in which the embryo is actually embedded inside the wall of the uterus. However, the term is now commonly applied to any attachment of the embryonic membranes to the wall of the uterus, and this is the most practical usage. The less widely used term nidation can be reserved for cases in which embedding into the wall of the uterus takes place.

The simplest form of implantation consists of little more than the very close contact of the cell membranes of the trophoblast and uterine luminal epithelium with retention of the integrity of all the intervening cell layers. Nutrient and other substances pass across the membranes from the maternal to fetal blood circulation and vice versa. In order to ensure the efficiency of the system, the surface area of the apposing membranes is increased enormously by the formation of microvilli on the trophoblast and luminal epithelium which interdigitate with each other. Furthermore the non-embryonic part of the embryo increases massively in size just before implantation. This is particularly prominent in the pig, where the blastocyst increases by a factor of 300 just before implantation.[2] As the pig also produces very large litters, not surprisingly, it has a massive uterus.

Many, if not most, species go through this first stage of implantation which Enders and Schlafke[3] divide into two parts, apposition and adhesion. In the first stage the blastocyst is positioned passively against the luminal surface of the uterine epithelium, whilst the second stage involves active processes in the apposing cell membranes. It is fairly easy to wash out blastocysts in the apposition stage, but they can only be washed out with difficulty after adhesion has taken place.

Some animals are able to temporarily halt implantation at the apposition stage and thus regulate, to some extent, the length of their gestation. This process has been extensively studied in rats and mice, where it has been shown that it is the absence of sufficient estrogen brought about by suckling of pups which causes the delay of implantation during lactation. In other species, other outside environmental factors are responsible for the delay.

In many species, e.g., pigs and horses, simple attachment of the trophoblast to the luminal surface of the uterus produces a very effective functional union between the mother and offspring. However, during the course of evolution other species have developed stratagems to increase the closeness of the fetal and maternal tissues. These may involve cell fusion, cell death, or migration of cells. For example, in the cow the trophoblast develops binucleate cells which pass into the uterine epithelium and fuse with the columnar cells to form giant cells, and for a short period the epithelium consists mostly of these cells.[4] Subsequently, the giant cells die off and the remaining uterine epithelial cells proliferate to reform the maternal epithelium. Multinucleate cells also form in the uterine epithelium of the goat, although there is no evidence at present that the trophoblast contributes to these.[5] A syncytium of cells also forms in the uterine epithelium of the ewe, but this appears to be formed largely from trophoblast binucleate cells and is not removed but is continuously replaced from the trophoblast throughout pregnancy.[6]

In the rabbit, both the trophoblast epithelium and the uterine cells form symplasma by cell fusion.[7] In fact, the uterine epithelial symplasmum forms also in pseudopregnancy and is not dependent on the presence of the trophoblast. At implantation the two symplasma fuse to form a single tissue originally containing both maternal and fetal nuclei. Later the former disappear leaving only the fetal nuclei.

In all the species discussed so far the extraembryonic part of the blastocyst expands considerably just before implantation to fill the center of the uterine lumen. This is known as central implantation. In other species the blastocyst remains small and becomes located at one side of the lumen where it forms a more intimate association with the vessels of the endometrium. This is eccentric implantation. Sometimes the blastocyst passes into the wall of the uterus so that the embryo develops inside the uterine stroma with the lumen reforming above it. This is referred to as invasive implantation, although strictly speaking, it is only in a few species that it is the active movements of the blastocyst that places the embryo in the uterine stroma. In rats and mice, the blastocyst is positioned at the antimesometrial side of the slit-shaped uterine lumen and then the epithelial cells surrounding it die off by a process of programmed cell death thus giving the blastocyst access to the uterine stroma. Once inside the stroma the trophoblast cells become giant cells by a process of endoreduplication and penetrate into the stroma, but this occurs after implantation. However, in the guinea pig,[8] chimpanzee,[9] and probably other primates including the human, the trophoblast appears to actively penetrate the uterine epithelium by passing between the epithelial cells with little cell death. This is referred to as interstitial implantation. Prior to this event the trophoblast becomes syncytial. In some way the fusion of the trophoblast cells seems to facilitate the passage between the epithelial cells. Enders states that it increases the flow characteristics of the tissue.

In all animals in which the blastocyst comes to lie within the wall of the uterus, the cells of the stroma are prepared in advance so as to limit the intrusion. The fibroblasts, which are unconnected free cells situated loosely in the connective tissue matrix, increase considerably in size and become connected to neighboring cells by gap junctions, thus forming a solid mass of tissue in which the blastocyst implants. This tissue contributes to the placenta and is shed with it at birth. It is known as decidual tissue and its formation is called the decidual cell reaction.

From the evolutionary point of view the decidual cell reaction is particularly interesting. It did not appear, even in viviparous mammals, until mechanisms had developed in the blastocyst and uterus to permit entry of the blastocyst into the uterine stroma. Theories on how it evolved must be largely speculative. One possible explanation is that the decidual reaction has gradually evolved from some more primitive response, already present in lower animals.[10]

Very early in evolution animals had developed mechanisms for getting rid of or overcoming the effects of foreign material which entered the body. First, there is the inflammatory reaction, followed closely by the immune response. The blastocyst is foreign to the mother and it would be expected that the mechanisms for its rejection would be brought into play as soon as it starts to enter into the uterine tissues. If development of the embryo inside the wall of the uterus was to evolve then mechanisms had to evolve to overcome the effects of inflammation and immunity.

The similarity of the uterine-response-to-a-blastocyst to the inflammatory-response-to-a-foreign-body has been noted by many workers. In particular, the similarity of the decidual cell reaction with the granulation tissue response has been examined.[11,12] It was suggested many years ago that the decidual response had evolved as a protection against the injurious effects of the invasion of the wall of the uterus by the blastocyst. Following this theme, Loeb,[13] a pathologist by training, showed that traumatization of the uterus of a guinea pig at the correct stage of the estrous cycle would cause the development of decidual tissue.

Other similarities between implantation and inflammation have also been noted. The demonstration of the pontamine sky blue reaction in the uterus at the time of blastocyst attachment by Psychoyos[14] was particularly relevant, and the more recent finding that some of the cells associated with implantation originate in the bone marrow is very interesting.

It is suggested that the uterus reacts in a similar way to the blastocyst as it would to a foreign body or injury. Somehow or other this potentially lethal mechanism has been adapted to protect the uterus against the effects of the blastocyst instead of causing its rejection and maybe at the same time, by forming a barrier between the mother and fetus, protect the latter against the secondary immune response of the mother. The mechanisms to bring this about seem to have evolved around the ovarian hormones, especially progesterone which had, of course, already made its appearance as a hormone of pregnancy. Without progesterone, injury to the uterus causes an inflammatory response with no decidual reaction.

Decidualization will be discussed in more detail later in this volume, but it is important to note from the point of view of species variation, that it probably only occurs in a minority of species.

Even in those species that are deciduate there is a difference in the mechanism for bringing about decidualization. Rodents, and probably most other deciduate species, still need the stimulus of the blastocyst to initiate the response. A few of the higher primates including women, however, have gone a stage further in evolution and are no longer dependent on any foreign stimulus but only the hormonal preparation which occurs with every ovarian cycle, fertile or infertile. This presumably confers some advantage to the mother in terms of preparation of the uterus but has the disadvantage that because the decidual cells are formed during every ovarian cycle, even with no pregnancy, they have to be shed with resulting tissue destruction and bleeding every cycle. Menstruation thus appears to be the penalty paid for the evolution of the decidual reaction.[15]

From this very brief discussion it can be seen that species vary considerably in the complexity of uterine response to the implanting blastocyst. Obviously, all methods are successful and it is certainly not possible to correlate complexity of implantation and placenta formation with the degree of development of the fetus before birth. Animals seem to have gone in the direction either of providing a huge area of exchange by expansion of the trophoblast or of keeping the blastocyst small but with a more intimate relationship with the maternal tissues. Nevertheless, the first stage of implantation, apposition and adhesion, probably occurs in most species, even if what follows varies considerably.

LOCATION OF THE BLASTOCYST

Before adhesion of the trophoblast to the wall of the uterus, the blastocyst has to be positioned in the lumen. In those species in which the blastocyst expands greatly in size and fills the luminal cavity before attachment either over the entire lumen or at specialized areas, there is probably little need for locating mechanisms, especially when only one blastocyst is present. However, in species in which there are many blastocysts, they have to be spaced along the length of the uterus. Furthermore, in those species in which the blastocyst remains small it usually implants in a certain part of the lumen to which it is directed, and before attachment the embryonic knob is orientated in a specific manner relative to the mesometrium. Thus location of the blastocyst involves three mechanisms, (1) spacing along the length of the uterus, (2) positioning in the correct part of the lumen, (3) orientation of the blastocyst.

The species in which most work has been done is the mouse, although more recently, the spacing of embryos along the length of the uterus in the pig has attracted attention, but even in this species the information available is not really adequate to explain any of the mechanisms.

1. Spacing along the length of the uterus.

With regard to spacing along the length of the uterus it should be stressed that whatever the mechanism, it does not necessarily produce even spacing. Rather it seems to prevent blastocysts from implanting too close together. Thus, if there are a large number of blastocysts then they will be spaced more or less evenly but with only a few blastocysts the spacing is adequate to get separation of the conceptuses.

Several suggestions have been put forward to account for the distribution of the blastocysts along the length of the uterus. McLaren and Michie[16] and Boving[17] suggested that the activity of the myometrium exerts pressure on the blastocyst which moves then along the uterus. More recent evidence for a role for muscular activity comes from the work of Pusey et al.[18] These workers injected relaxin, a hormone known to interfere with uterine contractions, into pregnant rats before the expected time of attachment. They then separated the uterine horns into three segments and by washing out the blastocysts from each determined their distribution in the three segments. In control animals, given saline, the distribution between the three segments was more or less equal. However, after relaxin the blastocysts were unevenly distributed, with the majority of ova appearing in the top segment. If the animals were not killed until day 10, that is after implantation, then the implantation sites were more equally spaced. Thus either the blastocysts had become spaced due to muscular activity after the effect of the relaxin has worn off or some other mechanism comes into operation at the time of attachment or later. Work on the pig also points to a churning up of blastocysts prior to implantation by muscular activity, and it has been suggested that the local production of a hormone, possibly estradiol or prostaglandin, by the embryo may be involved.[19]

It is difficult to see how the contraction of the muscle layers surrounding the lumen brings about movement of the blastocysts. The latter is very small in comparison with the size of the uterine lumen. At the time of blastocyst spacing the lumen is beginning to close down from the ballooning effect found at estrus by removal of intraluminal fluid.[20] There is nevertheless still a small amount of fluid left in the lumen in which the blastocyst is suspended. Presumably, muscular forces would act through currents set up in this fluid rather than directly on the blastocyst.

Myometrial contractility alone, however, might not be sufficient to prevent blastocysts encroaching on each other, and it has been proposed that other mechanisms are involved in bringing about a further fine adjustment following the rough churning by muscular activity. Mossman[21] suggested that, as each blastocyst implanted, an inhibition zone was set up around it which prevented other blastocysts from implanting close by. Whilst this idea sounds superficially attractive, it is difficult with the knowledge we have at present to suggest an inhibitory mechanism, especially as the spacing mechanisms are probably complete before any of the blastocysts have started implanting. McLaren and Michie[16] challenged Mossman's idea of an inhibitory zone. They increased the number of blastocysts by either using superovulating mice or tying one of the oviducts, which had the effect of increasing the number of implantations in the other horn. In these circumstances, the blastocysts implanted closer together and occasionally, two blastocysts implanted so close that the decidua merged and a common placenta was formed.

Injection of oil into the uterus very often causes the formation of a continuous decidual cell reaction along the length of the uterus, producing a sausage-like appearance.[22] This suggests that there is no mechanism to prevent the uterus from responding continuously to blastocysts in the mouse.

Another possible mechanism which might prevent blastocysts from developing too close together is rapid differential growth or stretching of the uterus between implantation sites. This was originally suggested by Hammond[23] in sheep and Reynolds[24] in rabbits. A rapid increase in length of the uterus at the time of implantation has since been demonstrated in the mouse.[25] Whether this is due to real growth (cell division) or tissue hydration following a local increase in vascular permeability at the implantation site[26] is undecided.

2. Positioning in the correct part of the uterus.

Once correctly spaced along the length of the uterus, the blastocyst, in species in which it remains small, becomes positioned with reference to the cross sectional diameter of the uterine lumen. This is very clearcut in the mouse. In this animal the uterine lumen, just before implantation, appears in cross section as a slit orientated in a mesometrial-antimesometrial direction. The blastocyst always implants at the antimesometrial side of this slit.

Again, the mechanism involved is not known. The most detailed discussion of a possible mechanism is by Martin.[27] He proposed that under the influence of the high levels of progesterone at the time of implantation the circular myometrial layer is preferentially active. He postulates that in cross section the antimesometrial side of the lumen is usually nearer the center of the circle enclosed by the muscle layers and that on muscular contraction the force exerted on the blastocyst would tend to push it towards the center, that is, towards the antimesometrial side of the lumen.

The injection of oil into the uterine lumen stimulates a decidual reaction which always starts in the stroma encircling the antimesometrial side of the lumen.[22] Recently, in collaboration with Marion Pope, I have carried out a detailed study of the distribution of the oil after injection into the uterine lumen of mice prepared hormonally for decidualization.

Immediately after the injection, the oil appears as a mass, usually filling the entire lumen. This then splits up into droplets which up to 24 hours after injection are distributed randomly across the lumen. There does not appear to be any preferential distribution of oil towards the antimesometrial side. This is in spite of the fact that the pontamine sky blue reaction can be demonstrated at ten and a half hours and by 24 hours the uterine reaction is under way. It is not until the decidual reaction is well developed, by 36 hours, that there is a definite location of oil in the antimesometrial end of the lumen. These results suggest that the antimesometrial side of the uterus responds preferentially to the stimulus given by the oil, but that at the time when the uterus is responding to the stimulus, the oil has not been preferentially placed there. Once the decidual cell reaction (DCR) is under way, however, there does appear to be some mechanism locating the oil antimesometrially.

It is difficult to relate these results to the situation that exists in implantation. Possibly before attachment the blastocyst is free to move within the lumen, but can only stimulate a DCR when contact is made with the antimesometrial side. The onset of the DCR then fixes the blastocyst at that end. Alternatively, perhaps the luminal surface of the uterine epithelium at the antimesometrial side, in addition to being specialized for the induction of the DCR, is also specialized for attachment so that when the blastocyst touches this point it becomes attached and fixed there. On the other hand, the oil droplets, although capable of mimicking the decidual trigger given by the trophoblast when at the antimesometrial side of the uterus, are not actively attached there and are, unlike the blastocyst, still free to move along the luminal slit. This would imply that they lack some specific attachment property of the trophoblast.

3. Orientation

The final location mechanism which has to take place is orientation of the blastocyst. In the mouse the blastocyst positions itself so that the embryonic disc is facing towards the mesometrium. The embryonic knob is surrounded by the trophoblast and Kirby et al.[28] proposed that the embryonic part can move around within the trophoblast shell. They suggested that orientation occurred after attachment of the blastocyst due to some directive force acting on the embryonic knob causing it to change its position within the trophoblast.

Gardner[29] tested this hypothesis in an ingenious series of experiments. He grew blastocysts in culture and labeled the cells abutting the embryo with melanin. He then transferred the blastocysts to recipient mice and killed them after attachment. He found that the embryonic knobs were orientated as expected but that the melanin particles were still in cells abutting the embryo. From this he concluded that there is no movement of the embryonic part relative to the trophoblast and that whatever causes the orientation must act on the whole blastocyst. Possibly, the surface of the trophoblast is differentiated in some way so as to cause attachment in the correct position.

It appears that the attachment reaction between the trophoblast and luminal epithelium may play a crucial role in bringing about correct positioning of the blastocyst within the uterus.

ATTACHMENT

Upon arrival in the uterus and during the early part of its sojourn there, the ovum is surrounded by the zona pellucida. Before the trophoblast can attach to the wall of the uterus the zona must be removed. The exception to this is the guinea pig in which tongues of trophoblast pass through the zona and then penetrate through the epithelial cells. In this invasive method of implantation, attachment over large areas of trophoblast is probably of less importance. Unfortunately, this stage has not, to my knowledge, been seen in chimpanzees and humans, which are also thought to implant invasively.

Breakdown and removal of the zona is brought about by the secretion of enzymes by the uterus.[30,31] Although this is the most important mechanism, under normal circumstances the blastocyst is able to hatch out of the zona without the aid of uterine enzymes. This appears to happen in delayed implantation when empty zonas can sometimes be found in the uterus.[32]

Attachment can be defined as the stage at which a functional close relationship is formed between the outer membrane of the trophoblast cells and the luminal membrane of the epithelial cells. Detailed study of the cellular relationships only became possible with the introduction of electron microscopy. It has been most studied in rodents, and the pioneering work of Ove Nilsson[33] and his group in Upsalla, Sweden should be mentioned. Mice and rats are particularly suitable models due to the sharp distinction between the preattachment and the attachment phases, and the possibility of holding the former for an extended period of time as in delayed implantation. If mated females are ovariectomized before day 4 of pregnancy and given progesterone, the blastocyst will remain in the preattachment stage until a small quantity of estrogen is administered. The blastocysts then attach.[34,35] If areas of the uterus are studied in which there are no blastocysts, a very distinct change can be seen in the surface of the luminal epithelium. Up to day 4 of pregnancy, the lumen under the influence of progesterone closes down so that the microvilli from apposing sides interdigitate closely. There is, however, still a small luminal space. At the time of implantation under the influence of the nidatory estrogen there is a pronounced change on the surface of the epithelial cells so that the regular microvillous arrangement is replaced by a more irregular surface with the surfaces from the two sides coming very close together to leave a gap of about 15 nm. This has been referred to as the second stage of closure. It can be mimicked in ovariectomized animals by the administration of progesterone and estrogen in an appropriate schedule of injections.[36] Although the first stage of closure can be seen with the light microscope, the change to the second stage can only be seen with the electron microscope.

This surface change is presumably necessary for attachment of the trophoblast. An equivalent change is probably induced on the surface of the trophoblast, but how it is brought about is at present not known. It is known that during delayed implantation the trophoblast rests on the uterine luminal surface without attaching and it is only when the second stage of closure has been induced in the uterus by estrogen that attachment takes place. This then leads to the resumption of development of the blastocyst, but whether there is a specific and necessary change on the surface of the trophoblast at attachment is not certain.

The mechanisms that are involved in bringing about this close relationship, either between apposing uterine luminal membranes or between the trophoblast and uterine luminal epithelium, are being extensively studied. Cells are normally held apart by negative charges on their surface and reduction of this is presumably necessary for them to come close together. Attempts have been made to assess changes in negativity using electron dense probes, for example, ruthenian red, alcian blue, colloidal ion hydroxide, and polycationic ferritin.[37-42] The results have been equivocal, some animals showing a change, some not.

Any change on the surface of the cells leading to attachment is probably associated with the complex carbohydrate moieties of the glycoprotein, glycolipids, and glycosaminoglycans located at the cell surface in the glycocalyx.[43-45] Possibly, reduced negativity could be caused by decreased amounts of sialic acid residues.[37,38]

Some authors have reported a loss of surface coat material before attachment while others have been unable to show such a change.[46,47] The binding of lectins has been used to study changes in the chemical nature of the surface carbohydrates (human;[48] cow;[43] rat;[49] mouse[50,51]).

Chavez[45] tested the binding of several lectins to both surfaces and showed changes at the time of adhesion in only one lectin, succinylated wheat germ agglutinin. From the studies he concluded that at the time of attachment there is a change in N-acetyl glucosamine on the cell surface.

Another approach to the investigation of changes involved in attachment is the isolation and purification of the plasma membranes from the luminal epithelial cells and investigation of their protein content (rabbit;[52] pig[53]). Changes have been demonstrated and Lampello et al.[52] have suggested that there may be a shift in the number, distribution, or configuration of some of the protein molecules on the surface. Similarly, Anderson et al.[54] have shown that three new polypeptides can be identified in endometrial epithelial cells from rabbit uteri at the time of sensitivity to implantation.

The rest of this section is devoted to detailed study of some of the problems I have mentioned.

References

1. Amoroso EC. Viviparity. In: Glasser SR, Bullock DW, eds. *Cellular & molecular aspects of implantation*. New York: Plenum Press, 1981:3-25.
2. Perry JS, Rowlands IW. Early pregnancy in the pig. *J Reprod Fert* 1962; 4:175-188.
3. Enders AC, Schlafke S. A morphological analysis of the early implantation stages in the rat. *Am J Anat* 1967; 120:185-226.
4. Wathes DC, Wooding FBP. An electron microscope study of implantation in the cow. *Am J Anat* 1980; 159:285-306.
5. Dent J. Ultrastructural changes in the intercotyledonary placenta of the goat during early pregnancy. *J Anat* 1973; 114,2:245-259.
6. Wooding FBP, Staples LD, Peacock MA. Structure of trophoblastic papillae on the sheep conceptus at implantation. *J Anat* 1982; 134:507-516.
7. Larsen JF. Electron microscopy of nidation in the rabbit and observations on the human trophoblast invasion. In: Hubinot PO, Leroy F, Robyn C, Leleux P, eds. *Ovoimplantation*. Basel, Munchen, New York: Karger, 1970;38-51.
8. Samson GS, Hill JP. Observations on the structure and mode of implantation of the blastocyst of Cavia. *Trans Zool Soc* 1931; 3:295-355.

9. Heuser CH. The chimpanzee ovum in the early stages of implantation (about 10-1/2 days). *J Morph* 1940; 66:155-173.
10. Finn CA. Implantation, menstruation and inflammation. *Biol Rev* 1986; 61:313-328.
11. Turner W. Report on the progress of anatomy. *J Anat Phys* 1873; 8:159-178.
12. Creighton C. On the formation of the placenta in the guinea pig. *J Anat Phys* 1878; XII:534-590.
13. Loeb L. Wounds of the pregnant uterus. *Proc Soc Exp Biol Med* 1907; 4:93-94.
14. Psychoyos A. Permeabilité capillaire et decidualization utérine. *CR Acad Sci Paris* 1961; 252:1515.
15. Finn CA. Why do women and some other primates menstruate? *Persp Biol Med* 1987; 30:566-574.
16. McLaren A, Michie D. The spacing of implantations in the mouse uterus. In: Eckstein P, ed. Implantation of ova. *Mem Soc Endocr* 1959; 6:65-74.
17. Boving B. Blastocyst-uterine relationships. *Cold Spr Harb Symp Quant Biol* 1954; 19:9-25.
18. Pusey J, Kelly WA, Bradshaw JMC, Porter DG. Myometrial activity and the distribution of the blastocysts in the uterus of the rat: interference by relaxin. *Biol Reprod* 1980; 23:394-397.
19. Pope WF, First NL. Factors affecting the survival of pig embryos. *Theriogenology* 1985; 23:91-105.
20. Nilsson O, Lindqvist I, Ronquist G. Decreased surface charge of mouse blastocyst at implantation. *Exp Cell Res* 1974; 83:421-423.
21. Mossman HW. Orientation and site of attachment of the blastocyst: a comparative study. In: Blandau RJ, ed. *The biology of the blastocyst*. Chicago: University of Chicago Press, 1971:49-57.
22. Finn CA, Hinchliffe JR. Reaction of the mouse uterus during implantation and deciduoma formation as demonstrated by changes in the distribution of alkaline phosphatase. *J Reprod Fert* 1964; 8:331-338.
23. Hammond J. The changes in the reproductive organs of the rabbit during pregnancy. *Trans Dynamics of Growth* 1935; 10:93.
24. Reynolds SRM. *The physiology of the uterus*. New York: Hoeber, 1949.
25. Finn CA. Increase in length of the uterus at the time of implantation in the mouse. *J Reprod Fert* 1968; 17:69-74.
26. Rogers PAW, Murphy CR, Gannon BJ. Changes in the spatial orgnaization of the uterine vasculature during implantation in the rat. *J Reprod Fert* 1982; 65:211-214.
27. Martin L. Early cellular changes and circular muscle contraction associated with the induction of decidualization by intrauterine oil in mice. *J Reprod Fert* 1979; 55:135-139.
28. Kirby DRS, Potts DM, Wilson IB. On the orientation of the implanting blastocyst. *J Embryol* 1967; 17:527-532.
29. Gardner RL. Analysis of determination and differentiation in the early mammalian embryo using intra- and interspecific chimeras. In: Markert CL, Papaconstantinou J, eds. *The developmental biology of reproduction*. New York: Academic Press, 1975:207-236.
30. Orsini MW, McLaren A. Loss of the zona pellucida in mice and the effect of tubal ligation and ovariectomy. *J Reprod Fert* 1967; 13:485-499.
31. Rosenfeld MG, Joshi MS. Effect of a rat uterine fluid endopeptidase on lysis of the zona pellucida. *J Reprod Fert* 1981; 62:199-203.
32. Alloiteau JJ, Psychoyos A. Y a-t-il pour l'oeuf de Ratte deux façons de pendre sa zone pellucide? *CR Acad Sci* Paris, 1966; 262:1561-1564.
33. Nilsson O. Attachment of rat and mouse blastocysts onto uterine epithelium. *Int J Fert* 1967; 12:5-13.
34. Canivenc R, Laffargue M. Suvie des blastocystes de Rat en l'absence d'hormones ovariennes. *CR Acad Sci* Paris, 1957; 245:1752-1754.
35. Cochrane RL, Meyer RK. Delayed nidation in the rat induced by progesterone. *Proc Soc Exp Biol* NY, 1957; 96:155-159.
36. Pollard RM, Finn CA. Ultrastructure of the uterine epithelium during the hormonal induction of sensitivity and insensitivity to a decidual stimulus in the mouse. *J Endocr* 1972; 55:293-298.
37. Nilsson O. Changes of the luminal surface of the rat uterus at blastocyst implantation. Scanning electron microscopy and ruthenium red staining. *Z Anat Entw-Gesch* 1974; 144:337-342.
38. Jenkinson EJ, Searle RF. Cell surface changes on the mouse blastocyst at implantation. *Exp Cell Res* 1977; 106:386-390.
39. Hewitt K, Beer AE, Grinnell F. Disappearance of anionic sites from the surface of the rat endometrial epithelium at the time of implantation. *Biol Reprod* 1979; 21:691-707.
40. Holmes PV, Dickson AD. Estrogen-induced surface coat and enzyme changes in the implanting mouse blastocyst. *J Embryol* 1973; 29:639-645.
41. Anderson TL, Hoffman LH. Alterations in epithelial glycocalyx of rabbit uteri during early pseudopregnancy and pregnancy and following ovariectomy. *Am J Anat* 1984; 171:321-334.
42. Guillomot M, Guay P. Ultrastructural features of the cell surfaces of uterine and trophoblastic epithelia during embryo attachment in the cow. *Anat Rec* 1982; 204:315-322.

43. Wordinger RJ, Amsler KR. Histochemical identification of the glycocalyx layer in the bovine oviduct and endometrium. *Anim Reprod Sci* 1980; 3:189-193.
44. Whyte A, Allen WR. Equine endometrium at pre-implantation stages of pregnancy has specific glycosylated regions. *Placenta* 1985; 6:537-542.
45. Chavez DJ. Cell surface of mouse blastocysts at the trophectoderm-uterine interface during the adhesive stage of implantation. *Am J Anat* 1986; 176:153-158.
46. Enders AC, Schlafke S, Welsh AO. Trophoblastic and uterine luminal epithelial surfaces at the time of blastocyst adhesion in the rat. *Am J Anat* 1980; 159:59-72.
47. Guillomot M, Flechon JE, Wintenberger-Torres S. Cytochemical studies of uterine and trophoblastic surface coats during blastocyst attachment in the ewe. *J Reprod Fert* 1982; 65:1-8.
48. Lee MC, Damjanov I. Pregnancy-related changes in the human endometrium revealed by lectin histochemistry. *Histochemistry* 1985; 82:275-280.
49. Murphy CR, Rogers AW. Effects of ovarian hormones on cell membranes in the rat uterus. III. The surface carbohydrates at the apex of the luminal epithelium. *Cell Biophys* 1981; 3:305-320.
50. Wu JT, Chang MC. Increase in concanavalin A binding sites in mouse blastocysts during implantation. *J Exp Zool* 1978; 205:447-453.
51. Lee MC, Wu TC, Wan YJM, Damjanov I. Pregnancy related changes in the mouse oviduct and uterus revealed by differential binding of fluoresceinated lectins. *Histochemistry* 1983; 79:365-375.
52. Lampelo SA, Ricketts AP, Bullock DW. Purification of rabbit endometrial plasma membranes from receptive and non-receptive uteri. *J Reprod Fert* 1985; 75:475-484.
53. Mullins DE, Horst MN, Bazer FW, Roberts RM. Isolation and characterization of a plasma membrane fraction derived from the luminal surface of the pig uterus during the estrous cycle and early pregnancy. *Biol Reprod* 1980; 22:1181-1192.
54. Anderson TL, Olson GE, Hoffman LH. Stage specific alterations in the apical membrane glycoproteins of endometrial epithelial cells related to implantation in rabbits. *Biol Reprod* 1986; 34:701-720.

COMPARISONS OF THE ABILITY OF CELLS FROM RAT AND MOUSE BLASTOCYSTS AND RAT UTERUS TO ALTER COMPLEX EXTRACELLULAR MATRIX *IN VITRO*

Alerick O. Welsh and Allen C. Enders

Department of Human Anatomy
University of California School of Medicine
Davis, California 95616 USA

IMPLANTATION of mammalian blastocysts is a series of cooperative events that involves both the conceptus and maternal tissues. During implantation, the conceptus becomes fixed within an area of the uterus that it will occupy throughout the duration of normal pregnancy. The continuation of this interaction, *placentation*, leads to the establishment of an area of metabolic exchange between dissimilar tissues that are closely associated. In chorio-allantoic placentation, the intimacy of this association can vary from epitheliochorial to hemochorial arrangement, depending on the species being studied. In the case of hemochorial placentation, extensive alteration of maternal tissues eventually makes it possible for extraembryonic cells of the conceptus, *trophoblast*, to come into direct contact with maternal blood. In several species, including rats and mice, trophoblast is brought into contact with maternal blood in two distinct arrangements that occur at different places and at different times. The first instance is the establishment of the yolk sac placenta that allows maternal blood to circulate in juxtaposition to trophoblast cells as early as day 8 of pregnancy in the rat. This is followed by the second association of maternal and extraembryonic tissues, the hemochorial placenta, that begins to function by day 12. To achieve such intimate associations, tissues that lie between trophoblast and maternal blood must either be removed or invaded. These tissues include the uterine luminal epithelium and its basal lamina, the cells and matrix of the uterine stroma, and the basal lamina and endothelium of maternal vessels. The cellular mechanisms that are involved in this juxtaposition of trophoblast and maternal blood are not clearly understood. Since the morphology of these events varies a great deal from species to species it is likely that the cellular mechanisms involved in implantation and placentation will also vary.

In order to examine some of the mechanisms of implantation, investigators have recently turned their attention to *in vitro* studies. For example, Lindenberg et al.[1] found that trophoblast cells from human blastocysts were able to displace cells of a uterine cell monolayer and contact the underlying surface. Fisher et al.[2] concluded that first trimester human cytotrophoblast cells were able to dissolve complex extracellular matrices derived from different cell lines. Some *in vitro* studies have suggested that mouse trophoblast cells are cytolytic when grown on cellular monolayers[3] and that proteases are active in the process,[4] whereas others have suggested that trophoblast cells displace the cultured monolayer.[5-7] More recent studies have looked at the interaction of mouse trophoblast cells with complex extracellular matrix, derived from a vascular smooth muscle cell strain, and found that the matrix was removed by the cells and that radioactively labeled components were released from the matrix.[8] On the other hand, one study[7] found that mouse trophoblast was unable to penetrate lens capsule matrix *in vitro*.

Recent *in vivo* studies of yolk sac placentation in the rat have suggested that maternal tissues may play an active role in allowing trophoblast access to maternal blood.[9] In particular, cells of the rat endometrium develop and regress in a manner that removes maternal tissues that were between maternal blood vessels and trophoblast cells. It has also been shown that decidual cells are the first cells to penetrate the uterine luminal basal lamina[10] and are capable of occupying walls of maternal vessels before they undergo apoptotic degeneration and are replaced by trophoblast cells.[9] Because of these observations and because some sort of alteration of uterine extracellular matrix seems essential during implantation, we decided to compare the ability of the cells from rat and mouse blastocysts and cells from the rat uterus to alter different complex extracellular matrices *in vitro*.

MATERIALS AND METHODS

Blastocyst Preparation

Late in the afternoon of day 5 of pregnancy, primigravid rats were anesthetized with ether, laparotomized, and the uterine horns removed and cleared of fat. (The morning that spermatozoa were found in the vaginal cell smear was designated day 1.) The horns were separated just above the cervix and blastocysts were flushed from the uterus with Hank's Balanced Salt Solution (HBSS; Gibco Laboratories, Grand Island, NY) or culture medium. Culture medium was Dulbecco's Modified Eagles Medium (Gibco Laboratories) with 10% fetal bovine serum (Hyclone Labs, Logan, UT), and penicillin (100 U/ml)-streptomycin (100 mg/ml)(Gibco Laboratories). Blastocysts were counted, examined for presence of zona pellucidas, transferred to fresh culture medium, and incubated overnight. Any blastocyst that was not free of its zona pellucida the next morning was pipetted in and out of a small-bore pipet until free of the zona. Zona-free blastocysts were placed on various substrates the afternoon of the day following their collection.

Nulliparous Swiss Albino mice were induced to superovulate by intraperitoneal injection (i.p.) of 5 IU of pregnant mare's serum gonadotropin (Sigma Chemical Co., St. Louis, MO) followed 48 hrs later by an i.p. injection of 5 IU human chorionic gonadotropin (Sigma Chemical Co.). At the time of the second injection males were placed in cages with the females, and the following morning the females were checked for vaginal plugs. Mouse blastocysts were treated essentially the same as rat blastocysts except they were flushed from the uterus on day 4 instead of day 5 and their culture medium was supplemented with 1% MEM amino acids, 50X concentrate (Gibco Laboratories).

Uterine Cell Preparation

Uterine stromal cells were harvested from primigravid rats on the afternoon of day 5 or from ovariectomized animals treated with 5 mg of progesterone (Sigma Chemical Co.), in 0.25 ml sesame oil, per day for four days and on the fourth day, 0.15 µg of estradiol (Sigma Chemical Co.), in 0.15 ml sesame oil. Uterine horns were removed 18 hours after the estrogen injection, and blastocysts were flushed as described above. The horns were then slit longitudinally along the antimesometrial border with irridectomy scissors and placed in 15 ml conical centrifuge tubes.

Preparation of cell suspensions. Suspensions of rat uterine cells were prepared according to modifications of a method developed by Glasser and Julian.[11] Briefly, a dispase type II (Boehringer Mannheim Biochemical, Indianapolis, IN) pancreatin (Gibco Laboratories) mixture was used to remove the epithelial cells from the uterine luminal basal lamina. The dispase solution was made with Dulbecco's phosphate buffered saline (PBS) without Ca^{++} and Mg^{++} (Gibco Laboratories), filtered with a 0.2 µm Millipore filter and added to the pancreatin solution. The final dispase concentration was 4.8 mg/ml PBS without Ca^{++}, Mg^{++} and pancreatin was 2.5%. The slit uterine horns were incubated in the dispase:pancreatin solution for one hour at 4° C, one hour at room temperature, and ten minutes at 37° C. Two ml were used for 2 horns, 3 ml for 4 horns, or 4 ml for 6 horns. The enzyme solution was removed and HBSS without Ca^{++}, Mg^{++} was added. The horns were then vortexed (10 sec at setting 5) and the supernate removed and saved. This was repeated twice. The supernates were pooled and set aside in an ice bath. Although this was an epithelial fraction, it apparently contained many stromal cells as well. Both cell types were identified by cytological characteristics when they were in suspension, grown on plastic, or on the particular substrates studied.

Dispase was then used to remove the stromal cells from the muscularis. The horns were incubated in a dispase solution (4.8 mg/ml PBS without Ca^{++}, Mg^{++}) for 15-20 minutes at 37 °C. They were vortexed for 10 sec and the supernate saved. HBSS without Ca^{++}, Mg^{++} was added, they were vortexed, and the supernate saved. This was repeated once and the supernates pooled. This stromal cell fraction also contained glandular epithelium and some luminal epithelium. When examined with a phase contrast microscope, the glandular epithelium appeared as small tubes of cells whereas luminal epithelium appeared as sheets of cells. In addition, there were many individual cells, probably of mixed stromal and epithelial origin. If the tube containing the supernate was permitted to sit for 5 minutes, the tubes of glandular epithelium and sheets of luminal epithelium settled to the bottom in large clumps and could be removed with a pipet.

The luminal epithelial cell fraction and the stromal cell fraction were pelleted and rinsed twice in HBSS without Ca^{++}, Mg^{++}. The studies of uterine cells on smooth muscle cell matrix, cornea matrix, Matrigel (Collaborative Research, Inc., Lexington, MA), and some early studies on amnion matrix were done with the epithelial and stromal cell fractions. Since there were no apparent differences in the abilities of the two fractions to alter the matrices, perhaps because these cell fractions were only enriched and not pure, and because this study was primarily concerned with the potential of uterine cells as compared to trophoblast cells to alter complex extracellular matrix, most of the studies on amnion matrix were done with pooled epithelial and stromal cell fractions. The separate or combined fractions were filtered through several layers of sterilized gauze, repelleted, and resuspended in culture medium. The final suspension of cells was divided, counted, and placed on the substrate of choice. Cells were seeded onto Matrigel-coated coverslips at a density of 2×10^6 to 7×10^6 cells per cm^2 and onto human amnion matrix at a density of 3×10^5 to 7×10^7 cells per cm^2. Although direct cell counts were not done for the cells placed on smooth muscle cell matrix and rat cornea, the method of cell harvesting was the same as that for the Matrigel studies. The size of the coverslips coated with smooth muscle cell matrix was the same as that coated with Matrigel, and the size of the culture vessels holding these coverslips and cornea matrix were the same, so the cell density was probably similar. In later studies with amnion matrix, cell density was varied to see if the time course of matrix disintegration would also vary. It did not.

Culture of blastocysts and uterine cells on matrix.
Blastocysts were cultured for 5 to 7 days and rat uterine cells were cultured for 2 or 3 days on the substrate of choice. Control cells were cultured for up to 7 days. The cultures were fixed in a dilute Karnovsky's fixative,[9] rinsed in phosphate buffer, and postfixed in 1% OsO_4 in phosphate buffer, dehydrated in ethanol, and embedded in araldite. Sections were cut for light microscopy and for transmission electron microscopy. Some specimens were prepared for scanning electron microscopy.

Controls

When each type of matrix was cultured for 4 days in complete medium without cells, there was no visible degeneration of the matrix. Although several matrices were studied we decided, for reasons covered later in this paper, that amnion matrix was the most suitable, and control experiments with cloned human placental fibroblasts and diestrous rat uterine cells were carried out on amnion matrix. Human placental fibroblasts were the kind gift of Dr. Gordon Douglas (Department of Human Anatomy, University of California, Davis, California) and were seeded onto human amnion matrix at a density of 2×10^5 cells per cm^2. Diestrous rat uterine cells were harvested according to the methods outlined above and seeded onto amnion matrix at a density of 2×10^6 cells per cm^2.

Preparation of Matrices

Four types of complex extracellular matrices were used: smooth muscle cell matrix, rat corneal matrix, Matrigel, and human amnion matrix. Vascular smooth muscle cell matrix appears to be rather loosely arranged and is composed primarily of glycoproteins, elastin, and collagen types I and III.[8] Rat corneal matrix without Descemet's membrane is highly organized and is composed primarily of type I collagen, Descemet's membrane is a very dense basal lamina that contains the usual components: type IV collagen with laminin, nidogen, entactin, and heparan sulfate proteoglycan, and, in addition, other collagen molecules that vary with different species. For example, type VIII collagen is a major component of bovine Descemet's membrane[12] while type II collagen predominates in avian species.[13] The predominant components of rat Descemet's membrane have not been referred to in the literature. Matrigel is a basement membrane matrix derived from Englebreth-Holm-Swarm (EHS) mouse tumor and is composed primarily of laminin, type IV collagen, heparan sulfate proteoglycan, and entactin (Collaborative Research literature). Human amnion matrix is composed of a basement membrane with type IV collagen, laminin, fibronectin and heparan sulfate proteoglycan[14,15] and a stroma composed primarily of type III collagen and fibronectin.[16] Type V collagen may serve as a link between the basement membrane and type I collagen in the stroma.[17]

Smooth muscle cell matrix was derived from rat vascular smooth muscle cells of the R22 strain that were kindly provided by Dr. Judith Aggeler (Department of Human Anatomy, University of California, Davis, CA). The cells were grown on Thermanox coverslips (Miles Scientific,

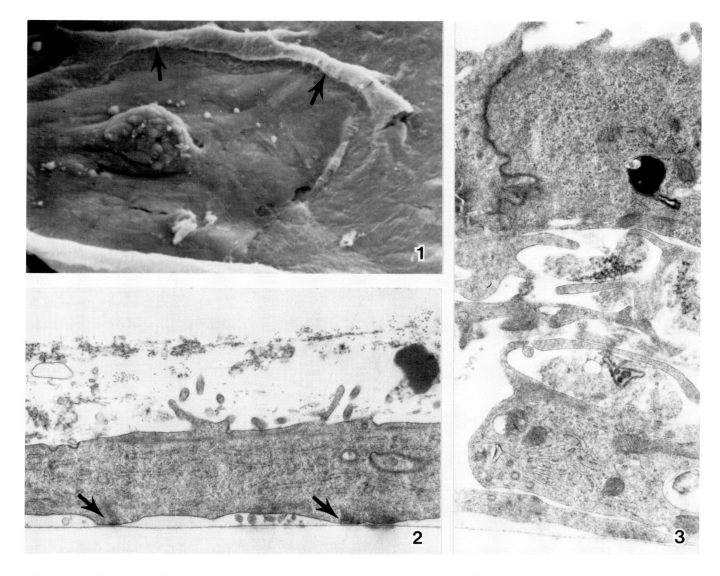

Figure 1. Mouse trophoblast that is growing out on the surface of smooth muscle cell matrix is shown in this scanning electron micrograph. At the outer edge of the trophoblast, the matrix is thrown up into a fold (arrows). Four days in culture. X270.

Figure 2. Mouse trophoblast cells often migrate between smooth muscle cell matrix and the surface of the petri dish as shown in this transmission electron micrograph. Notice the cellular processes and coated pits on the upper, apical surface and cellular modifications (arrows) at the surface where the cell comes into contact with the petri dish. Seven days in culture. X15,310.

Figure 3. When uterine cells are cultured on smooth muscle cell matrix, epithelial cells form a monolayer at the surface and stromal cells invade the matrix beneath the epithelium. After six days in culture very little smooth muscle cell matrix remains between the stromal cells. Six days in culture. X25,000.

Naperville, IL) until they formed a thick mat of matrix and were prepared according to the method used by Glass et al.[8] Adult rat corneal matrix was prepared from freshly removed corneas. Descemet's membrane was sometimes removed from the body of the cornea with fine forceps. Human amnion matrix was prepared from term placentas. The amnion was carefully peeled away from the chorion and was rinsed several times in phosphate buffer. In all three cases cells were lysed with 0.25M NH_4OH and the cell-free matrix was rinsed in running water and stored at $4°$ C in 10% EtOH until ready for use. Just prior to use the matrix was sterilized in 70% EtOH, rinsed in PBS then in culture medium prior to the introduction of blastocysts or uterine cells. The amnion matrix was fitted into holders made from sections of two different sizes of Tygon tubing before the entire unit was sterilized in 70% EtOH. In some experiments the amnion was placed in the holder with the basal lamina side up and in other cases with the stromal side up.

Matrigel was thawed at $4°$ C, then transferred with a precooled Pasteur pipet onto precooled 13 mm round Thermanox coverslips in Nunclon 4-Well Multidishes (Vanguard International, Inc., Neptune, NJ). For uterine cell studies, Matrigel was coated over the entire surface of the coverslip. For blastocyst studies Matrigel was either coated over the surface of the coverslip or small droplets of Matrigel were placed on the coverslip and blastocysts were placed in the droplet. This made it considerably easier to find the blastocysts later. The dishes were placed in an incubator and, after the Matrigel had gelled, culture medium was added.

RESULTS

Interaction of Blastocysts and Complex Matrices

Blastocysts on vascular smooth muscle cell matrix. When rat blastocysts were placed on complex smooth muscle cell matrix, they grew out onto the matrix, but there appeared to be little alteration of the matrix even after 8 days of culture. Mouse blastocysts altered the matrix. Not only did trophoblast that detached from the matrix during processing for SEM leave a distinct impression in the matrix, but, in addition, electron microscopy revealed that mouse trophoblast cells migrated both along the surface of the matrix (Fig. 1) and between the matrix and the Thermanox coverslip (Fig. 2). When examined with a phase contrast microscope, the matrix under mouse trophoblast often appeared to be clearer or smoother than the surrounding matrix. The matrix under rat trophoblast did not appear to change. There was a slight degree of polarity in both rat and mouse trophoblast cells with microvilli at the apical surface. Surprisingly, mouse cells retained this polarity even when they grew beneath the matrix onto the plastic coverslip; that is, the apical surface was against matrix while the smoother basal surface formed specialized attachments to the plastic (Fig. 2). Trophoblast cells of both rat and mouse developed ectoplasmic flanges, filopodia, lobopodia, and lamellipodia, and larger cell organelles were restricted to the area around the nucleus. The cells became very flat and heterogeneous. Although some cells appeared to detach from the other cells, they did not migrate far from the central mass. There were some signs of continued differentiation such as the appearance of fenestrations in flanges that protruded into areas between cells. Mouse cells often had processes extending into the matrix but there was little indication of phagocytosis of matrix. In both the rat and mouse, desmosomes and areas of close apposition were evident between some of the trophoblast cells. In both species there were often cytoplasmic vacuoles of various shapes and sizes and a few secondary lysosome-like structures.

Blastocysts on rat corneal matrix. Both rat and mouse blastocysts placed on corneal matrix grew out along the surface but the trophoblast cells did not penetrate the matrix with or without Descemet's membrane. The cells did follow the contours of the surface on which they were placed. Sometimes rat trophoblast cells were dislodged from the surface during processing, indicating that they were not very adherent. Trophoblast cells appeared polarized with microvilli at the apical surfaces and junctional complexes. On Descemet's membrane the cells developed microfilaments especially in the basal area. This was not seen to the same extent in the cells grown on corneal collagen. Sometimes there was material of moderate electron density between the trophoblast and Descemet's membrane. In a few cases fenestrated flanges were present and protruded into the areas between trophoblast cells. There were many more secondary lysosome-like vesicles and vacuoles in mouse cells than in rat cells but not as many vacuoles as occurred when these were grown on smooth muscle cell matrix.

Blastocysts on Matrigel. Rat and mouse blastocysts that were grown in small mounds of Matrigel or on its surface became disorganized (Fig. 4), but did not disrupt Matrigel or alter it to any appreciable extent even after 8 days in culture. Rat cells remained in the region where they were originally placed and did not appear to migrate through Matrigel. Some mouse cells did appear to move

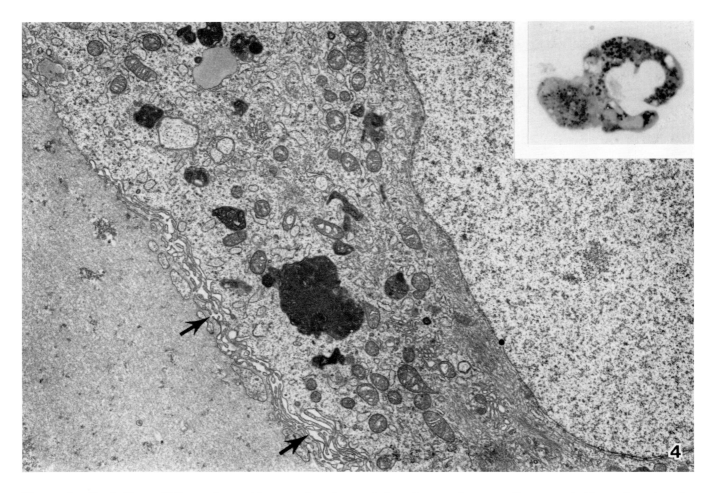

Figure 4. Trophoblast cell flanges become fenestrated and protrude into the areas between adjacent trophoblast cells or into the areas between the cells and the matrix, as illustrated in this micrograph of a mouse trophoblast cell. Notice that the area containing the flanges does not appear to have any Matrigel (arrows). The insert is a light micrograph of the same conceptus that illustrates how disorganized the blastocysts become. Five days in culture. X10,060; insert, X120.

a short distance into Matrigel; however, because the matrix was so malleable, it was difficult to determine whether the cells migrated into the matrix or whether the cells pulled the matrix around themselves. The cell surfaces bordering Matrigel were often irregular and cell processes protruded into Matrigel. Trophoblast cells developed fenestrated flanges that protruded into the spaces between adjacent cells or spaces between trophoblast cells and the matrix (Fig. 4). There was extensive development of secondary lysosome-like bodies and many vacuoles in both rats and mice. In mouse cell cultures, Matrigel in the immediate vicinity of cells often appeared denser and more organized than the rest of the Matrigel.

Blastocysts on human amnion matrix. When mouse or rat blastocysts were placed on human amnion matrix with either the basal lamina or stromal side up, they attached and grew out along the surface (Fig. 5a) and developed processes and filopodia similar to those seen during outgrowth on plastic (Fig. 5b). Trophoblast cells did not penetrate into the matrix (Fig. 6). Although trophoblast cell processes containing many microfilaments were present at the interface with matrix, these were short and did not appear to penetrate the matrix. Sometimes there was material of moderate electron density between trophoblast and matrix (Fig. 6). Although the basal lamina was often not present beneath trophoblast, it was also not always

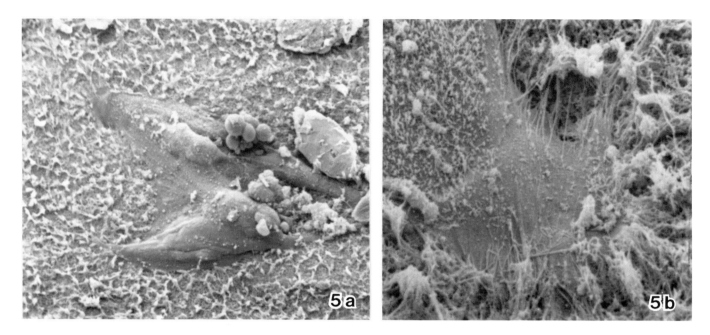

Figure 5a,b. *These scanning electron micrographs show mouse trophoblast growing on human amnion matrix. The leading edge of the outgrowth has numerous filopodia and fewer microvilli than other portions of the cell surface. Six days in culture. 5a, X380; 5b, X2500.*

present in areas without trophoblast so it is difficult to say that the trophoblast did or did not have an effect.

Interaction of Uterine Cells and Matrices

Uterine cells on vascular smooth muscle cell matrix. After three days in culture, uterine cells had disrupted smooth muscle cell matrix. Examination with the scanning electron microscope showed uterine cells covering and embedded in clumps of matrix that appeared to have been pulled away from the surface of the plastic. Surrounding these clumps were areas where uterine cells were growing on plastic. The uterine cells formed a monolayer of epithelial cells or a monolayer of epithelial cells overlying stromal cells (Figs. 7 and 8). In transmission electron micrographs, the epithelium was polarized with apical microvilli and junctional complexes (Fig. 3). It was squamous and very thin in places. There was a close association of these cells with underlying cells that sometimes had many intermediate filaments. The uterine cells readily penetrated (Fig. 6) the matrix and grew along the plastic coverslip. There was a tendency for cells with cytological characteristics of epithelial cells and cells with cytological characteristics of stromal cells to sort themselves out, that is, an epithelial component covered a stromal component (Figs. 7 and 8).

Uterine cells on rat corneal matrix. Cells grew along the surface sometimes surrounding the entire corneal matrix but did not disrupt the matrix even after 10 days in culture. With Descemet's membrane present there was no penetration by uterine cells. When Descemet's membrane was removed, there appeared to be some penetration of the matrix but this was probably limited to artifactual clefts or depressions created in the matrix when Descemet's membrane was removed (Fig. 9). There was sorting of epithelial and stromal cells as occurred with the uterine cells on smooth muscle matrix. The stromal cells had well-developed rough endoplasmic reticulum and Golgi complexes. There was some indication of intermediate filament development and some of the cells were binucleate, as is usually considered characteristic of decidualized stromal cells.

Uterine cells on Matrigel. Uterine cells harvested on day 5 of pregnancy and cultured on Matrigel disrupted the matrix after two or three days in culture (Fig. 11). The uterine cells formed several different arrangements

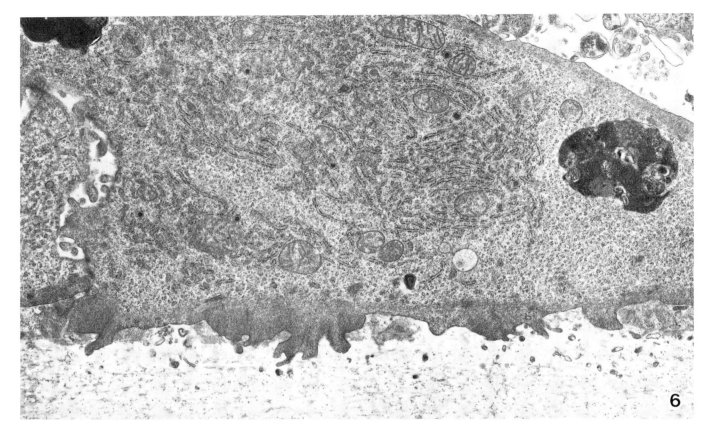

Figure 6. *Many cell processes protrude a short distance into amnion matrix from the surface of this mouse trophoblast cell. These processes contain many microfilaments. Six days in culture. X13,800.*

(Fig. 12). Epithelial cells formed a monolayer sheet at the surface of the Matrigel and were polarized. There were junctional complexes at the apex of these cells, apical vesicles, and basal lipid droplets (Fig. 13). The height of the cells varied from cuboidal to columnar. The epithelial sheets had a tendency to roll up and form tubes or spherical structures (Fig. 14). Matrigel remained attached to the epithelial cells and was pulled along, embedding the tubes or cysts in matrix.

Stromal cells penetrated Matrigel and formed clusters within the matrix (Figs. 12 and 15). These cells were often closely apposed and sometimes appeared to be connected by junctional structures, although no attempt was made to characterize the structures. The cells were larger than fibroblasts and sometimes contained two nuclei. Occasionally these cells also contained many clusters of intermediate filaments. As determined by these morphological criteria, they may have undergone partial decidualization. Stromal cells were often in proximity to spaces devoid of Matrigel and there was some indication that they phagocytosed matrix; that is, there were cell processes surrounding bits of Matrigel. The disruption of the matrix was not uniform. It appeared that areas underlying epithelial sheets were disrupted at a slower rate than the matrix in areas between these sheets, but, eventually, the entire matrix was disrupted.

Uterine cells on human amnion matrix. Uterine cells harvested on day 5 of pregnancy or uterine cells from ovariectomized rats given progesterone and estrogen produced holes in, or caused alteration of, amnion matrix after two or three days in culture (Fig. 16). It made no difference whether the cells were placed on the basal lamina surface or the stromal or chorionic surface of the matrix. When viewed in the dissection microscope, disruption started as discrete small holes that grew larger and

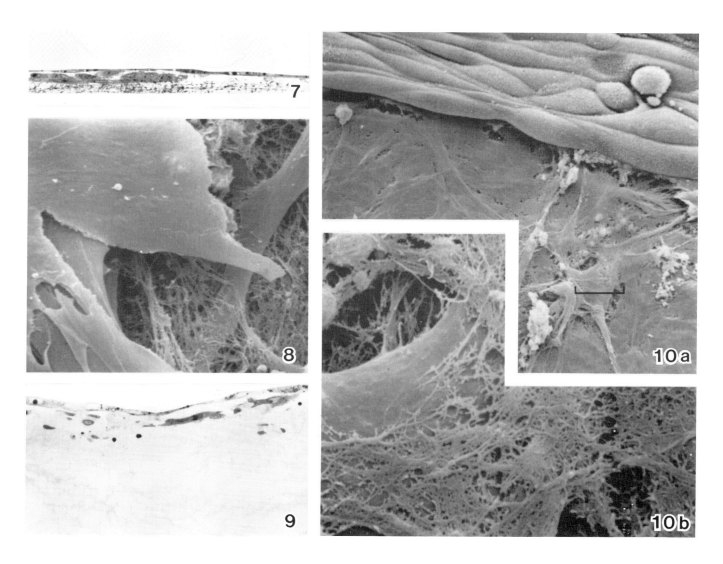

Figure 7. This light micrograph of uterine cells grown on smooth muscle cell matrix illustrates a monolayer of epithelial cells covering stromal cells. In this particular area the stromal cells have not penetrated the matrix. Three days in culture. X265.

Figure 8. In this scanning electron micrograph, from an area similar to the area shown in Fig. 7, tissue processing has caused the epithelial monolayer to split open revealing the underlying stromal cells and matrix. Notice, at the bottom of the micrograph, that matrix components cover the stromal cell indicating that this cell penetrates the matrix. Three days in culture. X2500.

Figure 9. When uterine cells are placed on rat cornea matrix stripped of Descemet's membrane the epithelial cells form a monolayer over the stromal cells. The penetration of the matrix by the stromal cells is very limited and is probably a result of the cells occupying spaces created during the removal of Descemet's membrane. Three days in culture. X265.

Figure 10. Uterine stromal cells are found penetrating amnion matrix when there is no epithelial covering. Fig. 10a shows the edge of an epithelial sheet and the surface of the amnion matrix. A portion of the matrix surface (brackets) is enlarged in Fig. 10b and illustrates a stromal cell that is penetrating the matrix. Three days in culture. Fig. 10a, X640; Fig. 10b, X5000.

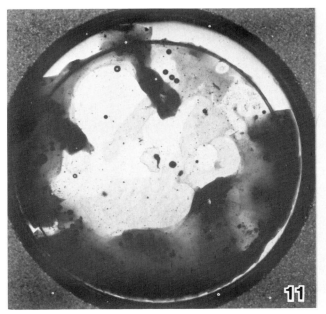 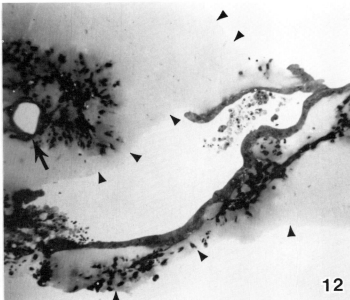

Figures 11 and 12. *When uterine cells are cultured on Matrigel, the matrix is disrupted within 3 days. In the whole mount, Fig. 11, there are clear areas where the matrix was removed and dark areas where the matrix is still intact. The darker thicker areas are often in proximity to an epithelial layer. The light micrograph, Fig. 12, is from a section of a uterine cell culture and illustrates how disorganized these cultures become. The surfaces of the Matrigel are indicated by arrowheads. In the upper left is a tube or cyst of epithelium (arrow) embedded within the Matrigel and surrounded by stromal cells that invade the matrix. Below that and to the right is a large space in the matrix with an epithelium covering part of the Matrigel surface and stromal cells within the matrix. Three days in culture. Fig. 11, X5; Fig. 12, X110.*

coalesced to form much larger holes. The matrix originally resisted the stress of handling but as alteration of the matrix continued it became very fragile. Even after fixation, matrix that was exposed to uterine cells for three days tended to fall apart during tissue processing if there were many large holes. When culture was continued for four days the amnion matrix was completely degraded in those areas exposed to uterine cells. In one case, uterine cells were placed within a glass ring holding the amnion matrix on the bottom of the petri dish. While the matrix within the ring disintegrated, the matrix outside the ring did not. Also, when amnion matrix was fitted in holders made from rings of Tygon tubing, some of the matrix was not exposed to cells and this matrix did not disintegrate.

In sections, cell distribution resembled that seen with Matrigel; that is, there were epithelial cells at the surface and stromal cells within the matrix. However, the surface of the amnion matrix was not distorted by the cells and hence was flatter than the Matrigel surface. When placed on either surface of the amnion matrix, uterine luminal epithelium grew out as a monolayer of cells that were polarized (Fig.18) with microvilli at their apical surface, junctional complexes on the apical-lateral surface, and a smooth basal surface that sometimes had processes that resembled those seen in the uterine luminal epithelium of a day 5 pregnant animal. The epithelial monolayer at the surface of the matrix covered groups of stromal cells that were found within the structure of the matrix (Fig. 18). Stromal cells were also present within the matrix when there was no epithelial covering (Fig. 10). Some amnion matrices prepared for SEM clearly showed these cells from the undersurface of the matrix, indicating that cells had migrated through the matrix (Fig. 17). Holes were usually but not always surrounded by epithelial cells that migrated around the lip of the hole and spread for a short distance along the undersurface of the amnion matrix.

Stromal cells were often in close contact with one another and occasionally appeared to have junctional connections. Many cells had processes that extended into the matrix and surrounded bits of matrix (Fig. 19). They usually had

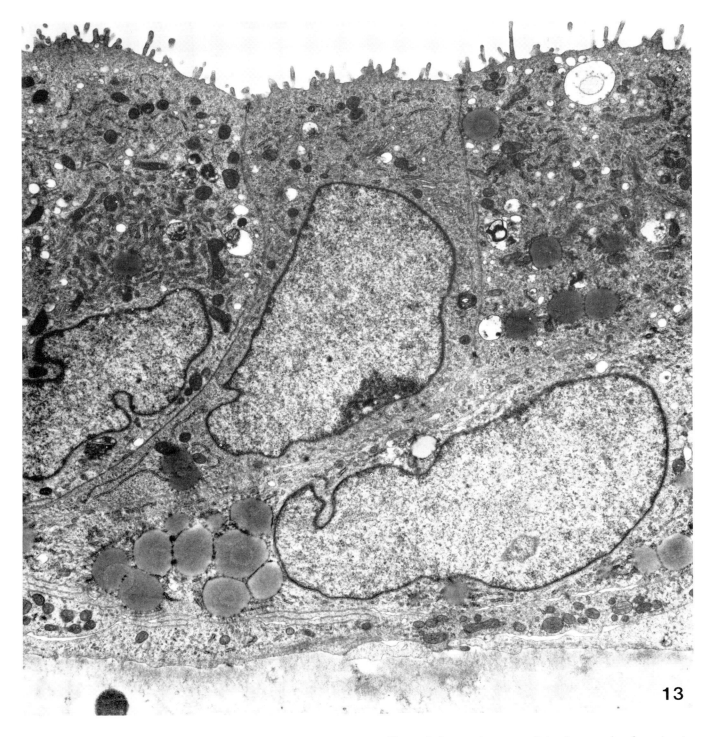

Figure 13. When uterine luminal epithelial cells are grown on Matrigel they retain many of the features they have in vivo. The epithelium is polarized with apical microvilli, junctional complexes, apical vesicles, and basal lipid droplets. Two days in culture. X10,000.

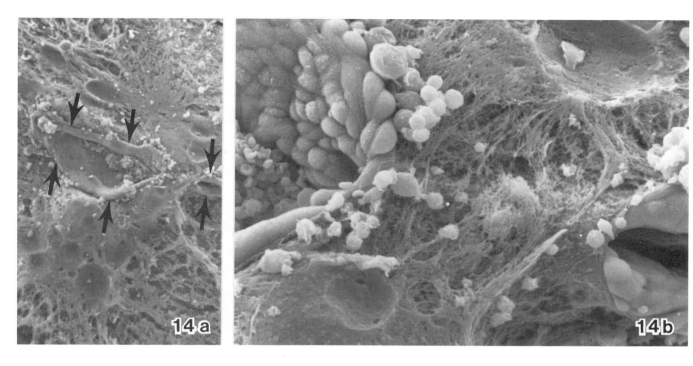

Figure 14a,b. *This scanning electron micrograph is of an area similar to that shown in Figs. 11 and 12. A sheet of epithelium folded over onto itself creating a tube (arrows), and it carried Matrigel with it so the tube is embedded in matrix. Two days in culture. Fig. 14a, X85; Fig. 14b, X640.*

only one nucleus and few intermediate filaments. These were similar to the stromal cells seen just beneath the basal lamina on day 7 of normal pregnancy.[10] Some stromal cells were in close contact with the basal surface of the epithelium (Fig. 18). Although spaces that were clear of amnion matrix occasionally surrounded stromal cells, the cells were usually in close contact with the matrix.

Controls

Scanning electron micrographs of amnion matrix that received diestrous rat uterine cells showed large continuous sheets of cells. Sections of this material revealed a continuous epithelial sheet with a few stromal cells between it and the amnion matrix. Few stromal cells appeared to penetrate the matrix. After 7 days of culture there were no holes through the amnion matrix. When cloned placental fibroblasts were placed on human amnion matrix they did not produce holes in the matrix after being in culture for up to six days. Matrices that were cultured without cells showed no apparent signs of degeneration within the normal times of culture.

DISCUSSION

These studies have shown that rat uterine cells harvested on day 5 of pregnancy, or equivalent (ovariectomized rats given progesterone and estrogen), had the ability to disrupt three of the four types of complex extracellular matrix that were studied: vascular smooth muscle cell matrix, Matrigel, and human amnion matrix. Mouse trophoblast cells clearly disrupted only one type of matrix, vascular smooth muscle cell matrix, and rat trophoblast did not disrupt any of the matrices studied. Although rat trophoblast attached and outgrew, the culture conditions may not have been as favorable for producing other results as they were for mouse trophoblast. In control cultures, without cells or with human placental fibroblasts or diestrous rat uterine cells, the human amnion matrix did not disintegrate. These results indicate that, in the rat, uterine cells have the potential to play an active role in remodeling the endometrial matrix during implantation. On the other hand, trophoblast cells of early blastocysts of rats and mice appear to have much less potential.

In order to bring trophoblast cells into contact with maternal blood, different types of uterine extracellular matrix,

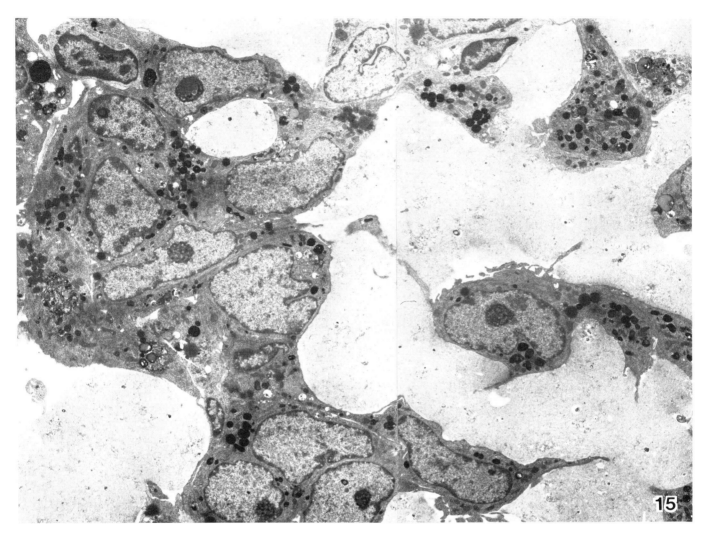

Figure 15. *Uterine stromal cells migrate into the matrix and form clusters or arrangements of single cells. Two days in culture. X4050.*

including the luminal epithelial basal lamina matrix surrounding stromal cells, and the basal lamina of an endothelium, must be removed. Because the composition of these matrices probably varies, we tested a variety of matrices to see whether uterine cells or trophoblast cells had the greatest potential to alter different matrices. Of course, cells grown on any other than endometrial matrix, provide only a limited model of cell-induced matrix changes. When considering the composition of the uterine matrix, however, there is a dual problem. It is likely that the composition of the matrix varies with the stage of the cycle or the stage of pregnancy,[18,19,23] and, during pregnancy, the composition of endometrial matrix probably varies with location; the matrix at an implantation site being different from that between implantation sites. If this is the case, studies with the endometrial matrix would require that the area of cell-matrix interaction be localized. Because of this uncertainty we initially used matrices that were fairly homogeneous over a large area rather than endometrial matrix.

There have only been a few studies concerning the composition of rat endometrial matrix. These include studies of post-partum involution of a rat endometrium,[20] biochemical studies of collagen synthesis in whole uteri during preg-

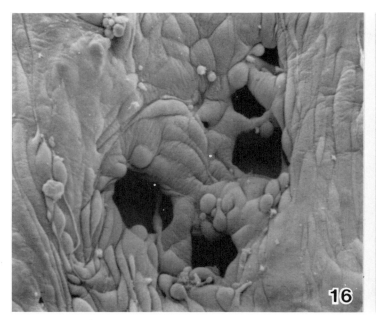
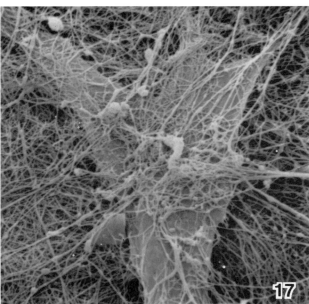

Figure 16. When rat uterine cells are cultured on human amnion matrix, holes are produced in the matrix on the third day of culture. In this scanning electron micrograph the surface of the matrix is covered with epithelial cells. X350.

Figure 17. This micrograph is from the reverse side of an amnion matrix similar to that shown in the previous figure. There are no epithelial cells here but a stromal cell is enmeshed in the matrix. Three days in culture X2500.

nancy,[21] histological studies of changes in dense collagenous connective tissue during various reproductive states,[22] and a study by Grinnell et al.[23] regarding fibronectin and cell shape during pregnancy. Although the basic components are probably similar to other connective tissues, the details of their proportions and arrangement are not well known. The endometrium is rich in type III collagen.[23]

Cell morphology and function are influenced by the type of matrix on which the cells are grown.[24-27] Thus, for *in vitro* studies, it is best to use a matrix that supports a cell morphology that closely resembles the morphology seen *in vivo*. When uterine cells were grown on smooth muscle cell matrix, corneal matrix, or plastic the epithelium was squamous or cuboidal, and the polarization of cytoplasmic constituents was not preserved. Epithelial cells grown on Matrigel retained many characteristics of epithelial cells seen *in vivo*, including basal lipid droplets and apical vesicles. Glasser et al.[28] have recently shown that immature rat uterine epithelial cells grown in the presence of Matrigel establish morphological and functional polarity. The uterine luminal epithelium grown on human amnion matrix did not resemble the epithelium seen *in vivo* as closely as that grown on Matrigel. We found, however, that there were some drawbacks in working with Matrigel. It was very malleable, and after the cells attached to it, they were able to distort it and possibly produce areas of thick and thin matrix by simple mechanical means. Mammary epithelial cells appear to have a similar effect on EHS matrix when they undergo morphogenesis *in vivo* to produce alveoli-like structures.[29] Also, because Matrigel is a basement membrane derivative it was not a good substrate for studying matrix changes in the stromal region. For the following reasons human amnion matrix was considered the most favorable model for future studies: it is readily available, gives fair retention of cell morphology, has a composition somewhat similar to endometrial matrix, including the presence of type III collagen, is not readily distorted by the cells growing on it, and can be suspended in a stable manner. Other conditions of cell culture, such as the composition of culture media, must also be considered when discussing the properties and potentials of any cell population *in vitro*. To monitor this sort of variable in trophoblast cells we examined the formation of fenestrations in

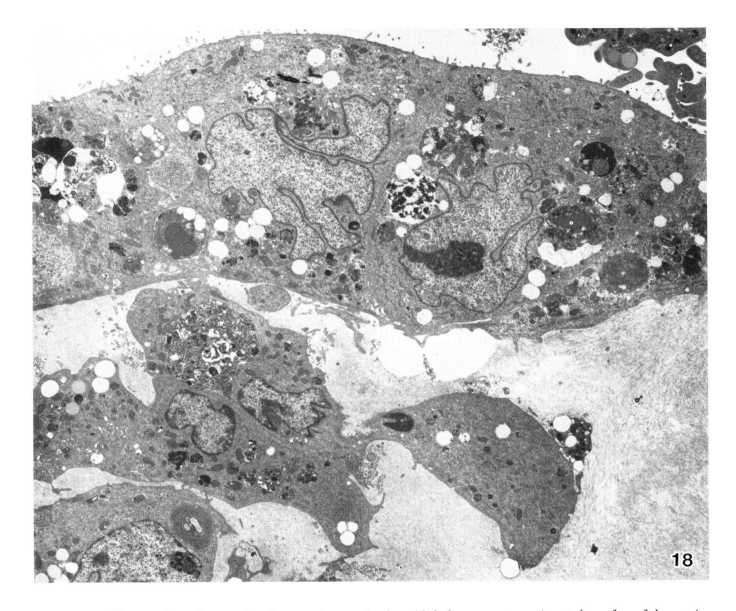

Figure 18. *When uterine cells are cultured on amnion matrix, the epithelial component remains at the surface of the matrix while the stromal component migrates into the matrix. Three days in culture. X5180.*

cell flanges and found that cell differentiation, in these terms, proceeded normally.[9]

Although several models have been developed to study the effect of trophoblast on cellular monolayers *in vitro*,[3-6,30] there have been only a few reports regarding the activity of trophoblast cells on complex extracellular matrix. The results reported here confirm those of Glass et al.,[8] who found that mouse trophoblast disrupted a complex extracellular matrix derived from vascular smooth muscle cells. Our results, however, also support those of Cammarata et al.[7] who found that mouse trophoblast cultured on bovine lens capsule did not infiltrate the lens capsule but was capable of attachment and outgrowth. These results were similar to our results with trophoblast not only on rat corneal matrix but also on human amnion matrix. Trophoblast cells from different stages or from

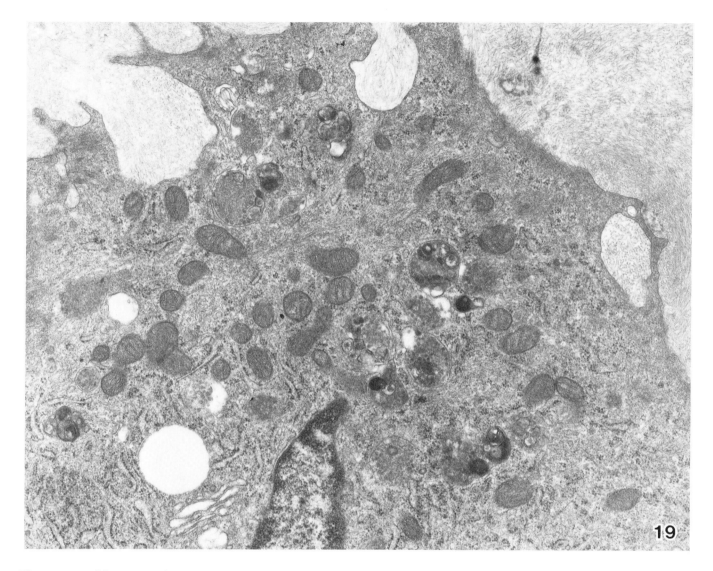

Figure 19. *Many stromal cells have surface processes that wrap around amnion matrix in a manner reminiscent of subliminal decidual cells from day 7 of normal pregnancy. Notice that this cell also has numerous intermediate filaments and a well-developed rough ER and Golgi apparatus similar to decidual cells. Three days in culture. X30,000.*

different species probably express different degradative potential on different types of matrix.

One possible reason that the degradative capacity of trophoblast cells varies on different matrices is that the components of the matrices vary and degradative enzymes for particular substrates may or may not be present. Also, the molecular arrangements of the components within different extracellular matrices may determine what cells are capable of disrupting them; that is, cells might be able to degrade a component as it appeared in one matrix but not in another. Cammarata et al.[7] suggested that mouse trophoblast cells could not penetrate the bovine lens capsule because of its high degree of organization rather than its composition. The same may be true of corneal matrix with or without Descemet's membrane since both layers are dense and highly organized. On the other hand, the amnion stromal matrix, which neither rat nor mouse trophoblast could penetrate, does not appear to be as regularly organized as corneal matrix.

The degradative potential of different trophoblast cell populations probably varies not only among species but also within the same cell population at different times during gestation. Fisher et al.[2] found that trophoblast of first-trimester human placentas degraded extracellular matrices derived from PF HR9 and PYS-2 cell lines whereas second-trimester human placental trophoblast did not. In rats and mice it is probable that trophoblast cells from later stages, such as Trager, have a greater invasive potential than the earlier mural trophoblast. It is interesting that the disruption of vascular smooth muscle matrix was evident in uterine cell cultures after 2-3 days but was not noticeable in mouse trophoblast cultures before 6-7 days. Glass et al.[8] reported a release of labeled peptides as early as day 5 of culture, a day or two before there was any visible sign of physical alteration of the matrix. Although we did not study the release of labeled peptides, there could have been a similar lag between the first release of label and microscopic evidence of disruption in the uterine cell cultures as well. This suggested that matrix disruption by uterine cells could have started as early as the first day of culture. At any rate, day 5 culture is long after the uterine cells would have completely disrupted the matrix. Although more information needs to be collected, our results suggest that trophoblast starts disrupting smooth muscle cell matrix later than uterine cells, and disruption by trophoblast cells should be associated with events later than those of early implantation.

The finding that rat uterine cells have a greater capacity to alter complex extracellular matrix than do trophoblast cells is not surprising since the uterine matrix of the pregnant rat undergoes a great many changes before trophoblast cells are in contact with it.[9,10,31,32] By day 6 the luminal epithelium lines the surface of a depression in the stroma, called the implantation or gestation chamber, that becomes longer and more cylindrical in shape during the next three days.[33-35] At the same time, the stroma that forms the wall of the chamber becomes more cellular as stromal fibroblasts decidualize. During this process, extracellular matrix surrounding decidual cells is reduced to very small quantities, and the decidualized stromal cells adjacent to trophoblast become apoptotic. By the time trophoblast cells reach the uterine stroma, on the afternoon of day 7, they are confronted by apoptotic decidual cells and very little extracellular matrix.[9] In normal pregnancy, chamber formation and decidualization are inseparable. Although the luminal epithelium may play a role during the initial stages of chamber formation, it is gone before chamber formation is complete. Implantation chambers, albeit somewhat abnormal, also form when stromal decidualization is artificially induced without a blastocyst present.[36] So it is likely that uterine stromal cells are primarily responsible for this reorganization.

In the rat, decidual cells probably alter the extracellular matrix that surrounds them, and, in addition, they extend processes that penetrate the uterine luminal basal lamina on the afternoon of day 7.[10] Decidual cells also penetrate the basal lamina of maternal blood vessels and interact with endothelial cells by becoming part of the vascular wall.[9] These observations suggest that stromal cells or cells derived from stromal cells are capable of altering different types of extracellular matrix.

Although our experiments have not directly addressed the question of which uterine cell type or types disrupt complex extracellular matrix *in vitro*, it seems reasonable that stromal cells occupying the matrix would be responsible. Our observations that uterine epithelial cells remain at the surfaces of matrices while stromal cells invade matrices are similar to the results of studies in which isolated corneal epithelial cells remained at the surface of collagen gels whereas isolated corneal fibroblasts invaded the gels.[26] Since uterine stromal cells are capable of invading matrices and since fibroblasts and macrophages are the primary cells involved in matrix formation and remodeling in other tissues,[35] uterine stromal cells are probably responsible for degradative changes in complex extracellular matrix, both *in vitro* and *in vivo*. It is possible that the uterine luminal epithelium also plays a role. In order to produce deciduomata in the uterine stroma, the inductive stimulus must be transmitted through the luminal epithelium.[37] Similarly, stromal cells may require the presence of epithelial cells in order to produce the effects observed in the present study. Experiments are now under way to improve the purity of the epithelial and stromal cell fractions and to test the ability of isolated cell populations to alter human amnion matrix.

It is difficult to draw conclusions about the nature of matrix degradation by uterine cells. When examined with transmission electron microscopy, human amnion matrix was usually in close contact with both stromal cells and epithelial cells, but occasionally there were clear spaces between stromal cells and surrounding matrix. If these clear spaces represent areas where matrix was degraded, it would suggest that there is local protease secretion or membrane-bound protease activity. When uterine cells were cultured on amnion matrix that was held in place by a glass ring, the matrix that was outside the ring, away from uterine cells, was not degraded. Similarly, when amnion matrix was held in Tygon tube rings, matrix that was a short distance away from the uterine cells was not degraded. This differs from the results of Werb et al.[38] who found that smooth muscle cell matrix floated above cultured macrophages degraded at the same rate as matrix in contact with the macrophages, indicating that a secreted protease was active. Although we did not float the amnion matrix above the uterine cells, the total distance up and over the glass ring was comparable. There appeared to be generalized weakening of the matrix in the areas surrounding holes, but only a few distinct holes usually formed in any one amnion matrix. Once holes were formed, they may have been enlarged by mechanical action of the cells contracting on a weakened matrix. When epithelial cells were at the margins of holes, both cells and matrix folded under suggesting some mechanical movement. When uterine cells were grown on amnion matrix, there was a tendency for the matrix to roll up if it was not held in place. This also suggests that the cells produced some tension on the matrix.

The identification of stromal cells in these cultures as fibroblasts, decidual cells, or other stromal cell types is not clear. Some cells were not characteristic stromal fibroblasts, but neither were they clearly decidual cells. Many of the cells beneath the epithelium in human amnion matrix closely resembled the decidual cells just beneath the uterine luminal basal lamina on day 7 of pregnancy. Although several studies have examined "*in vitro* decidualization" of rat uterine cells,[11,39,40] or mouse uterine cells,[41] it is difficult to interpret this phenomenon. The single designation, decidual cell, does not describe the variety of modified stromal cells in the pregnant rat uterus.[32] Bell and Searle[41] have described differences in cultured mouse uterine stromal cells and attempted to explain those differences. Also, some of the changes that are observed in stromal cells *in vitro* are characteristic of many types of cells cultured on plastic, for example, filament accumulation and multiple nuclei, and do not necessarily constitute decidual transformation. Glasser and Julian[11] have examined intermediate filaments common to decidual cells *in vivo* and *in vitro* and suggested that the appearance of desmin in uterine stromal cells may serve as a marker of decidualization. Should these markers prove consistent, this type of approach could be very useful.

The uterine cell-amnion matrix model provides an opportunity to examine interactions of uterine cells with extracellular matrix *in vitro*. Separation of epithelial and stromal cells of the rat endometrium should enable us to determine which cell type (or types) is responsible for matrix degradation, and immunocytochemical techniques will be helpful for identifying the isolated cells. Electrophoretic examination of culture media and inhibitors of proteolytic enzymes can be used to help determine what types of enzymes are involved, and antibodies against such enzymes can be used to localize them *in utero*.

SUMMARY

These studies have shown that rat uterine cells have a greater capacity to degrade a variety of complex extracellular matrices *in vitro* than either rat or mouse trophoblast cells. This observation is consistent with current information regarding implantation and placentation in normal pregnancy and indicates that a cautious approach be taken to *in vitro* studies of trophoblast invasiveness in these species. The uterine stroma is not a passive participant during implantation and placentation.

ADHESION / OUTGROWTH / PENETRATION / DISRUPTION
OF COMPLEX EXTRACELLULAR MATRIX BY RAT AND MOUSE TROPHOBLAST AND RAT UTERINE CELLS

	Rat Trophoblast	Mouse Trophoblast	Rat Uterine Cells
Smooth Muscle Cell Matrix	+ / + / − / −	+ / + / + / +	+ / + / + / +
Rat Cornea Matrix	+ / + / − / −	+ / + / − / −	+ / + / − / −
Matrigel	+ / + / * / *	+ / + / * / *	+ / + / + / +
Human Amnion Matrix	+ / + / − / −	+ / + / − / −	+ / + / + / +

*Because it is so malleable, when blastocysts are grown in Matrigel, it is difficult to determine whether the cells penetrate and disrupt the matrix or simply rearrange it.

References

1. Lindenberg S, Hyttel P, Lenz S, Holmes PV. Ultrastructure of the early human implantation *in vitro*. *Hum Reprod* 1986; 1:533-538.
2. Fisher SJ, Leitch MS, Kantor MS, Basbaum CB, Kramer RH. Degradation of extracellular matrix by the trophoblastic cells of first-trimester human placentas. *J Cell Biochem* 1985; 31:31-41.
3. Sherman MI, Salomon DS. The relationships between the early mouse embryo and its environment. In: Markert CL, Papaconstantinou J, eds. *The developmental biology of reproduction.* New York: Academic Press, 1975;277-309.
4. Kubo H, Spindle A, Pedersen RA. Inhibition of mouse blastocyst attachment and outgrowth by protease inhibitors. *J Exp Zool* 1981; 216:445-451.
5. Glass RH, Spindle AI, Pedersen RA. Mouse embryo attachment to substratum and interaction of trophoblast with cultured cells. *J Exp Zool* 1979; 208:327-336.
6. Van Blerkom J, Chavez DJ. Morphodynamics of outgrowths of mouse trophoblast in the presence and absence of a monolayer of uterine epithelium. *Am J Anat* 1981; 167:143-155.
7. Cammarata PR, Oakford L, Cantu-Crouch D, Wordinger R. Attachment of blastocysts to lens capsule: a model system for trophoblast-epithelial cell interaction on a natural basement membrane. *Cell Tissue Res* 1987; 250:633-640.
8. Glass RH, Aggeler J, Spindle A, Pedersen RA, Werb Z. Degradation of extracellular matrix by mouse trophoblast outgrowths: a model for implantation. *J Cell Biol* 1983; 96:1108-1116.
9. Welsh AO, Enders AC. Trophoblast-decidual cell interactions and establishment of maternal blood circulation in the parietal yolk sac placenta of the rat. *Anat Rec* 1987; 217:203-219.
10. Schlafke S, Welsh AO, Enders AC. Penetration of the basal lamina of the uterine luminal epithelium during implantation in the rat. *Anat Rec* 1985; 212:47-56.
11. Glasser SR, Julian J. Intermediate filament protein as a marker of uterine stromal cell decidualization. *Biol Reprod* 1986; 35:463-474.
12. Sage H. Type VII Collagen. In: Mayne R, Burgeson RE, eds. *Structure and function of collagen types.* Orlando: Academic Press, Inc. 1987:173-194.
13. Hendrix MJC, Hay ED, von der Mark K, Linsenmayer TF. Immunohistochemical localization of collagen types I and II in the developing chick cornea and tibia by electron microscopy. *Invest Ophthalmol Vis Sci* 1982; 22:359-375.
14. Alitalo DM, Kurkinen M, Vaheri A, Krieg T, Timpl R. Extracellular matrix components synthesized by human amniotic epithelial cells in culture. *Cell* 1980; 19:1053-1062.
15. King B. Distribution and characterizaton of anionic sites in the basal lamina of developing human amniotic epithelium. *Anat Rec* 1985; 212:57-62.
16. Aplin JD, Campbell S, Allen TD. The extracellular matrix of human amniotic epithelium: ultrastructure, composition, and deposition. *J Cell Sci* 1985; 79:119-136.
17. Modesti A, Kalebic T, Scarpa S, Togo S, Grotendorset G, Liotta A, Triche TJ. Type V collagen in human amnion is a 12 nm fibrillar component of the pericellular interstitum. *Euro J Cell Biol* 1984; 35:246-255.
18. Aplin JD, Charlton AK, Ayad S. An immunohistochemical study of human endometrial extracellular matrix during the menstrual cycle and first trimester of pregnancy. *Cell Tissue Res* 1988; 253:231-240.
19. Martello EMVG, Abrahamsohn PA. Collagen distribution in the mouse endometrium during decidualization. *Acta Anat* 1986; 127:146-150.
20. Padykula H. Cellular mechanisms involved in cyclic stromal renewal of the uterus II. The albino rat. *Anat Rec* 1976; 184:27-48.
21. Harkness MLR, Harkness RD. The distribution of the growth of collagen in the uterus of the pregnant rat. *J Physiol* 1956; 132:492-501.
22. Fainstat T. Extracellular studies of the uterus. I. Disappearance of the discrete collagen bundles in endometrial stroma during various reproduction states in the rat. *Am J Anat* 1963; 112:337-369.
23. Grinnell F, Head JR, Hoffpauir J. Fibronectin and cell shape *in vivo*: studies on the endometrium during pregnancy. *J Cell Biol* 1982; 94:597-606.
24. Gospodarowicz DJ. Extracellular matrices and the control of cell proliferation and differentiation *in vitro*. In: Kimball FA, Buhl AE, Carter DB, eds. *New approaches to the study of benign prostatic hyperplasia.* New York: Alan R. Liss, Inc., 1984:103-128.
25. Hay ED. Cell-matrix interaction in the embryo: cell shape, cell surface, cell skeletons, and their role in differentiation. In: Trelstad RL, ed. *The role of extracellular matrix in development.* New York: Alan R. Liss, Inc. 1984:1-31.
26. Hay ED. Matrix-cytoskeletal interactions in the developing eye. *J Cell Biochem* 1985; 27:143-156.
27. Reid LM, Jefferson DM. Cell culture studies using extracts of endometrial matrix to study growth and differentiation in mammalian cells. In: Mather JP, ed. *Mammalian cell culture.* New York: Plenum Publishing Corp., 1984: 239-280.
28. Glasser SR, Julian J, Decker GL, Tang J-P, Carson DD. Development of morphological and functional polarity in

primary cultures of immature rat uterine epithelial cells. *J Cell Biol* 1988; 107:2409-2423.
29. Barcellos-Hoff MH, Aggeler J, Ram TG, Bissell MJ. Functional differentiation and alveolar morphogenesis of primary mammary cultures on reconstituted basement membrane. *Development* 1989; 105:223-235.
30. Enders AC, Chavez DJ, Schlafke S. Comparison of implantation *in utero* and *in vitro*. In: Glasser SR, Bullock DW, eds. *Cellular and molecular aspects of implantation*. New York: Plenum Press, 1981:365-382.
31. Enders AC, Schlafke S. A morphological analysis of the early implantation stages in the rat. *Am J Anat* 1967; 120:185-227.
32. Welsh AO, Enders AC. Light and electron microscopic examination of the mature decidual cells of the rat with emphasis on the antimesometrial decidua and its degeneration. *Am J Anat* 1985; 172:1-30.
33. Enders AC. The implantation chamber, blastocyst and blastocyst imprint of the rat: a scanning electron microscope study. *Anat Rec* 1975; 182:137-150.
34. Enders AC, Schlafke S. Comparative aspects of blastocyst endometrial interactions at implantation. In: *Maternal recognition of pregnancy* (Ciba Foundation Series 64, new series). Amsterdam: Excerpta Medica, 1979:3-32.
35. Welsh AO, Enders AC. Occlusion and reformation of the rat uterine lumen during pregnancy. *Am J Anat* 1983; 167:463-477.
36. Finn CA, Hinchliffe JR. Histological and histochemical analysis of the formation of implantation chambers in the mouse uterus. *J Reprod Fertil* 1965; 9:301-309.
37. De Feo VJ. Decidualization. In: Wynn RM, ed. *Cellular biology of the uterus*. New York: Appleton-Century-Crofts, 1967:191-290.
38. Werb Z, Bainton DF, Jones PA. Degradation of connective tissue matrices by macrophages. III. Morphological and biochemical studies on extracellular, pericellular, and intracellular events in matrix proteolysis by macrophages in culture. *J Exp Med* 1980; 152:1537-1553.
39. Sananes N, Weiller S, Baulieu EE, Le Goascogne C. *In vitro* decidualization of rat endometrial cells. *Endocrinology* 1978; 103:86-95.
40. Vladimirsky F, Chen L, Amsterdam A, Zor U, Lindner HR. Differentiation of decidual cells in cultures of rat endometrium. *J Reprod Fert* 1977; 49:61-68.
41. Bell SC, Searle RF. Differentiation of decidual cells in mouse endometrial cell cultures. *J Reprod Fert* 1981; 61:426-433.

ISOLATED ENDOMETRIAL CELLS AS *IN VITRO* MODELS TO STUDY THE ESTABLISHMENT OF PREGNANCY

J.K. Findlay, L.A. Salamonsen and R.A. Cherny

Medical Research Centre
Prince Henry's Hospital Campus
Monash Medical Centre
St. Kilda Road
Melbourne, Victoria, 3004
Australia

SUCCESSFUL implantation and the establishment of pregnancy requires preparation of the uterine endometrium to become receptive to the blastocyst, maintenance and extension of the function of the corpus luteum, and sustainment of pre-embryonic growth and differentiation during early pregnancy. In both the human and sheep, evidence is accumulating that endometrial- and blastocyst-derived secretory products, e.g, proteins and prostaglandins, are involved in a paracrine regulatory manner to bring about these changes. In many cases, however, the identity, regulation, and time and mechanism of action of the regulators have not been established.

Several years ago we chose to use sheep as a model to study paracrine regulation at the level of the blastocyst and endometrium. Sheep have a characteristically long preimplantation period of 16 days during which the trophectoderm undergoes massive elongation (up to 10 cm length) and there is synchronous development of the endometrium brought about partly by maternal steroids and partly by the presence of the blastocyst.[1] A blastocyst-derived antiluteolytic factor(s) is responsible for preventing the action of the endometrial luteolysin, prostaglandin F$_2\alpha$ (PGF), and it was shown that this signal must reach the maternal organism by day 12 of pregnancy (day 0 = estrus), 4 days before implantation.[1] In addition to influencing prostaglandin synthesis and release, the preimplantation blastocyst can also influence protein synthesis by endometrial tissue.[1-4]

At this stage, it was decided that a thorough investigation of paracrine interactions within the endometrium, through stromal cell-epithelial cell interactions, and between endometrial and trophectoderm cells, required isolation and culture of the individual cell types. As a consequence, we have established primary cell cultures of ovine epithelial and stromal cells and examined the influence of ovarian steroids and blastocyst-derived factors on protein and prostaglandin production. More recently, we have investigated systems for primary culture of epithelial cells which maintain their polarity and can be adapted to study stromal-epithelial or trophectoderm-epithelial cell interactions.

ISOLATION AND CULTURE OF OVINE ENDOMETRIAL CELLS

Isolation and Enrichment of Cells

The endometrium can be dissected cleanly from the myometrium of intact or estrogen-replete, ovariectomized ewes. If required, it is also possible to separate by gross dissection the non-glandular areas of attachment of the trophoblast on the endometrium (caruncles; C) from the glandular, intercaruncular region (IC). We generally obtain 10-20 g of endometrial tissue per uterus which yields between 10 and 50 x 10^6 epithelial cells/5 g.[5] At first we routinely separated C from IC, but no longer do so because we have not observed any major differences in the protein synthetic activities of epithelial cells from the respec-

PREPARATION OF PURIFIED ENDOMETRIAL CELLS

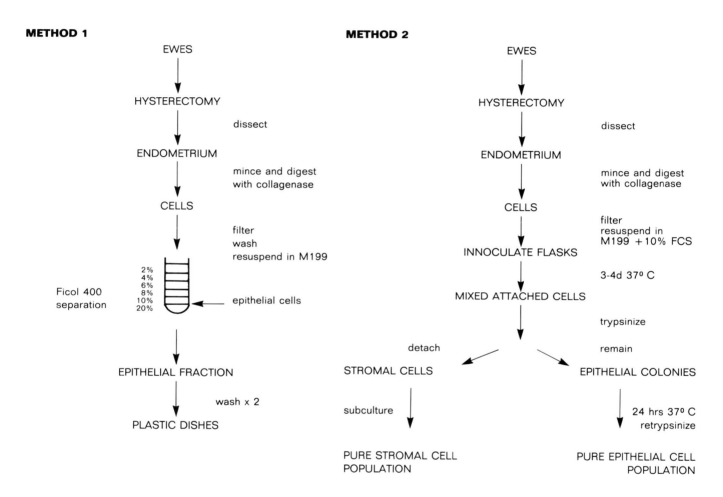

Figure 1. *A summary of the steps for isolation and separation of epithelial and stromal cells from sheep endometrium by Ficoll gradient (Method 1) and selective plating techniques (Method 2).*

tive tissues.[5] In addition to stromal cells, the C contains only luminal epithelial cells, whereas IC contains luminal plus glandular epithelial cells. It is possible that our method is selecting primarily for luminal epithelial cells.

The original method used to isolate epithelial and stromal cells from endometrial tissue involved collagenase treatment of chopped tissue and enrichment of epithelial cells on a Ficoll gradient.[5] Whilst providing much valuable data on protein[5-8] and prostaglandin[8] production by epithelial cells, the method suffers two major disadvantages. First, contamination of epithelial cells with stromal cells although low (<20%, generally 5-10%), was unacceptable for studies of stromal-epithelial cell interactions. Second, stromal cells prepared in this way did not attach and grow in primary culture on plastic dishes. Recent modification of the original method omits the Ficoll gradient step and uses selective trypsination and replating of stromal cells from epithelial cells in primary culture,[9] resulting in cultures of highly purified epithelial and stromal cells which appear stable over longer periods than cells obtained by the original method (3-5 days). The respective methods are summarized in Figure 1.

Identification of Isolated Cells

A major requirement of studies using separated cells is proper identification of the cell types. Ideally, a combination of several methods should be used, in our case, phase contrast and electron microscopy and specific immunohistochemical staining.

Under transmission electron microscopy, luminal epithelial cells of both the C and IC regions *in situ* are simple columnar cells with junctional complexes containing desmosomes in the lateral walls.[5] Glandular epithelial cells are similar but can be ciliated. All the epithelial cells are characterized by having microvilli and prominent nucleoli and are sometimes surrounded by a glycocalyx. Often abundant glycogen and polyribosomes can be seen together with bundles of microfilaments in the marginal cytoplasm. Isolated epithelial cells retain these *in situ* morphological characteristics and differ markedly from stromal fibroblasts, which have irregular nuclei, no surface microvilli, and no desmosomes at mesenchymal cell junctions. In addition, stromal cells have a higher nuclear-to-cytoplasmic ratio than epithelial cells, and *in situ*, are not polarized. The epithelial cells are polarized *in situ*, but polarity appears to be lost when they attach to plastic.

The intermediate filament proteins are characteristic of individual cell types, and immunohistochemical staining using specific antisera to the filament proteins offers a simple means for positive identification. Cytokeratin, ubiquitous in epithelial cells, has been used to identify ovine endometrial epithelial cells.[5] For the stromal cells, we use fibronectin, a component of the extracellular matrix secreted exclusively by fibroblasts, as a positive marker.[9] The absence of endothelial cells has been established by lack of staining with antiserum to Factor VIII.

Culture of Isolated Cells

In our original method, 1×10^6 epithelial cells are cultured in duplicate 35 mm plastic dishes in 1 ml Medium 199 (M199) containing 5% (vol/vol) charcoal- and heat-treated fetal calf serum.[5] The cells do not attach and spread in the absence of serum. Once attached in the presence of serum, the epithelial cells can be maintained satisfactorily for several days in serum-free medium. Increases in serum concentration up to but not beyond 5% resulted in increased spreading on the dishes and higher incorporation rates of ^{35}S-methionine into protein.[5] Routinely, the epithelial cells are initially plated in the presence of 5% charcoal- and heat-treated serum in M199 for 20 hrs at 37° C. The medium is removed and after washing, the cells are incubated for a further 24 hrs in methionine-free Dulbecco's modified Eagle's Medium containing 100 μCi ^{35}S-methionine. Subsequently, incorporation of labeled methionine into cellular and secreted protein can be analyzed. Cells cultured for up to 3 to 4 days give similar patterns of newly synthesized protein, but thereafter, the pattern changes,[10] suggesting dedifferentiation, culture senescence, or an increasingly significant contribution from contaminating (fibroblastic?) cells.

In an attempt to create culture conditions more closely approximating those *in vivo*, we conducted parallel experiments using collagen-coated microcarrier beads (Pharmacia, Uppsula, Sweden). The beads offer the advantages of increased surface area, permeability to growth medium, and a substrate (collagen) that is more interactive with the cell surface than the plastic. Data obtained suggest that both the level of incorporation of label and the pattern of protein secretion are affected substantially by the culture substrate.[11]

With our modified method[9] we plate separated stromal or epithelial cells on Millicell culture well inserts (Millipore, Bedford MA). The nitrocellulose membrane which forms the attachment surface is precoated with rat sarcoma extracellular matrix (Matrigel; Collaborative Research, Bedford, MA). Epithelial colonies maintained on plastic in the absence of stromal cells quickly flatten and lose their characteristic cobblestone appearance, cell size increases dramatically, vacuoles appear in the cytoplasm, and cell borders contract. When grown in Matrigel-coated inserts, the epithelial cells retain their characteristic morphology for over two weeks. Similarly, highly purified stromal preparations grown on plastic commonly, though not invariably, aggregate in large detached clumps after several days in culture. This aggregation and detachment is prevented when the cells are cultured on Matrigel-treated inserts. This culture method is now being used to examine the directionality and cellular source of endometrial secretions, to search for evidence of putative stromal-epithelial interactions and to examine the relationship between trophoblast and epithelium. It may prove valuable as well to reevaluate the microcarrier system[11] using these highly purified cell preparations.

CONTROL OF PROTEIN SYNTHESIS AND SECRETION BY OVINE ENDOMETRIAL EPITHELIAL CELLS

In the first experiments, we examined the effects of treating ovariectomized ewes *in vivo* with either nothing or implants of estrogen (E), progesterone (P), or E plus P, on incorporation of ^{35}S-methionine into cellular and secreted proteins of epithelial cells *in vitro*.[5] The extent to which individual proteins are steroid dependent was determined by analysis of the profiles of newly synthesized protein on two-dimensional sodium dodecyl sulfate, polyacrylamide gel electrophoresis (2D-PAGE) after autoradiography. It was found that epithelial cells from E-treated ewes had higher uptake and incorporation of ^{35}S-methionine into cellular and secreted protein than ewes treated with nothing or with P alone. However, the effects of E were significantly reduced in the presence of P. When secreted protein was expressed as a percent of total incorporated labeled amino acid, P treatment alone or with E increased the proportion of labeled protein secreted by epithelial cells. Analysis of individual proteins by 2D-PAGE revealed that the treatment E plus P, which represents the hormonal status in the luteal phase ewe and at implantation, induced 5 secreted proteins, including a 46,000 dalton protein which was a major component of the secretions. The protein was subsequently shown to be P-dependent.[7] Five other secreted proteins were inhibited by steroid treatment.[5] Many of the secreted proteins had considerable charge heterogeneity and were susceptible to neuraminidase treatment, indicating that they were glycosylated. Both induction and inhibition of cellular proteins were also apparent, although of a lesser magnitude than secreted proteins.

Attempts to reproduce these *in vivo* steroid effects by treating epithelial cells with steroids *in vitro* were only partly successful.[7,10] We attributed this to inappropriate cell culture conditions, the possibility of *in vivo* refractoriness to *in vivo* steriods carried over *in vitro* and/or the absence of stromal cells. It was at this stage that we decided to develop coculture systems for stromal and epithelial cells.

Meanwhile, the epithelial cell primary culture system was used to determine whether or not the presence of a conceptus *in vivo* or *in vitro* influenced protein secretion.[6] Previous studies[3,4] had demonstrated a quantitative increase in the rate of leucine incorporation into cellular protein by endometrium of pregnant (Pr) ewes before implantation. Secreted proteins were not examined. Furthermore, Godkin et al.[12] demonstrated that ovine trophoblast protein-1 (oTP-1), the antiluteolysin secreted by the trophectoderm, bound specifically to ovine endometrium and increased the rate of protein release by endometrial explants of non-pregnant (NPr) ewes. We showed that incorporation of ^{35}S-methionine into secreted protein was significantly higher in cells from Pr than NPr ewes on day 13.[6] Secretion by epithelial cells from NPr ewes was increased in 3 out of 4 cases by addition of media conditioned by 15-day blastocysts (BM). 2D-PAGE analysis showed 5 secreted proteins (mol wt range 74,000 - 120,000; isoelectric point < 6.5), which were either absent or present in only small amounts in secretions from cells from NPr ewes, were greatly enhanced in secretions of cells from Pr ewes. The addition of BM to cultures from NPr ewes enhanced the secretion of these same proteins, even after heat treatment (80° C/15 min) of BM. We concluded that endometrial epithelial cells from Pr ewes are metabolically more active than those from NPr ewes, and that the blastocyst and its secretions induce secretion of several specific proteins by epithelial cells, some of these proteins being the same as those controlled by the E plus P treatment.

The secreted polypeptides whose concentrations were enhanced in pregnancy were similar in molecular weight and acidic nature to some observed by Godkin et al.[12] to be stimulated when purified oTP-1 was added *in vitro* to endometrial explants from day 12 NPr ewes. We therefore examined the effects of pure oTP-1 on proteins secreted by primary cultures of enriched epithelial cells from E plus P treated ovariectomized ewes.[8] At about this time, it was revealed that oTP-1 and interferon-α were members of the same gene family[13,14] so the comparison was extended to include recombinant human-α$_2$ interferon (IFN: Roferon-A, Hoffman-La Roche, Basel). It was shown that oTP-1 and IFN stimulated synthesis and secretion of the same "pregnancy-related" proteins seen in the previous study, with the exception of one protein which was only found to be induced by oTP-1/IFN in the later study[8] (Fig.2).

CONTROL OF PROSTAGLANDIN SYNTHESIS AND SECRETION BY OVINE ENDOMETRIAL EPITHELIAL CELLS

oTP-1 is a major secretory product of the ovine blastocyst during the period immediately prior to implantation. Its infusion into the uterine lumen of cyclic ewes delays luteal regression[12] and suppresses the *in vivo* production of uterine PGF in response to exogenous E and oxytocin.[15] We compared the actions of oTP-1 and IFN on prostaglandin release from ovine endometrial cells in primary culture.

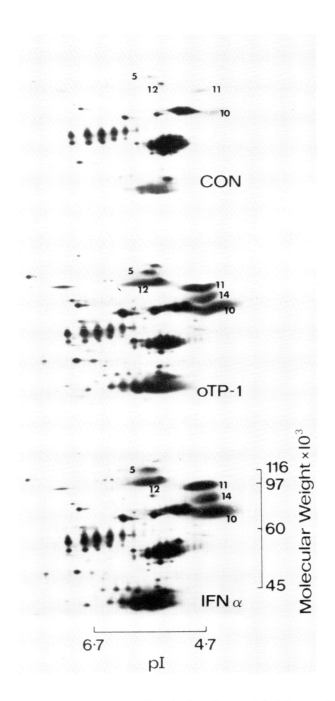

Figure 2. 2D-PAGE profiles of ^{35}S-methionine-labeled secreted proteins, following culture of endometrial cells from ovariectomized, estrogen- and progesterone-treated ewes with either no in vitro treatment (CON), with oTP-1 (30 ng/ml) or IFN (500 U/ml). From Salamonsen et al.[8] Reproduced with permission of the Journal of Endocrinology Ltd.

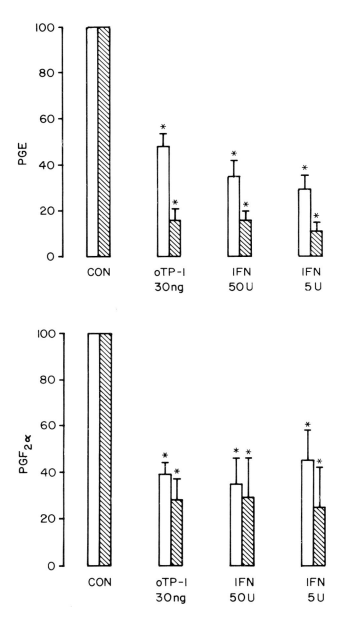

Figure 3. Effect of oTP-1 and human IFN in vitro on PGE and $PGF_2\alpha$ secretion by cultured endometrial cells derived from ovariectomized, estrogen- and protesterone-treated ewes (N= 4), on day 0-1 (open bars, + fetal calf serum) and day 1-2 (hatched bars, no fetal calf serum) of culture. Results are expressed as % of control (CON, no in vitro treatment, 100%) for each batch of cells. Mean ± SEM *P <0.05 compared with CON. From Salamonsen et al.[8] Reproduced with permission of the Journal of Endocrinology Ltd.

Both oTP-1 (30 ng/well) and IFN (50 or 5 µ/well) significantly attenuated release of PGE and $PGF_2\alpha$ by these cells (Fig. 3). In both cases, the inhibition was greater on the second day of culture in the absence of serum than on the first day. We have now demonstrated these effects of oTP-1 and IFN to be time and dose-dependent.[16] This action of oTP-1 on PG release supports its hypothesized role in the antiluteolytic process, although a role for PGE in this process has not been defined. The inhibition of both PGE and PGF suggests that oTP-1 (and IFN) exerts its control at a point prior to the formation of the endoperoxidase intermediate which is common to both products. Studies are in progress to identify the point at which oTP-1 controls synthesis and metabolism of arachidonic acid. It has been postulated that this occurs subsequent to formation of arachidonic acid in early pregnancy in the cow.[17]

It appears likely that oTP-1 is an ovine homolog of interferon-α_2 and that it is an important paracrine regulator of the production of proteins and prostaglandins. Whether or not an interferon-related peptide is important in the establishment of human pregnancy has never been reported. However, because PG's have been implicated in control of menstruation, it is possible that an endometrial oTP-1-like or interferon-α_2 peptide could regulate onset of menstruation.

CONCLUSION

There are several advantages gained by using isolated cell systems to study endometrial function *in vitro*.[18] These include the opportunity to study the functions and responses to stimuli of one cell type over prolonged periods, and to examine the interactions between different cells of the endometrium and between cells of the endometrium and the trophectoderm. At a technical level, the sheep model provides relatively large quantities of cells which are readily identifiable. The limitations of these methods include the effects of cell isolation and culture conditions which may result in cellular functions different from those *in vivo*, and the need to maintain polarity, particularly for epithelial cells in culture. The dual chamber systems have much to offer in this regard, particularly for investigations of paracrine interactions.

A number of questions remain to be addressed, such as those concerning proliferation of endometrial cells and the need to develop serum-free culture systems in which cells can be passaged without loss of function or dedifferentiation.

Meanwhile the sheep model system described here provides a useful and practical method to study paracrine interactions at the level of the endometrium and trophoblast.

Acknowledgment

We thank the National Health and Medical Research Council of Australia and the Buckland Foundation for financial support, and Faye Coates for secretarial assistance.

References

1. Findlay JK, Maule Walker FM, Heap RB. The sheep as model to study embryo-maternal relationships in the preimplantation period. In: Serio M, Martini L, eds. *Animal models in human reproduction.* New York: Raven Press, 1980:283-297.
2. Findlay JK. The endocrinology of the preimplantation period. In: Martini L, James VHT, eds. *The endocrinology of pregnancy and parturition. Current topics in experimental endocrinology.* Vol. 4, New York: Academic Press, 1981:35-67.
3. Findlay JK, Ackland N, Burton RD. Protein, prostaglandin and steroid synthesis in caruncular and intercaruncular endometrium of sheep before implantation. *J Reprod Fert* 1981; 62:361-377.
4. Findlay JK, Clarke IJ, Swaney J, Colvin N, Doughton B. Estrogen receptors and protein synthesis in caruncular and intercaruncular endometrium of sheep before implantation. *J Reprod Fert* 1982; 64:329-339.
5. Salamonsen LA, O WS, Doughton BW, Findlay JK. The effects of estrogen and progesterone *in vivo* on protein synthesis and secretion by cultured epithelial cells from sheep endometrium. *Endocrinology* 1985; 117:2148-2159.
6. Salamonsen LA, Doughton BW, Findlay JK. The effects of the preimplantation blastocyst *in vivo* and *in vitro* on protein synthesis and secretion by cultured epithelial cells from sheep endometrium. *Endocrinology* 1986; 119:622-628.
7. Salamonsen LA, Healy DL, Findlay JK. Progesterone *in vitro* stimulates secretion of a specific protein by ovine epithelial endometrial cells. *J Steroid Biochem* 1987; 28:285-288.
8. Salamonsen LA, Stuchbery SJ, O'Grady CM, Godkin JD, Findlay JK. Interferon-α mimics effects of ovine trophoblast protein 1 on prostaglandin and protein secretion by ovine endometrial cells *in vitro. J Endocr* 1988; 117:R1-R4.
9. Cherny RA, Findlay JK. Protein secretion patterns of separated ovine endometrial cells cultured in dual environment chambers. *Proc Aust Soc Reprod Biol* 1988; 20:50.

10. Salamonsen LA. Control of endometrial protein secretion during early pregnancy in the ewe. Ph.D. Thesis 1986, Monash University.
11. Cherny RA, Findlay JK. Comparison of protein secretion patterns by ovine endometrial epithelial cells grown on microcarriers and on plastic dishes. *Proc Aust Soc Reprod Biol* 1987; 19:112.
12. Godkin JD, Bazer FW, Thatcher WW, Roberts RM. Ovine trophoblast protein 1, an early secreted blastocyst protein, binds specifically to uterine endometrium and affects protein synthesis. *Endocrinology* 1984; 114:120-130.
13. Stewart HJ, McCann SHE, Barker PJ, Lee KE, Lamming GE, Flint APF. Interferon sequence homology and receptor binding activity of ovine trophoblast anti-luteolytic protein. *J Endocr* 1987; 115:R13-R15.
14. Imakawa K, Anthony RV, Kazemi M, Marotti KR, Polites HG, Roberts RM. Interferon-like sequence of ovine trophoblast protein secreted by embryonic trophectoderm. *Nature* 1987; 330:377-379.
15. Vallet JL, Bazer FW, Fliss MFV. Effects of ovine conceptus secretory protein and ovine trophoblast protein-one on uterine production of prostaglandins. *Biol Reprod* 1987; 36, Suppl 1:327.
16. Salamonsen LA, Manikhot J, Findlay JK. Studies on the inhibitory action of interferons on prostaglandin release by ovine endometrial cells *in vitro*. *Proc Soc Study Fertil* 1988; in press.
17. Gross TS, Thatcher WW, Hansen PJ, Johnson JW, Helmer SD. Presence of an intracellular endometrial inhibitor of prostaglandin synthesis during early pregnancy in the cow. *Prostaglandins* 1988; 35:359-379.
18. Findlay JK, Salamonsen LA, Cherny RA. The use of isolated cells to study endometrial function *in vitro*. In: Milligan SR, ed. *Oxford reviews of reproductive biology.* in press.

IMPLANTATION: *IN VITRO* MODELS UTILIZING HUMAN TISSUES

Harvey J. Kliman,* Christos Coutifaris,† Ronald F. Feinberg,†
Jerome F. Strauss III,*† and Julia E. Haimowitz*

*Departments of Pathology and Laboratory Medicine, and
†Obstetrics and Gynecology
University of Pennsylvania School of Medicine
Philadelphia, Pennsylvania 19104 USA

THE mechanism by which trophoblastic elements penetrate into the human endometrium is not known. To date, most studies examining nidation have been performed in a variety of non-human mammalian systems.[1-4] These animal studies have provided insight into the possible mechanisms of human implantation.[4-7] On the basis of electron microscopic studies, Schlafke and Enders[8] proposed three possible mechanisms for implantation: (1) intrusive implantation, which is characterized by trophoblast penetration between cells of the uterine epithelium and adhesion to the basal lamina; (2) fusion implantation, where syncytial trophoblasts fuse with uterine epithelial cells; and (3) displacement implantation, where trophoblasts dislodge the uterine epithelium from their basal lamina and replace it. Since detailed *in vivo* biological and biochemical studies are not possible in the human, *in vitro* systems will be critical to select among these possible implantation mechanisms and to further our understanding of normal human nidation. In this paper we will review the available *in vitro* implantation models, present preliminary data utilizing our human trophoblast-endometrium co-culture model systems, and present our hypothesis for human implantation.

A MODEL FOR HUMAN IMPLANTATION

We are hypothesizing a four-step model for human nidation (Fig. 1): (1) trophoblast-endometrial epithelium interaction, (2) trophoblast-extracellular matrix (ECM) protein interaction, (3) controlled degradation of the ECM by a combination of proteases, and (4) resynthesis of the ECM. We are proposing that the initial step of implantation occurs between the trophoblast cell surface and an appropriately receptive endometrial epithelial cell surface through cell adhesion molecules (CAMs). Once this initial contact takes place, the trophoblasts interdigitate between the endometrial epithelial cells and make specific contact with the underlying supporting extracellular matrix proteins (fibronectin, laminin, types I and IV collagen, and proteoglycans) through substrate adhesion molecules (SAMs). At this point, the trophoblasts are stimulated to secrete proteases which degrade the preexisting extracellular matrix. The extent of degradation is controlled by membrane-associated and secreted protease inhibitors. At a later time, the trophoblasts are induced to synthesize new ECM proteins which permit firm adherence to the uterine stroma. We also propose that the trophoblasts which invade the uterus and reach the spiral arteries later in pregnancy are subject to these same basic control mechanisms.[9]

Our hypothesis makes a number of predictions: (1) trophoblasts can synthesize proteases capable of degrading extracellular matrix proteins, (2) trophoblasts can synthesize specific protease inhibitors which are capable of neutralizing the action of these proteases, and (3) trophoblasts are capable of synthesizing extracellular matrix proteins.

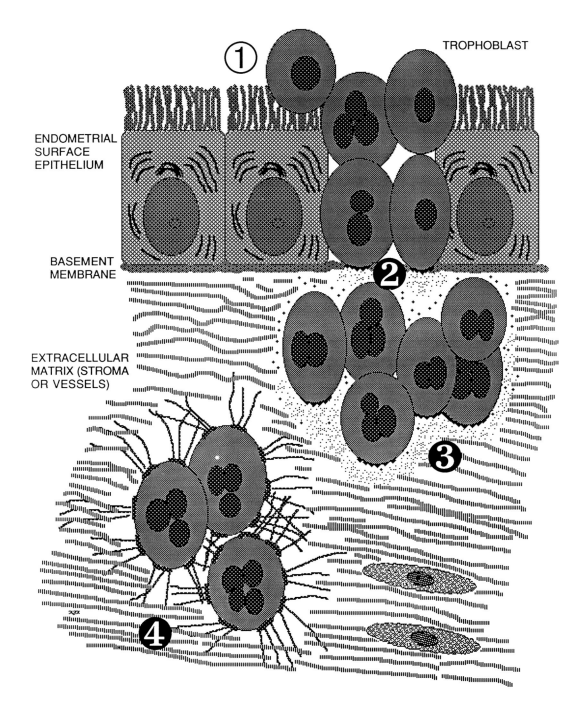

Figure 1. *Model of human implantation. Trophoblasts attach to the endometrial surface epithelium through cell adhesion molecules (CAMs) (1). The trophoblasts interdigitate between the epithelial cells. Eventually, the trophoblasts make contact with the basement membrane (2), initiating the secretion of proteases (3). The extent of proteolysis is regulated by membrane associated (▼) and secreted (+) protease inhibitors. Once the trophoblasts have reached their final destination (e.g., a maternal spiral artery), they synthesize ECM proteins which firmly attach them to their surroundings (4).*

Figure 2. *Immunoperoxidase staining for laminin (A,B) in cultured human trophoblasts. Purified human cytotrophoblasts were cultured in serum-free Dulbecco's modified Eagles' medium on an uncoated surface (A) or on a collagen-coated surface (B), fixed at 24 hrs with Bouin's and immunocytochemically stained. (A) Laminin is present in the cytoplasm with little membrane staining. (B) Less laminin cytoplasmic staining is apparent, but the membrane surfaces are laminin positive (arrows), particularly at the cell contact points between these two cells, suggesting that the collagen has induced cytoplasmic laminin to become membrane-associated laminin.*

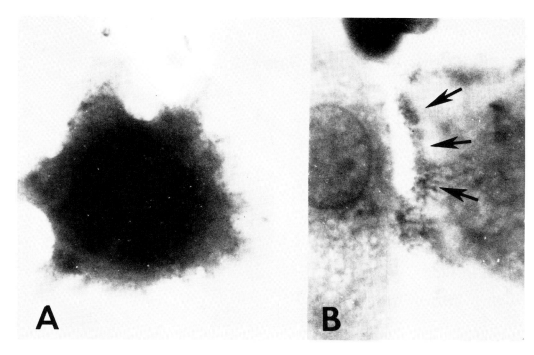

Experimental support for this model comes from a variety of sources. *Step one*, endometrium-trophoblast interactions: Cell surface glycoproteins have been implicated in the process of implantation by a number of workers. Guillomot et al.,[10] for example, have demonstrated that interactions between blastocysts and endometrium in the ewe involve glycoconjugates which interact with concanavalin A. *Step two*, trophoblast-ECM interactions: The importance of extracellular matrix protein interactions was reported by Armant et al.[11] who demonstrated that fibronectin and laminin promote the *in vitro* attachment and outgrowth of mouse blastocysts. In addition, we have demonstrated[12] that human trophoblasts have specific fibronectin receptors and that they attach firmly to laminin and a variety of collagens. *Step three*, ECM degradation: Proteases have been implicated in implantation,[13,14] and Fisher et al.[15] have demonstrated that chorionic villi from first trimester human placentae can degrade extracellular matrix proteins. Queenan and co-workers have recently demonstrated that cytotrophoblasts obtained from term placentae synthesize and secrete urokinase-type plasminogen activator (u-PA).[16] Furthermore, we have demonstrated that cultured trophoblasts also contain tissue plasminogen activator and plasminogen activator inhibitor (PAI) types 1 and 2,[17] proteins which may regulate protease activity during nidation.

We also have evidence that in placental beds *in situ*, invading trophoblasts contain both immunoreactive t-PA and a specific PA inhibitor, PAI-1.[17] And finally, *step four* ECM resynthesis: We have demonstrated that cultured trophoblasts synthesize fibronectin,[18] and laminin (Fig. 2).

IN VITRO IMPLANTATION MODELS

Since detailed biochemical studies cannot be performed in the human *in situ*, *in vitro* approaches are a necessity. Such systems would permit researchers to evaluate the cellular, biochemical, and molecular mechanisms involved in human implantation. Several laboratories have proposed *in vitro* models for implantation in which blastocysts from laboratory animals have been cultured on extracellular matrices, endometrial tissue, and lens capsules (Table I). Although researchers in the United States are not able to directly study human trophoblasts within the blastocyst, we suggest that the placental trophoblasts used in our model systems illuminate the mechanisms by which trophoblasts interact with the endometrium. While no *in vitro* model system could hope to completely recapitulate the *in vivo* processes of implantation and placentation, trophoblasts *in vitro* appear to share many morphologic and biochemical properties with trophoblasts *in situ*.

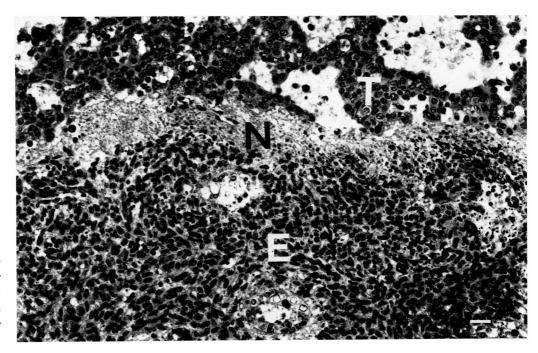

Figure 3. Contact necrosis. High-power view of zone of necrosis (N) induced by term-trophoblasts (T) co-incubated with endometrium (E) for 24 hrs. The bar represents 20 μm.

Manipulation of these cells *in vitro* should add fundamental information to our limited understanding of human implantation and placentation. Therefore, we have developed *in vitro* systems to explore the interactions of human trophoblasts with human endometrial explants and purified endometrial epithelial cells in culture[30,31] as models for human implantation.

We recently described a method to purify cytotrophoblasts from human placentae and have characterized their differentiation *in vitro*.[32,33] These human cytotrophoblasts: (1) produce steroidal (estrogen and progesterone) and protein (hCG, hPL, SP1) hormones typical of the human placenta; (2) fuse to form syncytial trophoblasts in culture and respond to 8-bromo-cAMP by producing increased amounts of these hormones;[34] (3) produce u-PA,[16] PAI-1 and 2;[17] and (4) synthesize fibronectin[18] and laminin (see Fig. 2). Therefore, by co-incubating these purified human cytotrophoblasts with tissue and cells from human endometrium, we expect to replicate *in vitro* the processes that occur during normal implantation and subsequent establishment of the placental bed.

Two *in vitro* model systems have been explored: trophoblast-endometrial explant co-incubation and trophoblast-endometrial monolayer co-culture. The explant system has the advantage of maintaining intact the cellular architecture of the endometrium, but the survival of the endometrial explants is limited to several days. On the other hand, the isolated endometrial cells in standard culture, which can last up to two weeks, offer the opportunity of examining prolonged interactions between specific cell types. Thus, these two methods complement each other.

Cytotrophoblast Interactions With Endometrial Explants

Cytotrophoblasts isolated from first or third trimester placentae bind to endometrial explants in suspension co-culture during a 24-48 hour incubation. The cytotrophoblasts preferentially attach to the cut surfaces of proliferative and secretory endometrium, where stroma and extracellular matrix proteins are exposed. The trophoblasts have only attached to the surface epithelium when the explant was derived from day-19 endometrium. After 24-48 hrs of co-incubation, a zone of tissue necrosis can be observed at the junction between the attached trophoblastic elements and the endometrium (Fig. 3). Histologically, this zone resembles Nitabuch's layer, which is made up of fibrinoid material and separates the cytotrophoblast cell columns from the decidua seen in normal human implan-

Table I. In vitro models for the study of implantation.

MODELS	DESCRIPTION	REFERENCES	
Blastocyst Outgrowth	Animal blastocysts cultured on ECM coated surfaces	Jenkinson Armant, et al. Farach, et al. Carson, et al.	1978 (19) 1986 (11) 1987 (20) 1988 (21)
	Animal blastocysts cultured on cell monolayers	Glass, et al.	1979 (22)
Endometrial Floating Collagen Gels	Endometrial epithelium cultured on floating collagen gels	Sengupta, et al.	1986 (23)
Attachment Model	Animal blastocysts cultured on lens capsule	Cammarata, et al.	1987 (24)
Endometrial Explant Co-culture	Animal blastocysts cultured with animal endometrial strips	Glenister, et al.	1961 (25)
Endometrial Organ Co-culture	Animal blastocysts cultured with whole animal uteri	Grant, et al.	1975 (26)
	Human blastocysts cultured with whole perfused human uteri	Bulletti, et al.	1988 (27)
Endometrial Monolayer Co-culture	Human chorionic villi cultured on endometrial gland monolayers	Kishimoto, et al.	1987 (28)
	Human blastocysts cultured on human endometrial gland monolayers	Lindenberg, et al.	1986 (29)
	Human trophoblasts cultured on endometrial gland monolayers	Coutifaris, et al.	1988 (30)
Endometrial-trophoblast Suspension Co-culture	Human trophoblasts co-cultured in suspension with endometrial explants	Kliman, et al.	1988 (31)

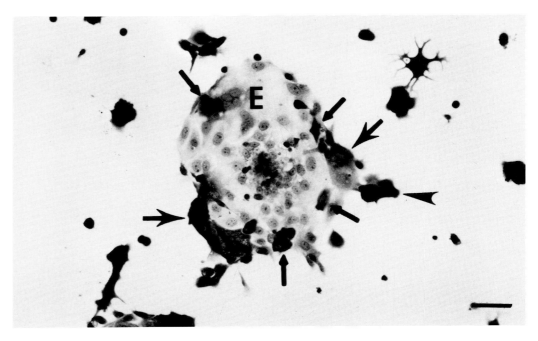

Figure 4. *Endometrial gland co-culture. Purified human endometrial glands were co-cultured with human cytotrophoblasts for 24 hrs, fixed with Bouin's solution and immunocytochemically stained with antibodies against alpha-hCG. Several darkly stained trophoblast groups can be seen around the endometrial gland (E). Note a trophoblast group making initial contact with the gland (arrowhead). Two large syncytial trophoblast groups can be seen adherent to the edge of the gland (large arrows). In addition, several trophoblasts have penetrated the glandular group (small arrows). The bar represents 50 μm.*

tation sites. Some cytotrophoblasts penetrate into the endometrial explants and can be clearly identified in tissue sections by the use of immunocytochemistry with antibodies against hCG subunits.

It is important to note that there appears to be no qualitative differences in the behavior of cytotrophoblasts isolated from first trimester and term placentae with respect to these interactions with endometrial explants. Like cytotrophoblasts, melanoma cells, endothelial cells, and amniocytes attach preferentially to the exposed extracellular matrix surfaces of the endometrial explants, but, unlike trophoblasts, do not induce a zone of necrosis (data not shown). Therefore, it appears that the endometrial surface epithelium is the component that imparts specificity to the initial interaction which takes place between trophoblast and endometrium.

Cytotrophoblast Interactions with Endometrial Glandular Epithelium and Stroma

Gurpide and colleagues[35] have developed methods to prepare human endometrial cells and maintain them in culture. These techniques have permitted us and others to examine the interaction of cytotrophoblasts with enriched endometrial cell types. Isolated endometrial glands form nests of epithelial cells after being established in culture. When added, cytotrophoblasts bind to the collections of glandular epithelial cells and then penetrate into the islands (Fig. 4).[30,28] Sequential observation reveals that the trophoblastic cells insinuate between the endometrial epithelial cells, in some cases dislodging them from the culture dish. In contrast, melanoma cells surround the nests of glandular epithelium but do not interact or invade them. Yet cytotrophoblasts, JEG-3 choriocarcinoma cells, and melanoma cells all adhere to established cultures of endometrial stromal cells and co-mingle with them.[36]

DISCUSSION

Our preliminary findings suggest that cytotrophoblasts have a proclivity for endometrial epithelial cells and are capable of penetrating through them in a process which resembles intrusive implantation. There seems to be specificity to this interaction since cytotrophoblasts do not exhibit the same type of behavior when presented with other epithelia.[36] However, cytotrophoblasts indiscriminately associate with stromal cells and a variety of extracellular matrix proteins. For as we have shown previously, a number of matrix proteins permit trophoblast attachment, flattening, and syncytium formation.[12] Therefore, we speculate that the specificity of attachment of trophoblasts is determined by the endometrial surface epithelium while the underlying extracellular matrix is always permissive. Thus under normal circumstances, implantation would occur only in the presence of a receptive endometrial epithelium. However, if the epithelium is eroded, exposing stroma and extracellular matrix, implantation (or even ectopic implantation) could occur in a variety of locations (e.g., sites where the oviductal epithelium is denuded).

Studies in laboratory animals suggest that a variety of proteases are involved in implantation, including plasminogen activator.[13,14] Axelrod[37] reported that the t^{W73} mouse produces blastocysts which are less invasive than controls and have an associated diminished production of plasminogen activator activity. Other proteases, such as stromelysin and collagenases, which degrade extracellular matrix, probably participate in trophoblast invasion, since a variety of proteins must be hydrolyzed in concert or sequence during implantation. Purified human cytotrophoblasts elaborate several proteases capable of digesting gelatin, among them urokinase.[16] Urokinase may have a direct role in the degradation of fibronectin, as well as activating other enzymes, including plasmin and collagenase, which hydrolyze matrix proteins.[15] The expressed activity of urokinase is determined not only by the amount of enzyme protein but also by levels of plasminogen activator inhibitors which covalently bind to and inhibit the enzyme.[38] The human trophoblast produces at least two different plasminogen activator inhibitors, plasminogen activator inhibitor types 1 and 2 (PAI-1 and PAI-2). PAI-1 is localized by immunocytochemistry primarily to trophoblasts invading into the endometrium whereas PAI-2 is found predominantly in the syncytial trophoblast of the chorionic villi.[17] Since trophoblast invasion must be controlled, mechanisms to restrict the site of protease action and to limit the activity of the enzymes are also expected to play a key function in implantation. Our work suggests that PAI-1 might serve the role of limiting protease activity of invasive trophoblasts, i.e., trophoblasts which penetrate the placental bed.[17]

The coordinated regulation of urokinase/tPA and PAIs provides one means by which trophoblast invasion could be tightly regulated.[39] Urokinase is also known to bind to cell surface receptors, fixing the site of its action. Thus, there are several levels at which plasminogen activator activity can be modulated, including (1) enzyme synthesis, (2) enzyme activation, (3) modulation of distribution by association with cell surface receptors for the enzyme, and (4) inactivation of enzyme by specific inhibitors. Plasminogen activators are not the only proteases with multiple loci for control. Stromelysin and collagenases are also produced as proenzymes and a specific inhibitor of these metalloproteinases (TIMP: Tissue inhibitor of metalloproteinases) is present in the uterine environment.[40]

The use of the *in vitro* model systems described here should permit us to begin to probe the cellular and biochemical processes which occur during human implantation and placentation, namely, (1) trophoblast attachment to endometrial surface epithelium, (2) penetration of the epithelial layer, (3) degradation of the ECM to permit invasion into the endometrial stroma, and (4) resynthesis of ECM proteins to permit firm attachment of trophoblasts to the endometrium.

References

1. Denker H-W. Basic aspects of ovoimplantation. *Obstet Gynecol Annu* 1983; 12:15-42.
2. Enders AC, Chavez DJ, Shlafke S. Comparison of implantation *in utero* and *in vitro*. In: Glasser SR and Bullock DW, eds. *Cellular and molecular aspects of implantation*. Plenum, 1981:365-382.
3. Enders AC, Hendricks AG, Schlafke S. Implantation in the Rhesus monkey: initial penetration of endometrium. *Am J Anat* 1983; 167:275-298.
4. Schlafke S, Welsh AO, Enders AC. Penetration of the basal lamina of the uterine luminal epithelium during implantation in the rat. *Anat Record* 1985; 212:47-56.
5. Hata T, Ohkawa K, Uchida K. Contact patterns between cytotrophoblast and decidual cells in human implantation site. *Acta Obst Gynaec Jpn* 1981; 35:529-536.
6. Hata T, Ohkawa K, Tomita M, et al. Phagocytosis of human cytotrophoblast cell invading into decidual tissue in early stage of gestation. *Acta Obst Gynaec Jpn* 1981; 33:537-544.
7. Glasser SR. Current concepts of implantation and decidualization. In: Hoszar G, ed. *The physiology and biochemistry of the uterus in pregnancy and labor*. CRC Press, 1986; 127-154.
8. Schlafke S, Enders AC. Cellular basis of interaction between trophoblast and uterus at implantation. *Biol Reprod* 1975; 12:41.
9. Robertson WB, Brosens I, Pijenborg R, et al. The making of the placental bed. *Europ J Obstet Gynec Reprod Biol* 1984; 18:255-266.
10. Guillomot M, Fléchon JE, Wintenberger-Torres S. Cytochemical studies of uterine and trophoblastic surface coats during blastocyst attachment in the ewe. *J Reprod Fert* 1982; 65:1-8.
11. Armant DR, Kaplan HA, Lennarz WJ. Fibronectin and laminin promote *in vitro* attachment and outgrowth of mouse

blastocysts. *Dev Biol* 1986; 116:519-523.
12. Kao L-C, Caltabiano S, Wu S, Strauss JF III, Kliman HJ. The human villous cytotrophoblast: interactions with extracellular matrix proteins, endocrine function, and cytoplasmic differentiation in the absence of syncytium formation. *Dev Biol* 1988; 130:693-702.
13. Denker H-W. Proteinases and implantation. *J Reprod Fert* Suppl 1981; 29:183-186.
14. Glass RH. Degradation of extracellular matrix by mouse trophoblast outgrowths: a model for implantation. *J Cell Biol* 1983; 96:1108-1116.
15. Fisher SJ, Leitch MS, Kantor MS, Basbaum CB, Kramer RH. Degradation of extracellular matrix by the trophoblastic cells of first-trimester human placentas. *J Cell Biochem* 1985; 27:31-41.
16. Queenan JT Jr, Kao L-C, Arboleda CE, Ulloa-Aguirre A, Golos TG, Cines DB, et al. Regulation of urokinase-type plasminogen activator production by cultured human cytotrophoblasts. *J Biol Chem* 1987; 262:10903-10906.
17. Feinberg RF, Strauss JF III, Wun T-C, Kliman HJ. Plasminogen activators (PAs) and plasminogen activator inhibitors (PAIs) in human trophoblasts: markers of trophoblast invasion [Abstract]. *Society for Gyn Invest* 1989.
18. Ulloa-Aguirre A, August AM, Golos TG, Kao L-C, Sukuragi N, Kliman HJ, et al. 8-Bromo-3′5′-adenosine monophosphate regulates expression of chorionic gonadotropin and fibronectin in human cytotrophoblasts. *J Clin End Metab* 1987; 64:1002-1009.
19. Jenkinson EJ. The *in vitro* blastocyst outgrowth system as a model for the analysis of peri-implantation development. In: Johnson M, ed. *Development in mammals*. Vol. 2, Amsterdam: North-Holland, 1978:151-172.
20. Farach MC, Tang JP, Decker GL, Carson DD. Heparin/heparan sulfate is involved in attachment and spreading of mouse embryos *in vitro*. *Dev Biol* 1987; 123:401-410.
21. Carson DD, Tang JP, Gay S. Collagens support embryo attachment and outgrowth *in vitro*: effects of the Arg-Gly-Asp sequence. *Dev Biol* 1988; 127:368-375.
22. Glass RH, Spindle AI, Pedersen RA. Mouse embryo attachment to substratum and interaction of trophoblast with cultured cells. *J Exp Zool* 1979; 208:327-336.
23. Sengupta J, Given RL, Carey JB, Weitlauf HM. Primary culture of mouse endometrium on floating collagen gels: a potential *in vitro* model for implantation. *Ann NY Acad Sci* 1986; 976:75-94.
24. Cammarata PR, Oakford L, Canta-Crouch D, Wordinger R. Attachment of blastocysts to lens capsule: A model system for trophoblast-epithelial cell interactions on a natural basement membrane. *Cell Tissue Res* 1987; 250:633-640.
25. Glenister TW. Organ culture as a new method for studying the implantation of mammalian blastocysts. *Proc Royal Soc B* 1961; 154:428-431.
26. Grant PS, Ljungkvist I, Nilsson O. The hormonal control and morphology of blastocyst invasion in the mouse uterus *in vitro*. *J Embryol Exp Morphol* 1975; 34:310.
27. Bulletti C, Jasonni VM, Tabanelli S, Gianaroli L, Ciotti PM, Ferraretti AP, et al. Early human pregnancy *in vitro* utilizing an artificially perfused uterus. *Fertil Steril* 1988; 49:991-996.
28. Kishimoto Y, Tominaga T, Aso T, Kinoshita M, Mori T. Human trophoblast and endometrial interactions *in vitro*. *Acta Obst Gynaec Jpn* 1987; 39:463.
29. Lindenberg S, Hyttel P, Lenz S, Holmes PV. Ultrastructure of the early human implantation *in vitro*. *Human Reprod* 1986; 1:533-538.
30. Coutifaris C, Kliman HJ, Strauss JF III. Development of an *in vitro* model system for human embryo implantation [Abstract]. Annual Meeting of the AFS, Atlanta, 1988.
31. Kliman HJ, Coutifaris C, Feinberg RF, Strauss JF III, Haimowitz JE. Interactions between human term trophoblasts and endometrium *in vitro*. 11th Roch Troph Conf, Rochester, 1988.
32. Kliman HJ, Nestler JE, Sermasi E, Sanger JM, Strauss JF III. Purification, characterization, and *in vitro* differentiation of cytotrophoblasts from human term placentae. *Endocrinology* 1986; 118:1567-1582.
33. Kliman HJ, Feinman MA, Strauss JF III. Differentiation of human cytotrophoblasts into syncytiotrophoblasts in culture. In: Miller R and Thied H, eds. *Trophoblast Research* Volume 2. New York, Plenum Medical, 1987; 407-422.
34. Feinman MA, Kliman HJ, Caltabiano S, Strauss JF III. 8-Bromo-3′,5′-adenosine monophosphate stimulates the endocrine activity of human cytotrophoblasts in culture. *J Clin Endocrinol Metab* 1986; 63:1211-1217.
35. Schatz F, Markiewicz L, Gurpide E. Effects of estriol on $PGF_2\alpha$ output by cultures of human endometrium and endometrial cells. *J Steroid Biochem* 1984; 20:999-1003.
36. Coutifaris C, Kliman HJ, Wu P, Strauss JF III. Specificity of trophoblast-endometrial interactions in a human *in vitro* implantation model system [Abstract]. 36th Annual Meeting of the Society for Gynecologic Investigation, San Diego, 1989.
37. Axelrod HR. Altered trophoblast functions in implantation-defective mouse embryos. *Dev Biol* 1985; 108:185-190.
38. Blasi F, Vassalli J-D, Keld D. Urokinase-type plasminogen activator: proenzyme, receptors, and inhibitors. *J Cell Biol* 1987; 104:801-804.

39. Feinberg RF, Kao L-C, Ringler G, Murray S, Queenan JT Jr, Kliman HJ, et al. Coordinate regulation of urokinase and plasminogen activator inhibitors in human cytotrophoblast [Abstract]. 35th Annual Meeting of the SGI, Baltimore, 1988.

40. Bunning RA, Murphy G, Kumar S, Phillips P, Reynolds J. Metalloproteinase inhibitors from bovine cartilage and body fluids. *E J Biochem* 1984; 139:75-80.

SECTION III: ENDOMETRIAL INVASION

IS TROPHOBLASTIC INVASION HEMOTROPIC IN THE RABBIT?

Loren H. Hoffman and Virginia P. Winfrey

Department of Cell Biology
Vanderbilt University School of Medicine
Nashville, Tennessee 37232 USA

IN the 1960's, Dr. Bent Boving offered a view of early implantation events in the rabbit in which the site of trophoblast attachment and invasion through uterine epithelium was proposed to be dependent on the location of underlying endometrial blood vessels, i.e., "hemotropic" invasion.[1,2] Aspects of this hypothesis were received with skepticism by some, but a good deal of interest in early implantation events was generated (see discussion related to Dr. Boving's presentation in ref. 2). The subject has received relatively little attention in recent years, although a variety of observations pertinent to the argument have emerged in the literature. A number of features of rabbit uterine epithelium, vasculature, and trophoblast have been described which bear, directly or indirectly, on the problem. It seemed to us that a re-evaluation of this "hemotropic" mechanism might be instructive in light of findings since Boving's original presentation.

THE HYPOTHESIS ON HEMOTROPIC INVASION

Anatomical Evidence

The conclusion that a correlation exists between specific sites of trophoblast attachment and the location of subepithelial blood vessels was derived in part from a quantitative analysis based on histological sections from 7 and 8 day implantation sites in which statistical analysis of vessel size, spacing, and distances between trophoblast attachment sites and such vessels was presented.[2] Observations were made on the antimesometrial aspect of implantation chambers where the apposed trophoblast of pre-implantation embryos is aggregated in "knobs" of syncytiotrophoblast. The chorio-allantoic placenta develops on the opposite, or mesometrial, aspect of implantation chambers and attachment events on this surface are delayed relative to those focused upon by Boving. The only factor judged to be positively correlated with trophoblast knob attachment was proximity to the subepithelial vessels; other conceivably favorable factors such as glycogen deposits, gland openings, or structural features of the knobs showed no such correlation. It was inferred from these findings "that the uterine epithelium promotes penetration in some places but not in others," the preferred sites being epithelial regions immediately overlying vessels.[2]

Experimental Evidence

In support of the anatomical observations, experimental results were cited which related trophoblast attachment and penetration to local changes in pH.[1] These observations included the following: (1) At 7 days post coitum (p.c.) chemical exchange across the uterine epithelium is channeled almost exclusively through the cells that have a vessel at their base; the epithelial surface thus presents to the trophoblast a chemical image of the vessels at its base; (2) An aspect of chemical exchange probably significant for attachment is loss of bicarbonate from the blastocyst through uterine epithelium to maternal circulation with accompanying reactions that generate a high pH; and (3) At high pH, trophoblast gets sticky and uterine epithelium dissociates. Taken together, the results suggested to Boving "that bicarbonate loss and pH rise are restricted to epivascular epithelium and thereby first generate trophoblast adhesiveness selectively at such sites and then cause uterine epithelium to come apart selectively at such sites, forming a path for trophoblast penetration directly to the vessel."[2] The earlier notion of Assheton[3] that trophoblast knobs were wedges driven through epithelium by blastocyst turgor was refuted. Nonetheless, a modified version of a hydraulic mechanism of penetration was formulated. Namely, unattached knobs were reported to be comprised of a shell of cytotrophoblastic cells surrounding a core of syncytiotrophoblast. The localized rise in pH reported to create gaps in uterine epithelial cells could also cause a separation between cytotrophoblast cells of the knobs creating a path for "extrusion" of the syncytiotrophoblast directly into the existing epithelial lesion. Extrusion of knob contents in isolated blastocysts following localized application of a sodium carbonate solution was offered as indirect evidence for the extrusion mechanism. The localized (epivascular) nature of these chemical changes was supported by histochemical results demonstrating the presence of a substance in epivascular epithelium which precipitated silver in epivascular epithelial cells following vascular perfusion of silver nitrate solution. The blastocyst was proposed as the origin of bicarbonate ions, and endometrial carbonic anhydrase activity, stimulated by high progesterone levels, was viewed as a necessary participant in the bicarbonate/carbon dioxide exchange.[2] Also, exposing the lining of 7 day pregnant uteri to alkaline solutions resulted in epithelial dissociation, an event considered to mimic the localized alkaline changes of epivascular regions.

MORE RECENT OBSERVATIONS PERTINENT TO THE ARGUMENT

Various aspects of rabbit implantation with possible relevance to the attachment/penetration mechanism proposed by Boving have been reported since 1966.

Trophoblast Knob Structure

The syncytial nature of the pre-implantation trophoblastic knobs was challenged by Glenister (Discussion, pp. 86-87, ref. 2), who believed the trophoblast to represent an "undifferentiated type of syncytium." Similarly, Steer[4] considered his ultrastructural observations on trophoblast knobs to be directly contradictory to those of Boving. Steer described two types of knob structures, neither of which had a syncytial core surrounded by a capsule of cellular cytotrophoblast or endoderm. Although Enders and Schlafke[5] observed pre-attachment knobs with centrally located syncytial trophoblast and cytotrophoblast around or beneath the syncytium, they added that the cellular layer did not appear to form a complete "cone" around the syncytium.

Trophoblast Interaction with Uterine Epithelium

Larsen[6,7] described the fusion of trophoblast of the knobs with uterine epithelial cells at attachment sites in the rabbit. This was confirmed by Enders and Schlafke[5] who also provided considerable detail on the fusion/invasion process. These authors found no evidence for dissociation of uterine luminal epithelial cells, tending to rule out a facilitated sloughing mechanism as reported for the rat[8] as well as the pH-related epithelial dissociation as postulated by Boving.[2] Thus, gaps between sloughing epithelial cells would be lacking as potential pathways for trophoblast penetration in the rabbit. The exclusive attachment of trophoblast knobs at epivascular epithelial sites would appear to be contradicted by a report on findings using scanning electron microscopy (EM) to localize knob attachment sites. Segalen and Chambon[9] concluded that trophoblastic knobs show a preferential attraction to gland openings on the antimesometrial wall. It should be noted here that the "gland openings" are, in fact, crypts forming the lateral walls of the numerous minor mucosal folds of the progestational endometrium in rabbits as has been documented elsewhere.[10] With blastocyst-induced distension of the uterine wall, the mucosal folds are reduced in depth, bringing the true glands closer to the surface. Glandular epithelium, however, is never in immediate apposition to the blastocyst surface.

Results from a number of studies have potential relevance to the issue of directed invasion of trophoblast in the rabbit. Several examinations employing scanning EM of rabbit endometrium or vascular casts of rabbit endometrial vessels have been published as well as studies on changes in epithelial surface properties which correlate with receptivity to an implanting embryo. Most such studies have not focused directly on the problem of hemotropic invasion of trophoblast. Nevertheless, indirect information on this process may be gleaned from such results. We chose to re-examine specimens available in this laboratory which had been employed for implantation-related experiments in an attempt to derive such information and to survey the published results of others with regard to this event. These will be reviewed as two categories: (1) light micro-

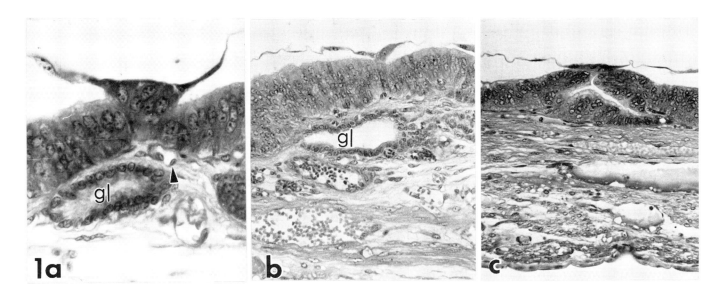

Figure 1. Light micrographs of early trophoblast knob attachment sites. In 1a, the trophoblast has fused with uterine epithelium and reached the basement membrane overlying a small vessel (arrowhead). 1b and 1c illustrate knob attachment to epithelium not underlain by blood vessels and to the surface of a flattened crypt, respectively. The uninucleate appearance of cells lining the uterine glands (gl) is apparent.

scopic observations on early trophoblast attachment to luminal epithelium and distribution of potential trophoblast-uterine recognition factors on the uterine surface, and (2) scanning and transmission EM views of the uterine epithelial and vascular structures during attachment and invasion of trophoblast.

Light microscopy of trophoblast knob attachment and of uterine surface properties: Specimens available for examination included samples of implantation sites from over 30 females (>200 implantation sites) fixed in various solutions for paraffin embedding and light microscopic examination or in glutaraldehyde-osmium for transmission or scanning EM. Implantation stages represented included samples obtained between 6.75 and 7.75 days p.c. Additional samples from pseudopregnant females at "receptive" (e.g., 6-7 day) and "non-receptive" (estrous) stages were examined as well. The first component of our survey was to examine the sites of trophoblast attachment to uterine epithelium with reference to the proximity of underlying vessels. Our observations did not include measurements of trophoblast-to-vessel distances or vessel-to-vessel distances, etc., as did those of Boving;[2] results were categorized only as to whether a subepithelial vessel was present immediately under the site of attachment and whether attachment occurred preferentially on the surface of uterine folds or over openings into the crypts. Observations were confined to samples from early stages of implantation (through 7.5 days p.c.) and thus do not include the trophoblast-endometrial attachment and invasion on the mesometrial surface, the site of future chorio-allantoic placentation.

Our survey suggested that early knob attachment and fusion sites were indeed located primarily on the surface of flattened folds of the mucosa (approximately 70% of sites), and in over one-half of such attachment sites, a subepithelial vessel was present immediately beneath the epithelium of the uterine cells involved. As will be shown later, vessels are always present near the base of these cells whether or not they are visible on an individual section. Attachment to the epithelium lining the flattened crypts was not uncommon, and was seen in nearly one-third of the attachment sites. This epithelium undergoes the same transition to multinucleated cells (later to symplasma) as seen on the more exposed luminal surface. The glandular epithelium, located at a deeper level, remains uninucleate throughout the implantation period as it does during pseudopregnancy.[10] In none of the samples was direct attachment of trophoblast to the uninucleate glandular epithelium noted. Examples of knob attachment on the luminal surface, with or without underlying vessels, and of crypt epithelium attachment are illustrated in Figure 1.

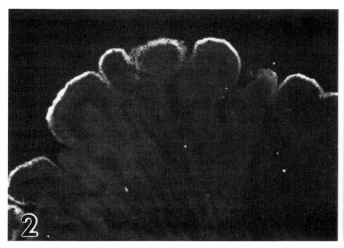
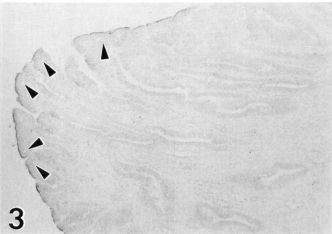

Figure 2. Fluorescence micrograph showing uniform binding of RCA-I to the apical membrane of receptive stage endometrium, irrespective of underlying vessels.[12]

Figure 3. Immunolocalization of a 42 kDa glycoprotein to the apical membrane.[13] Subepithelial vessels are present at arrowheads.

Thus, our survey suggests that initial attachment of trophoblast is somewhat more random than implied by previous reports. Preferential attachment over either crypts ("gland openings")[9] or to epivascular epithelium[1,2] was not apparent.

The mechanism of implantation proposed by Boving[1] included the view that the epithelial surface over vessels presented to the blastocyst a "chemical image" of the underlying vessels. The chemical change was believed to be due to localized alkalinity related to bicarbonate/carbon dioxide exchange. Studies in recent years have revealed several properties of rabbit uterine epithelial cells which are believed to correlate with the receptive condition of the uterus. Such alterations in surface properties would presumably be candidates for directed attachment and may be expected to show variable distribution with respect to underlying vessels. Specimens from some of these studies[11-12] were available for re-examination with regard to such preferential distribution of surface properties. The apical plasmalemma of rabbit uterine epithelial cells has a well-developed glycocalyx which is demonstrable ultrastructurally after staining with periodic acid-alkaline bismuth (PABi) and which demonstrates affinity for cationic ferritin.[11] The surface negativity (cationic ferritin affinity) is gradually lost on the surface epithelium as the receptive period approaches (i.e., day 6-7). Although the affinity for ferritin was recorded by transmission EM, the loss of negativity was, in fact, observed uniformly over the plasma membrane, i.e., no patches of cells, as would be present immediately over a vessel, were seen to have different properties than adjacent cells. Similarly, we observed changes in the nature of saccharide components in membrane glycoconjugates of this epithelium using fluorescent-labeled lectins.[12] A battery of labeled lectins was tested and, of these, only *Ricinus communis* I (RCA-I; binds D-galactose) appeared to exhibit increased binding which correlated with the acquisition of receptivity. The changing patterns of lectin binding were illustrated for all lectins tested, but the darkfield images published do not permit identification of underlying vessels. An examination of photomicrographic negatives printed to permit exposure of endometrial features revealed an absence of correlation of surface saccharide distribution with subepithelial blood vessels. An example is illustrated in Figure 2, in which RCA-I affinity is visualized in a relatively uniform layer at the surface of mucosal folds irrespective of proximity to vessels. The decreased reaction along the walls of crypts is believed to be due to the fact that the epithelium was exposed to lectin solutions by luminal incubation, precluding access of the lectins to cryptal epithelium. Another epithelial property which changes with acquisition of receptivity is the profile of apical membrane polypeptides or glycoproteins. At least three polypeptides are present in the membranes of receptive (day 6-7) uteri which are missing, or present in trace quantities, in non-receptive (estrus, day 1-2) uteri.[12] It should be noted that, to date, none of these membrane constituents has been positively identified as having affinity for trophoblastic surface components, although testing of this possibility is a goal of continued research in this area. The distribution of one of the surface markers of receptivity referred to above has been examined using immunolocalization. A polyclonal antiserum against the 42 kDa glycoprotein (RCA-I-binding) was prepared and used to map distribution of this stage-specific membrane marker.[13] The glycoprotein first appears on day 4 after ovulation and by days 6-7, when the uterus is receptive to blastocyst attachment, the glycoprotein is seen only on the apical membrane of luminal epithelial cells. It is not present on glandular epithelium nor on the lining of deeper areas of the crypts. Figure 3 illustrates this localization and reveals no correlative distribution with respect to underlying vessels.

Other investigators have reported stage-specific alterations in apical membrane or glycocalyx constituents of potential relevance to receptivity. A monoclonal antibody was prepared by Lampelo and coworkers[14] which had high affinity for the cell surface of luminal epithelial cells during the receptive state (day 6 p.c.). Also, Classen-Linke et al.[15] reported changes in the activity of a number of apical membrane-bound enzymes of luminal epithelium using histochemical methods. The changes in membrane composition were regarded as correlates of development of the receptive state. Illustrations accompanying these two reports reveal relatively uniform apical membrane staining (or loss of staining reactions). No indications were given that any pattern of reaction was obtained which might reflect the presence of underlying vessels. A review of such surface features in the rabbit uterus and in other species is presented elsewhere in this volume (T. Anderson).

Also available for examination with reference to directed invasion of trophoblast was a series of samples prepared for scanning electron microscopy of the epithelial surface, basement membrane, and underlying vessels of rabbit implantation sites. The epithelial surface and vascular casts of rabbit uteri at the time of implantation have been examined but, to our knowledge, no correlation of vessel location with potential attachment sites has been identified. As with the light microscopic observations, attention has been directed toward events on the antimesometrial and lateral surfaces of implantation chambers in samples obtained between 6.75 and 7.5 days p.c. Figure 4 illustrates the flattened mucosal folds where the endometrium was apposed to the expanded blastocyst. The epithelial surface is relatively uniform, only an occasional ciliated cell is present (not obvious at low magnification), although differences in the apical surface area may reflect the ongoing process of multinucleate cell formation at this time (7.25 days p.c.). Epithelial cells were removed from the surface of implantation and adjacent non-implantation regions of the uterine segments to expose the underlying basement membrane. The method of epithelial removal employed was to evert uteri and stir these in a solution containing 4 mM EDTA for several hours, followed by sonication and osmication of remaining tissue. The results are similar to those obtained by Highison et al. on various organs using boric acid-sonication methods.[16] The flattening and stretching of the surface at an implantation region (Fig. 5) can be compared with an adjacent non-implantation region (Fig. 6). It was anticipated that these basement membrane preparations would permit localization of trophoblast penetration sites, since they were obtained from uteri at 7.5 days p.c., at which time invasion to subepithelial tissue should have been accomplished.[5] Candidate sites for basement membrane penetration were indeed observed; these measured approximately 10 μm in diameter and were present exclusively in basement membranes located at or near the crown of mucosal folds. An additional feature noted was a qualitative difference in appearance of the basement membrane when examined at higher magnifications (not illustrated). The surface of the membrane from implantation sites often presented a somewhat mottled and thinned appearance relative to non-implantation regions. These defects would not be confused with potential trophoblast penetration sites, but may reflect indirect disruptive effects of the blastocyst on epithelial function with respect to maintenance of its basal lamina. It should be recalled that the luminal (and cryptal) epithelium at implantation areas begins changes leading to symplasma formation at about this time,[10] and within 2-3 days thereafter the symplasmic epithelium is sloughed into the lumen. Beneath the basement membrane, the stromal tissue is vascularized by a rich subepithelial plexus, best observed in scanning EM preparations of vascular casts. It is apparent that the epithelium is underlain by an extremely rich series of seemingly anastomotic arcades. Figure 7 represents the vascular network available to the trophoblast after penetrating the epithelial basal lamina. It is tempting to observe that it might be difficult for the trophoblast to miss a vessel as it penetrated into the stromal tissue. The vessels of the plexus do not form simple loops as they reach the surface, but course in a serpentine pattern along the minor folds in parallel with the crown regions of the minor mucosal folds (compare with Figs. 4 and 5). Transmission EM studies on the syncytiotrophoblastic penetration of the epithelial basement membrane have sug-

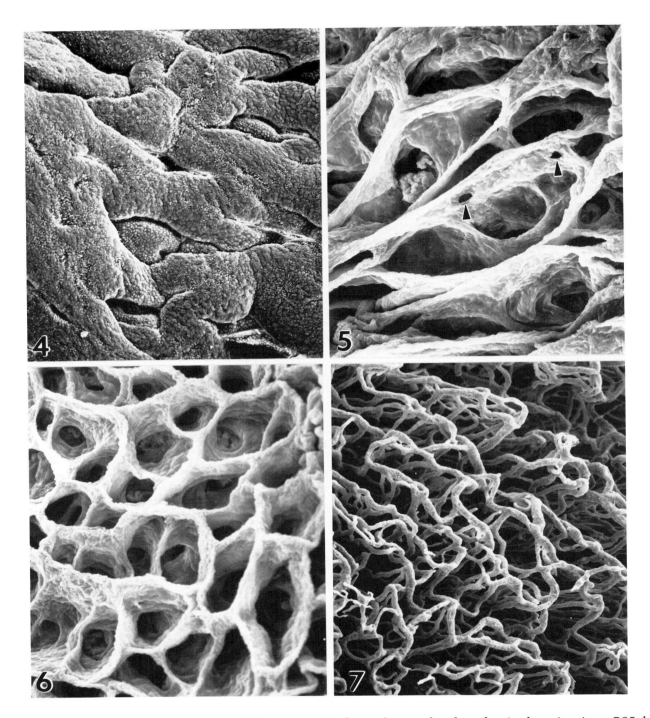

Figures 4-7. Scanning electron micrographs, X250. Fig. 4 is the flattened mucosal surface of an implantation site at 7.25 days p.c. A corresponding view of the basement membrane surface from a similar region (day 7.5) is seen in Fig. 5. Holes in the membrane which may represent trophoblast penetration sites are seen (arrowheads). Compare with the less distended basement membrane of an adjacent non-implantation region, Fig. 6. Fig. 7 is a vascular cast of the lateral wall of an implantation chamber at 7 days p.c.

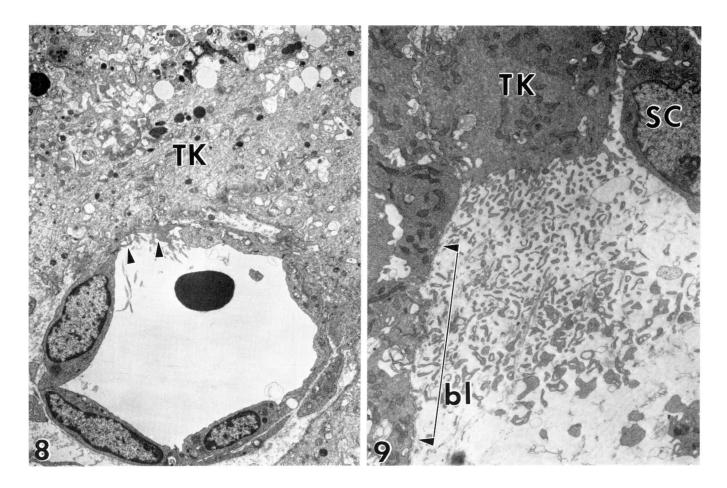

Figures 8 and 9. *Trophoblast knob (TK) penetration between endothelial cells of a subepithelial vessel at 7.25 days p.c. Note the membranous processes (arrowheads) projecting into the vessel lumen. The extent of the trophoblast processes is apparent in Figure 9. Here, on day 7, a knob (TK) has penetrated the epithelial basal lamina (still intact at "bl") and its processes project into stromal tissue in which no vessel was apparent. SC = stromal cell.*

gested that there exists at least a brief pause, or lag, at this level in invasion.[5-7,17] It was noted by Enders and Schlafke[5] that the plasma membrane of the trophoblastic knob is, at least potentially, a mosaic of epithelial and trophoblastic membranes. Thus, it may have properties different from either of these membranes alone. Furthermore, the knob can be considered to be penetrating its own basal lamina in a sense, since it is the original basement membrane of the epithelial cell(s) with which the syncytiotrophoblast has fused. Basement membrane penetration and subsequent advance of trophoblast is accomplished by a membranous fringe of irregularly shaped processes.[5,7,17] These long, branching processes probe the outer layers of subepithelial vessels, penetrate between endothelial cells, and then project into the vascular lumen (Fig. 8). Although vascular components, such as platelets, are ingested by the syncytiotrophoblast, the endothelial cells remain relatively undamaged by this process and a seal is formed between trophoblast and endothelial cells (Hoffman unpublished).[5] It is apparent in EM views of this process that the point of trophoblast invasion does not always coincide with the position of underlying vessels. Nevertheless, the branching trophoblastic processes appear to fan out to such an extent that the probability of encountering a vessel wall is maximized (Fig. 9). Perhaps the trophoblastic processes have affinity for components of the endothelial basal lamina or, as suggested originally by Boving, are chemotactically attracted to endothelium or blood-derived factors. Orientation of the inner cell mass and polar trophoblast in the rat along a gradient of unknown vascular factors has been suggested.[18] Parallels may be drawn between the directed growth of cell processes toward molecular constituents of a target cell (e.g., growth cone guidance).[19] Likewise, the behavior of trophoblast toward extracellular matrix constituents is being investigated in a number of laboratories.

The hypothesis of Boving regarding the hemotropic invasion of trophoblast in the implantation of the rabbit remains viable, although several specifics of the proposal may be unsubstantiated. The notion of explosive extrusion of trophoblast knobs between detaching epithelial cells has been negated by observations that the epithelium remains intact and that trophoblast attachment involves a fusion of cells. Similarly, the view that the luminal surface facing the blastocyst presents a chemical imprint of underlying vessels is not supported by preferential distribution of apical membrane constituents of the receptive phase epithelium. The focal alkalinity with respect to knobs and epivascular epithelium described by Boving,[1] has been neither supported nor conclusively negated by recent studies. This may be amenable to further study using antibodies to anion channel proteins, such as band 3, which are present in non-erythroid tissues as well as in red cell membranes.[20] The morphological observations on the endometrium and subjacent blood vessels as reported here give the impression that initial attachment of trophoblast to the uterine surface is random. Some knobs attach to the lateral margins of endometrial crypts and others to the more flattened surface of mucosal folds. Once fusion of syncytiotrophoblast and uterine epithelial cells occurs, the invading knob is necessarily directed toward the basement membrane and stromal tissue immediately beneath that epithelial cell or cells. The structure of the trophoblastic processes appears to allow contact with specific structures (vessels of subepithelial plexus) even at some distance from the initial lesion in the epithelial basement membrane. Furthermore, as seen in vascular casts, the array of vessels in the stroma of mucosal folds is extremely rich; again maximizing the chances for trophoblast-vessel interaction. What seems certain is that trophoblast does in fact reach the subepithelial vessels with a high percentage of success; perhaps even 100% success. Trophoblastic knobs, or the giant cells derived from them, are located more deeply in the endometrial stroma on days 8-9 p.c. and, in virtually every such structure, evidence of interaction with vessels is present (ingested platelets, red blood cells, etc.; unpublished observations). It seems quite possible that a chemotactic process could be involved in ensuring trophoblast interaction with endometrial vessels once the trophoblast has penetrated the basement membrane; substantiating, at least in part, the overall hemotropic nature of early implantation events. Potential chemotropic mechanisms associated with this process may be amenable to examination using *in vitro* trophoblast-uterine model systems modified appropriately to take into account the potential role of vascular structures or factors of vascular origin.

References

1. Boving BG. Implantation mechanisms. In: Hartman CG, ed. *Mechanisms concerned with contraception.* New York: Pergamon Press Ltd., 1963:321-396.
2. Boving BG. Some mechanical aspects of trophoblast penetration of the uterine epithelium in the rabbit. In: Wolstenholme GEW, O'Connor M, eds. *Egg implantation.* Boston: Little, Brown and Co., 1966:72-93.
3. Assheton R. On the causes which lead to the attachment of the mammalian embryo to the walls of the uterus. *Quart J Micro Sci* 1985; 37:173-190.
4. Steer HW. The trophoblastic knobs of the preimplanted rabbit blastocyst: a light and electron microscopic study. *J Anat* 1970; 107:315-325.
5. Enders AC, Schlafke S. Penetration of the uterine epithelium during implantation in the rabbit. *Am J Anat* 1971; 132:219-240.
6. Larsen JF. Electron microscopy of the implantation site in the rabbit. *Am J Anat* 1961; 109:319-334.
7. Larsen JF. Histology and fine structure of the avascular and vascular yolk sac placentae and the obplacental giant cells in the rabbit. *Am J Anat* 1963; 112:269-284.
8. Enders AC, Schlafke S. A morphological analysis of the early implantation stages in the rat. *Am J Anat* 1967; 120:185-226.
9. Segalen J, Chambon Y. Ultrastructural aspects of the antimesometrial implantation in the rabbit. *Acta Anat* 1983; 115:1-7.
10. Davies J, Hoffman LH. Studies on the progestational endometrium of the rabbit: I. Light microscopy, day 0 to 13 of gonadotropin-induced pseudopregnancy. *Am J Anat* 1973; 137:423-445.
11. Anderson TL, Hoffman LH. Alterations in epithelial glycocalyx of rabbit uteri during early pseudopregnancy and pregnancy, and following ovariectomy. *Am J Anat* 1984; 171:321-334.
12. Anderson TL, Olson GE, Hoffman LH. Stage-specific alterations in the apical membrane glycoproteins of endometrial epithelial cells related to implantation in rabbits. *Biol Reprod* 1986; 34:701-720.

13. Hoffman LH, Winfrey VP, Anderson TL, Olson GE. Uterine receptivity to implantation in the rabbit: evidence for a 42 kDA glycoprotein as a marker of receptivity. *Troph Res* 1989;4:in press.
14. Lampelo SA, Anderson TL, Bullock DW. Monoclonal antibodies recognize a cell surface marker of epithelial differentiation in the rabbit reproductive tract. *J Reprod Fert* 1986; 78:663-672.
15. Classen-Linke I, Denker H-W, Winterhager E. Apical plasma membrane-bound enzymes of rabbit uterine epithelium. *Histochem* 1987; 87:517-529.
16. Highison GJ, Johnson RB, McClugage SG, Low FN. Ultrasonic microdissection techniques for scanning electron microscopy. *Crit Rev Anat Sci* 1988; 1:193-227.
17. Enders AC, Schlafke S. Cytological aspects of trophoblast-uterine interaction in early implantation. *Am J Anat* 1969; 125:1-30.
18. Christofferson RH, Nilsson BO. Morphology of the endometrial microvasculature during early placentation in the rat. *Cell Tissue Res* 1988; 253:209-220.
19. Dodd J, Jessell TM. Axon guidance and the patterning of neuronal projections in vertebrates. *Science* 1988; 242:692-699.
20. Drenckhahn D, Schluter K, Allen DP, Bennett V. Colocalization of band 3 with ankyrin and spectrin at the basal membrane of intercalated cells in the rat kidney. *Science* 1989; 230:1287-1289.

EPITHELIAL CELL DEATH DURING RODENT EMBRYO IMPLANTATION

Earl L. Parr and Margaret B. Parr

Department of Anatomy
Southern Illinois University School of Medicine
Carbondale, Illinois 62901-6503 USA

IT is usually assumed that uterine epithelial cells die during embryo implantation in laboratory rodents,[1-4] and it has been well established that the epithelial cells are phagocytosed by the trophoblast. Ultrastructural studies of rat implantation sites have indicated that the epithelial cells are intact and exhibit normal morphologic features at the time of phagocytosis by the trophoblast.[5-7] In hamsters, most epithelial cells in the implantation chamber showed normal ultrastructure until the trophoblast invaded the epithelium, at which time cell death was indicated by the disruption of organelles in a few cells.[8] In mice, Poelmann[9] reported that there were few signs of degeneration in the epithelial cells at the time of trophoblast invasion, but El-Shershaby and Hinchliffe[4] reported extensive degeneration of epithelial cell organelles and suggested that cell death appeared to be due to an autolytic process involving autophagosomes and lysosomal enzymes before phagocytosis by trophoblast. Abraham et al.[10] concluded that autolysis was the basis of epithelial cell death in rabbits.

Since the original description of apoptotic cell death by Kerr and co-workers,[11] it has become widely accepted that all cell death occurs by one of two fundamentally different processes: necrosis or apoptosis.[12-17] Cell death by necrosis is characterized by surface membrane damage, osmotic swelling of the cells and mitochondria, disintegration of organelles, and a cellular inflammatory response.[13,18] In contrast, apoptosis is characterized by cell shrinkage, blebbing or fragmentation of the cells, condensation of chromatin and fragmentation of nuclei, intact cytoplasmic organelles, phagocytosis of the dying cell or its fragments by adjacent cells, and no cellular inflammation.[13] We recently conducted an ultrastructural study of mouse and rat implantation sites to determine whether uterine epithelial cells die by apoptosis or necrosis.[19]

METHODS

Pregnant female mice were killed at 10 a.m. on day 5 of pregnancy or at 8-10 p.m. on the same day; day 1 being the day that sperm were found in the vagina. Rats were killed at 10 a.m. on day 5, 6, or 7 of pregnancy. The uteri were fixed by vascular perfusion and processed by routine methods.[19]

RESULTS

On the evening of day 5 of pregnancy, the mouse blastocyst was present in an implantation chamber at the antimesometrial side of the uterus and was closely surrounded by luminal epithelial cells (Fig. 1). In the implantation sites studied at this time there was a variable loss of epithelial cells from the chamber, ranging from a few cells to nearly all of the cells adjacent to the abembryonic and mural trophoblast. Rat implantation sites on the morning of day 7 of pregnancy had a similar appearance. The structures that were of greatest interest in this study, the trophoblast cells and the luminal epithelial cells, were similar in mice and rats, and most of the ultrastructural charac-

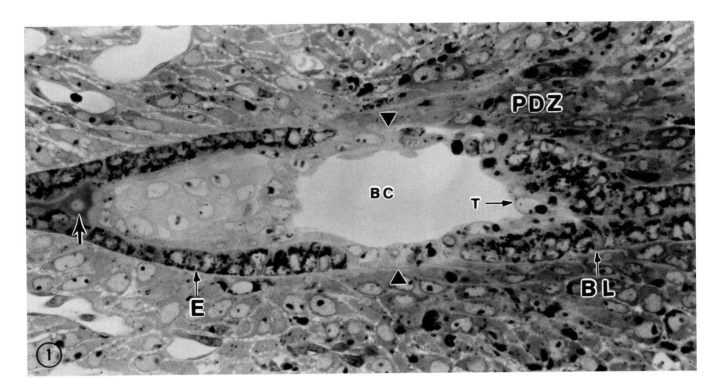

Figure 1. A transverse section of a mouse uterus at an implantation site at 8 p.m. on day 5 of pregnancy shows the embryonic pole of cells to the left of the blastocyst cavity (BC), while the mural and abembryonic trophoblast cells (T) surround the remainder of the cavity. The uterine luminal epithelium (E) adjacent to the embryonic pole of the blastocyst retains its polarity, but adjacent to the abembryonic pole the cells are rounded and stratified. Further to the right, the luminal epithelium at the antimesometrial side of the uterus again shows more polarity. At two sites (arrowheads) the epithelial layer is interrupted by the trophoblast, which has invaded to reach the epithelial basal lamina (BL). An amorphous material (arrow) was consistently observed in the uterine lumen adjacent to the developing ectoplacental cone of the embryo. The embryo and the uterine epithelium are surrounded by the closely packed cells of the primary decidual zone (PDZ), which is avascular. Capillaries and small venules are present around the periphery of the PDZ. X670.

teristics of epithelial cell death to be described were observed in both species. Therefore, the observations from the two species will be described together. All of the illustrations are from day 5, 8 p.m. for mice or day 7, 10 a.m. for rats.

Mouse and rat epithelial cells on the morning of day 5 of pregnancy were columnar in shape, and their nuclei were mainly oval, showing only a thin rim of peripheral heterochromatin. In contrast, the mouse epithelial cells that remained in the implantation chamber on the evening of day 5 were often not columnar in shape, and they appeared to be reduced in size. They were either rounded, irregular in shape, or flattened, and they often appeared to be layered so that there were several cells between the trophoblast and the epithelial basal lamina. The epithelial cell nuclei were more irregular in shape, often showing one or more deep indentations, and there was a more conspicuous condensation of chromatin around the periphery. Similar changes were seen in rat epithelial cells in implantation sites on day 6 of pregnancy, and these changes were more pronounced on day 7.

The apical ends of many of the epithelial cells adjacent to the trophoblast exhibited irregular projections that were located in corresponding recesses in the surface of trophoblast cells. The surface membranes of the two cell types were closely apposed throughout most of this region, but no cellular junctions were observed. Some of the epithelial cell projections were constricted at the base, and vesicles containing epithelial cytoplasm were often present within trophoblast vesicles, suggesting that the epithelial cell

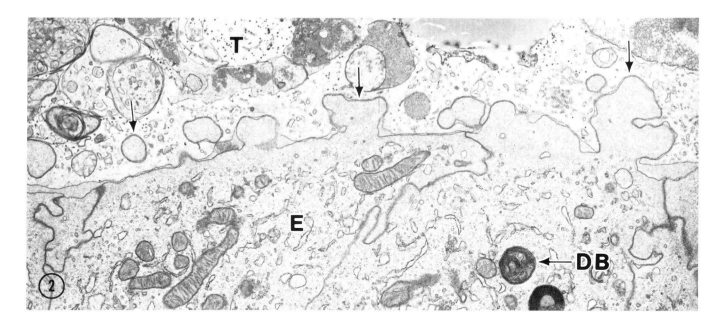

Figure 2. Uterine epithelial cells (E) in the mouse implantation chamber exhibited many irregularly shaped apical projections that indented the adjacent trophoblast (T) cells (arrows). The projections were often constricted at their point of attachment to the epithelium, and it appeared that some were detached and had been phagocytosed by the trophoblast. Such vesicles in trophoblast cells were bounded by two cell membranes. DB is dense body. X12,000.

projections pinched off and were phagocytosed by trophoblast cells (Fig. 2). Some luminal epithelial cells in the implantation chamber exhibited constrictions (Fig. 3), and these cells may undergo fragmentation. We frequently observed groups of small membrane-bounded structures between the epithelial basal lamina and trophoblast that appeared to be fragments of epithelial cells (Fig. 4). They were small, irregular in shape, closely packed, and contained dense cytoplasm similar to that of epithelial cells.

Trophoblast cells or processes penetrated the epithelial layer. In such locations the epithelial cells were sometimes detached from their basal lamina, but in most cases long, slender trophoblast processes were interposed between the epithelial cells and the basal lamina. The morphological appearance of cytoplasmic organelles in epithelial cells that were adjacent to trophoblast processes and presumably about to be phagocytosed by trophoblast is relevant to the mode of epithelial cell death. Epithelial cells adjacent to invading trophoblast processes invariably exhibited normal mitochondria (Figs. 3, 5). There was no swelling of the mitochondrial matrix or disruption of the cristae, and there were no matrix densities. The cell membrane and Golgi apparatus appeared to be intact, and the cytoplasm was either normal or slightly increased in staining density. Rough endoplasmic reticulum cisternae only rarely showed indications of slight swelling (Fig. 5). Dense bodies that ranged in size from 0.5 μm to a maximum of 3.0 μm in diameter were present (Figs. 5, 6). The dense bodies sometimes contained membrane or particles that resembled ribosomes (Fig. 6), but only rarely did they contain a recognizable mitochondrion. The nuclei were deeply indented in both species and had a more conspicuous rim of peripheral heterochromatin than on the morning of day 5 of pregnancy (Fig. 7). Occasionally, epithelial cell nuclei at this time were fragmented (Fig. 8).

Epithelial cells were phagocytosed by trophoblast cells (Figs. 4, 9). Some of the ingested epithelial cells exhibited recognizable nuclei and well preserved mitochondria. The chromatin of ingested epithelial cells was sometimes highly condensed. It appeared that a relatively larger amount of epithelial cell material was present in trophoblast heterophagosomes than in epithelial cell autophagosomes (Fig. 9). Other trophoblast phagosomes contained unrecognizable material that was either the remains of epithelial cells or cell fragments in more advanced stages of digestion, or could perhaps be autophagosomes.

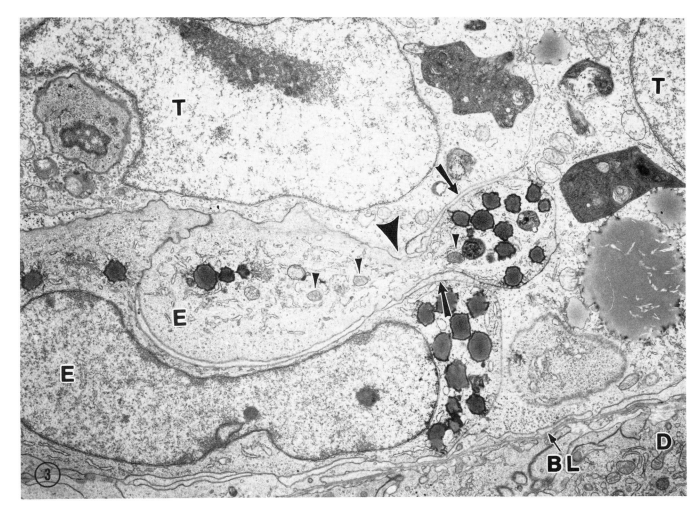

Figure 3. Two mouse uterine epithelial cells are oriented parallel to the basal lamina (BL), between trophoblast (T) and decidual cells (D). The upper epithelial cell has a constricted region (arrowhead), to the right of which its cytoplasm contains many lipid droplets. The trophoblast cell on the right is adjacent to the basal lamina, and it has processes (arrows) which surround the lipid-containing portion of the constricted epithelial cell. The mitochondria (small arrowheads) in the constricted epithelial cell are normal in appearance, similar to those in the decidual cell. X7,200.

During the period of our observations, the only epithelial cells that were lost from the implantation chamber were those that were adjacent to trophoblast cells. The epithelial cells that were present in crypts extending out from the implantation chamber were less closely associated with the trophoblast cells and were not lost. The main crypt is at the antimesometrial end of the implantation chamber, but other crypts were observed along the sides of the chamber in sections cut perpendicular to the long axis of the blastocyst. Such epithelial cells appeared to be reduced in size, and their nuclei had irregular shapes and increased staining of peripheral chromatin. However, most of the cells retained their polarity and there were not indications of fragmentation.

DISCUSSION

Uterine luminal epithelial cells in mouse and rat implantation sites exhibited all of the accepted morphologic characteristics of apoptotic cell death. These include surface blebbing, shrinkage and fragmentation of the cells, intact surface membrane and normal or increased cytoplasmic density, normal cytoplasmic organelles, condensation

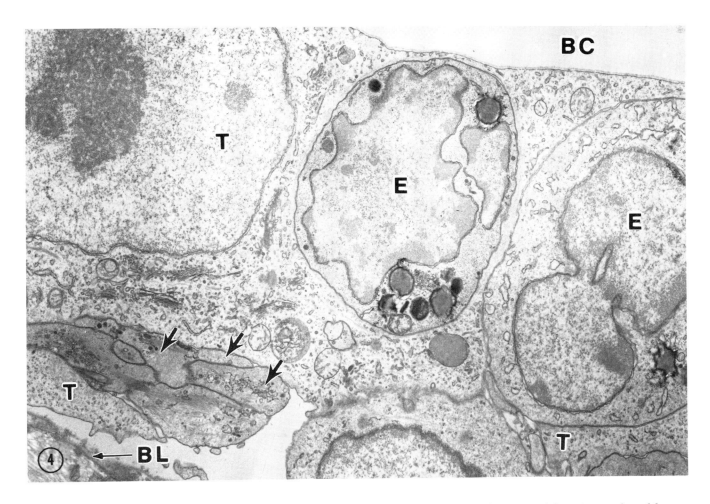

Figure 4. *A mouse trophoblast cell (T) has phagocytosed a uterine epithelial cell (E) at the center of the micrograph and has surrounded most of the cell to the right. Both epithelial cells contain recognizable nuclei that are irregular in shape and show somewhat increased staining of peripheral chromatin, and both are surrounded by their own surface membrane and that of the trophoblast heterophagosome. At the lower left there is a trophoblast cell process near the epithelial basal lamina (BL) and a group of what appear to be epithelial cell fragments (arrows). The blastocyst cavity (BC) is at the upper right. X11,000.*

of chromatin, indentation of nuclear envelope and nuclear fragmentation, and phagocytosis of the cells and their fragments by nearby cells.[13] In contrast, epithelial cells in the implantation chamber exhibited none of the morphologic characteristics of necrosis, such as swollen cells, loss of cytoplasmic density, swollen mitochondria and mitochondrial matrix densities, and disintegrated organelles.[13] Hence, we conclude that mouse and rat uterine luminal epithelial cells in the implantation chamber undergo apoptotic death.

Our ultrastructural observations of mouse and rat implantation sites are in good agreement with previous descriptions in rats,[5,7] hamsters,[8] and mice.[9] The common conclusion of these investigators was that the epithelial cells and their organelles were surprisingly well preserved when trophoblast cells invaded the epithelial layer. We confirm Poelmann's observation that the surface of epithelial cells was "bubbled," and Parkening's impression that trophoblast cells phagocytosed small portions of the apical ends of epithelial cells. We also confirm El-Shershaby and Hinchliffe's[4] description of loss of polarity and rounding of mouse epithelial cells, peripheral chromatin condensation, and fragmentation of some cells and nuclei. In particular, we confirm the suggestion of Smith and Wilson[3]

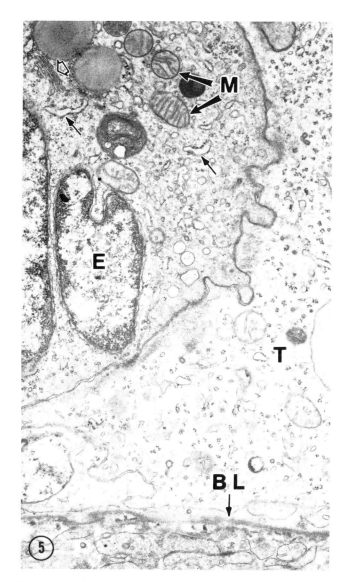

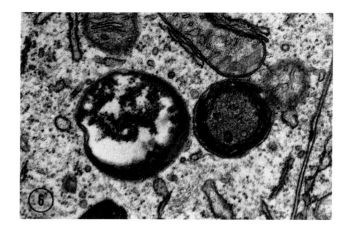

Figure 5. *A mouse uterine epithelial cell (E) adjacent to an invading trophoblast cell (T) is shown at higher magnification. The mitochondria (M) in the epithelial cell are well preserved, as are the rough endoplasmic reticulum cisternae (arrows) and Golgi apparatus (open arrow). The cytoplasm of the epithelial cell shows normal staining density, indicating that its surface membrane is intact, but the nucleus is deeply indented. Basal lamina (BL). X18,000.*

Figure 6. *Dense bodies that contain ribosomes (left) and membrane whorls (right) are shown in a mouse uterine epithelial cell before phagocytosis by trophoblast. The mitochondria and rough endoplasmic reticulum cisternae are well preserved. X35,000.*

that cell shrinkage, cytoplasmic condensation, and nuclear indentations in mouse epithelial cells are similar to the features described by Kerr et al.[11] as being characteristic of apoptotic cell death.

Several previous investigators have suggested that uterine epithelial cell death during implantation may be due to an autolytic process.[4,10,20-23] This view is based mainly on an ultrastructural study of epithelial cell degeneration in mouse implantation sites that emphasized the occurrence of autophagosomes, swollen mitochondria, distended rough endoplasmic reticulum cisternae, and disintegrated organelles in epithelial cells before their phagocytosis by trophoblast.[4] In contrast, we found that the mitochondria, rough endoplasmic reticulum, and other organelles of mouse epithelial cells remained intact and were not swollen, and that the cytoplasm maintained a normal or increased staining density. It is unlikely that we would have observed autolytic changes in epithelial cells if we had chosen a later time for our studies because the previously reported autolytic changes were observed before phagocytosis of the epithelial cells by trophoblast and there were numerous phagocytosed epithelial cells in all of the implantation sites we studied. Autophagic dense bodies containing recognizable cell organelles were present in mouse and rat epithelial cells in the implantation chambers, but autophagosomes are a normal component of many kinds of viable epithelial cells and there is no cogent evidence that they cause cell death. The amount of epithelial cell material in trophoblast heterophagosomes far exceeded that in epithelial cell autophagosomes, and hence the majority of the digestion of epithelial cells appeared to take place in the trophoblast cells. Furthermore, in other cell systems in which apoptotic death occurs it is gener-

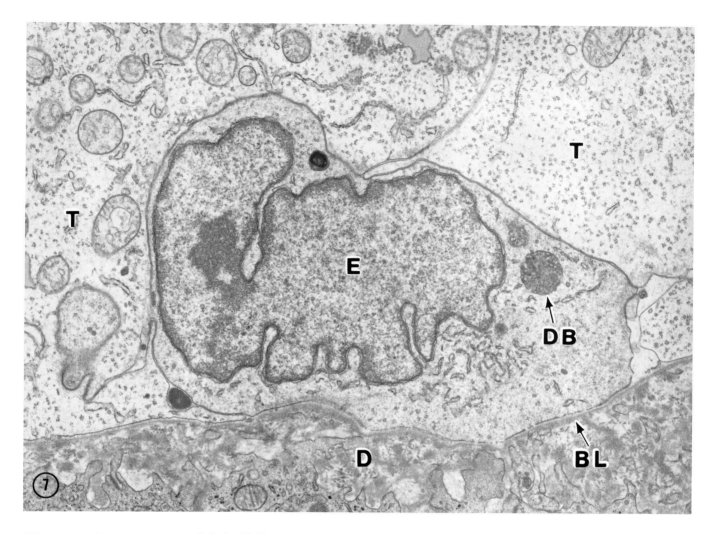

Figure 7. A mouse uterine epithelial cell (E) is in contact with the basal lamina (BL) but is otherwise surrounded by trophoblast (T). The epithelial cell appears to be reduced in size and its nucleus is indented, but its surface membrane is intact and its cytoplasm exhibits a normal staining density. D, decidual cell; DB, dense body. X14,000.

ally accepted that autophagosomes, lysosomal enzymes, and autolysis play no role in the death of the cells.[13] Our observations also differ from those of Wilson and Smith,[24] who reported that the whole epithelial layer around the mouse blastocyst sloughed off with the onset of decidualization and that the epithelial cells exhibited protoplasmic swelling and general dissolution, and from those of Smith and Wilson,[3] who reported that mouse epithelial cell organelles other than the nucleus disintegrated and became almost unrecognizable before phagocytosis by trophoblast. The differences between our ultrastructural observations and those of previous investigators are probably all due to better tissue fixation in the present study.

Apoptosis is regarded as a physiologic form of cell death.[13,15] It occurs in the liver during involution after cessation of various treatments that cause liver hyperplasia[17,25,26] in the adrenal cortex after withdrawal of ACTH,[27] in thymocytes in response to glucocorticoid treatment,[16,28] and in tissues undergoing remodeling during embryonic development.[29-32] Macromolecular synthesis is required for apoptosis, and inhibitors of RNA and protein synthesis block this form of cell death.[33,34] In contrast,

Figure 8. *A trophoblast cell (T) and flattened uterine epithelial cells (E) are adjacent to the epithelial basal lamina (BL) in a rat implantation site. The epithelial cell nucleus on the right is fragmenting (arrowheads), and there are two small pieces of nucleus (N) in the adjacent trophoblast cytoplasm. The nuclear fragments (N) are continuously bounded by two unit membranes, the epithelial cell surface and trophoblast heterophagosome membranes. The two nuclear envelope membranes can be detected in some places toward the periphery of the fragments, but they no longer form a continuous boundary for the chromatin. A nearby trophoblast vesicle (V) is bounded by two unit membranes and has a homogeneous content resembling the apical cytoplasm of epithelial cells; this suggests that it may be a heterophagosome containing a fragment of the apical portion of an epithelial cell. The epithelial cell on the left shows a narrow constriction (C) below its nucleus. The nucleus is irregular in shape and shows margination of chromatin. Mitochondria in both epithelial cells (arrows) are normal in appearance, as are the rough endoplasmic reticulum cisternae (open arrows). X13,000.*

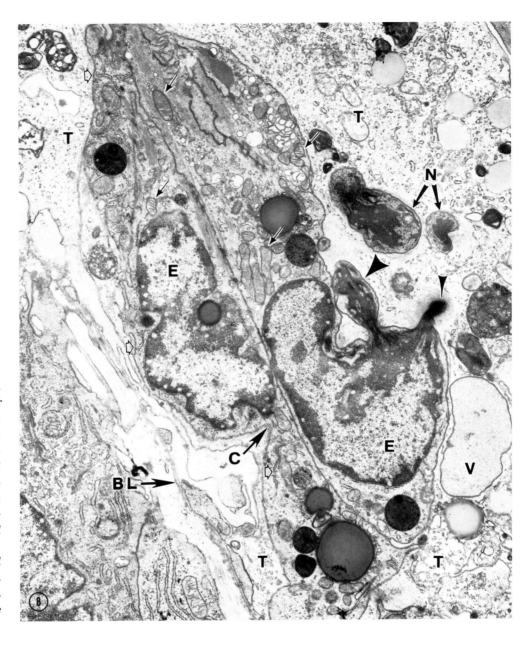

necrotic death is due to severely disturbed environmental conditions, such as anoxia, that are inconsistent with continued viability of the cells.[13] If epithelial cell death during implantation were due to a restriction of the flow of oxygen or nutrients to the implantation chamber by the closely packed cells of the primary decidual zone, as suggested by Smith and Wilson,[3] it should be expected that the dying epithelial cells would exhibit the morphologic characteristics of necrotic cells. Since they do not, it seems unlikely that this is the cause of epithelial cell death.

As mentioned above, inhibitors of RNA and protein synthesis block apoptosis. Finn and Bredl[2] reported that epithelial cell degeneration in mouse implantation sites was blocked by treatment with actinomycin D. Finn[35] has emphasized the involvement of cellular synthetic activity in epithelial breakdown by referring to the process as

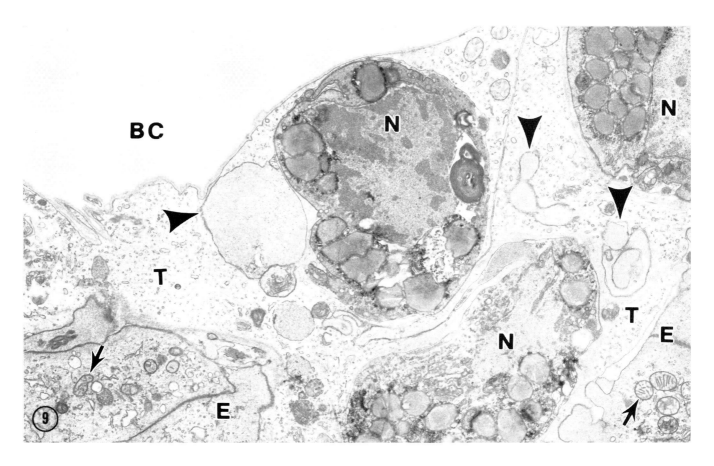

Figure 9. *Mouse trophoblast cells (T) contain partly or completely phagocytosed uterine epithelial cells whose nuclei (N) are still recognizable. The trophoblast cells also contain structures with the appearance of the apical projections from epithelial cells but surrounded by two cell membranes (arrowheads). These structures could be trophoblast heterophagosomes containing fragments of epithelial cells. The blastocyst cavity (BC) at the upper left and epithelial cells (E) that have not yet been phagocytosed are also indicated. The latter contain normal mitochondria (arrows) and exhibit apical projections. X10,000.*

"programmed cell death." Investigators studying apoptosis in other cell systems have also referred to the process as "programmed cell death."[16,17] The observations of Finn and Bredl thus provide support for the conclusion that uterine epithelial cells in mouse and rat implantation sites die by an apoptotic process.

One of the characteristic features of apoptotic cell death is phagocytosis of the dying cells by nearby cells. These are usually macrophages, which bind to and phagocytose apoptotic cells but not normal cells.[13] Wyllie[36] has reported that there are changes in the surface membrane carbohydrates of thymocytes undergoing apoptosis, and he suggested that these changes may account for the recognition of apoptotic cells by macrophages. Similar changes in the surface membrane of luminal epithelial cells undergoing apoptosis during implantation may account for trophoblast adhesion to these cells, and further biochemical studies of the surface changes in apoptotic cells may contribute to a better understanding of the adhesion stage of implantation.

SUMMARY

During embryo implantation in several laboratory rodents the loss of the uterine epithelium surrounding the blastocyst is important in bringing the the trophoblast into close association with the endometrial stroma. It is usually assumed that the epithelial cells die during this process, and it has been clearly established that the epithelial cells are phagocytosed by the trophoblast. The cause of epithelial cell death remains speculative.

Since the original description of apoptotic cell death by Kerr and co-workers, it has become widely accepted that all cell death occurs by one of two fundamentally different processes: apoptosis or necrosis. Apoptosis is regarded as a physiologic form of cell death, whereas necrosis is due to disturbed environmental conditions that are inconsistent with continued viability of the cells.

Each type of cell death is associated with characteristic ultrastructural features, and the purpose of a recent study in our laboratory was to determine whether the appearance of uterine epithelial cells in mouse and rat implantation chambers is consistent with apoptotic or necrotic death. We found that the epithelial cells exhibited all of the accepted morphologic characteristics of apoptotic death, including surface blebbing, shrinkage and fragmentation of the cells, intact surface membrane and normal or increased cytoplasmic density, normal cytoplasmic organelles, condensation of chromatin, indentation of the nuclear envelope and nuclear fragmentation, and phagocytosis of the cells and their fragments by nearby cells. In contrast, epithelial cells in the implantation chamber exhibited none of the morphologic characteristics of necrosis, such as swollen cells, loss of cytoplasmic density, swollen mitochondria and mitochondrial matrix densities, and disintegrated organelles. Hence, we conclude that mouse and rat uterine luminal epithelial cells in the implantation chamber undergo apoptotic death during embryo implantation.

References

1. Lawn AM. Uterine implantation of the mammalian ovum. *Proc of the Royal Society Med* 1969; 62:141-143.
2. Finn CA, Bredl JCS. Studies on the development of the implantation reaction in the mouse uterus: influence of actinomycin D. *J Reprod Fert* 1973; 34:247-253.
3. Smith AF, Wilson IB. Cell interaction at the maternal-embryonic interface during implantation in the mouse. *Cell and Tiss Res* 1974; 152:525-542.
4. El-Shershaby AM, Hinchliffe JR. Epithelial autolysis during implantation of the mouse blastocyst: an ultrastructural study. *J Embryol Exp Morphol* 1975; 33:1067-1080.
5. Enders AC, Schlafke S. A morphological analysis of the early implantation stages in the rat. *Am J Anat* 1967; 120:185-226.
6. Enders AC, Schlafke S. Cytological aspects of trophoblast-uterine interaction in early implantation. *Am J Anat* 1969; 125:1-30.
7. Tachi S, Tachi C, Lindner HR. Ultrastructural features of blastocyst attachment and trophoblastic invasion in the rat. *J Reprod Fertil* 1970; 21:37-56.
8. Parkening TA. An ultrastructural study of implantation in the golden hamster II. Trophoblastic invasion and removal of the uterine epithelium. *J Anat* 1976; 122:211-230.
9. Poelmann RE. An ultrastructural study of implanting mouse blastocysts: coated vesicles and epithelium formation. *J Anat* 1975; 119:421-434.
10. Abraham R, Hendy R, Dougherty WJ, Fulfs JC, Goldberg L. Participation of lysosomes in early implantation in the rabbit. *Exp Mol Pathol* 1970; 13:329-345.
11. Kerr JFR, Wyllie AH, Currie AR. Apoptosis: a basic biological phenomenon with wide-ranging implications in tissue kinetics. *Br J Cancer* 1972; 26:239-247.
12. Wyllie AH, Kerr JFR, Currie AR. Cell death: the significance of apoptosis. *Int Rev Cytol* 1980; 68:251-306.
13. Wyllie AH. Cell death: a new classification separating apoptosis from necrosis. In: Bowen ID, Lockshin RA, eds. *Cell death in biology and pathology*. London: Chapman and Hall, 1981:9-34.
14. Searle J, Kerr JFR, Bishop CJ. Necrosis and apoptosis: distinct modes of cell death with fundamentally different significance. *Path Annual* 1982; 17:229-259.
15. Kerr JFR, Bishop CJ, Searle J. Apoptosis. *Recent Adv Histopathol* 1984; 12:1-15.
16. Morris RG, Hargreaves AD, Duvall E, Wyllie AH. Hormone-induced cell death. 2. Surface changes in thymocytes undergoing apoptosis. *Am J Pathol* 1984; 115:426-436.
17. Columbano A, Ledda-Columbano GM, Coni PP, Faa G, Liguori C, Santa Cruz G, Pani P. Occurrence of cell death (apoptosis) during the involution of liver hyperplasia. *Lab Invest* 1985; 52:670-675.
18. Trump BF, Berezesky IK, Osornio-Vargas AR. Cell death and the disease process. The role of calcium. In: Bowen ID, Lockshin RA, eds. *Cell death in biology and pathology*. London: Chapman and Hall, 1981:209-242.
19. Parr EL, Tung HN, Parr MB. Apoptosis as the mode of uterine epithelial cell death during embryo implantation in mice and rats. *Biol Reprod* 1987; 36:211-225.
20. Schlafke S, Enders AC. Cellular basis of interaction between trophoblast and uterus at implantation. *Biol Reprod* 1975; 12:41-65.
21. Moulton BC, Elangovan S. Lysosomal mechanisms in blastocyst implantation and early decidualization. In: Glasser SR, Bullock DW, eds. *Cellular and molecular aspects of implantation*. New York: Plenum Press, 1981: 335-344.

22. Craig SS, Jollie WP. Epithelial ultrastructure during decidualization in rats. *Anat Embryol* 1981; 163:215-222.
23. Welsh AO, Enders AC. Light and electron microscopic examination of the mature decidual cells of the rat with emphasis on the antimesometrial decidua and its degeneration. *Am J Anat* 1985; 172:1-29.
24. Wilson IB, Smith MSR. Primary trophoblastic invasion at the time of nidation. In: Hubinont PO et al. eds. *Ovo-implantation human gonadotropins and prolactin*. Basel: Karger, 1970:1-8.
25. Kerr JFR. Shrinkage necrosis: a distinct mode of cellular death. *J Pathol* 1971; 105:13-22.
26. Bursch W, Lauer B, Timmermann-Trosiener I, Barthel G, Schuppler J, Schulte-Hermann R. Controlled death (apoptosis) of normal and putative preneoplastic cells in rat liver following withdrawal of tumor promoters. *Carcinogenesis* 1984; 5:453-458.
27. Wyllie AH, Kerr JFR, Macaskill AM, Currie AR. Adrenocortical cell deletion: the role of ACTH. *J Pathol* 1973; 111:85-97.
28. Wyllie AH. Glucocorticoid-induced thymocyte apoptosis is associated with endogenous endonuclease activation. *Nature* 1980; 284:555-557.
29. Crawford AM, Kerr JFR, Currie AR. The relationship of acute mesodermal cell death to the teratogenic effects of 7-OHM-12-MBA in the fetal rat. *Br J Cancer* 1972; 26:498-503.
30. Wyllie AH, Kerr JFR, Currie AR. Cell death in the normal neonatal rat adrenal cortex. *J Pathol* 1973; 111:255-264.
31. Young RW. Cell death during differentiation of the retina in the mouse. *J Comp Neurol* 1984; 229:362-373.
32. Furtwangler JA. Sutural morphogenesis in the mouse calvaria: The role of apoptosis. *Acta Anatomica* 1985; 124:74-80.
33. Wyllie AH, Morris RG, Smith AL, Dunlop DJ. Chromatin cleavage in apoptosis: Association with condensed chromatin morphology and dependence on macromolecular synthesis. *J Pathol* 1984; 142:67-77.
34. Cohen JJ, Duke RC. Glucocorticoid activation of a calcium-dependent endonuclease in thymocyte nuclei leads to cell death. *J Immunol* 1984; 132:38-42.
35. Finn CA. The implantation reaction. In: Wynn RM, ed. *Biology of the uterus*. New York: Plenum Press, 1977: 245-308.
36. Wyllie AH. The biology of cell death in tumors. *Anticancer Res* 1985; 5:131-136.

FETOMATERNAL CELL FUSION AT RUMINANT IMPLANTATION

F.B.P. Wooding and G. Morgan

AFRC Institute of Animal Physiology and Genetics Research
Babraham, Cambridge, CB2 4AT
United Kingdom

THE ruminant blastocyst enters the uterus at about 7-8 days post coitum (dpc), loses its zona pellucida and expands two or three times. In the sheep this produces a spherical 10 mm diameter blastocyst.[1]

If the uterine site of insertion of the umbilical cord is taken as indicating the original implantation site,[2] then most ruminant conceptuses implant in a predictable region, one-third the way up one horn of the bicornuate uterus from the cervix. Single conceptuses do not necessarily implant in the horn down which they enter the uterus, so presumably myometrial contractions are responsible for blastocyst mobility and eventual positioning prior to implantation. The blastocyst immobilizes itself at the preferred site by extending trophectodermal papillae, cellular protrusions, down the uterine glands[3,4] (Fig. 1).

In the non-pregnant ruminant uterus there are rows of *caruncles*, circular areas (approx. 5 mm diameter) without uterine glands. These are the initial sites of blastocyst attachment, implantation, and eventual villus elaboration which develop into the characteristic cotyledons.

Between 12 and 15 dpc in the sheep (15-19 dpc in the cow) the conceptus elongates more than ten-fold very rapidly and expands to fill the narrow uterine lumen. At the start of implantation the ewe conceptus is about 12 cm long and 2 cm wide.

As the blastocyst elongates it produces considerable amounts of specific proteins[5] which are thought to have important roles in both the maintenance of the corpus luteum and immunological defence of the blastocyst. In the absence of such trophectodermal proteins, luteolysis is induced by prostaglandins transferred from the uterus by lymphatic and venous countercurrent exchange to the ovarian artery.[6]

At 14-15 dpc in the sheep (goat 16-17 dpc; cow, 17-18 dpc) binucleate cells (BNC) of characteristic structure differentiate from and within the uninucleate trophectoderm as the trophectodermal microvilli come into close apposition to those of the uterine epithelium[7] (Fig. 1). There is evidence for some changes in surface charge[8] and alkaline phosphatase activity[9] as the long fetal microvilli modify into bulbous protrusions which flatten against the unchanged uterine epithelial microvilli. The trophectoderm protrusions then differentiate back into microvilli which now interdigitate with those of the uterine epithelium.[10]

Implantation can be defined in ruminants by the start of BNC migration to, and fusion with, the uterine epithelial cells (16 dpc sheep,[11] 19 dpc goat, 20 dpc cow.[12]) The BNC have differentiated below the trophectodermal tight junction seal and the migration referred to is their passage through this junction while fully maintaining its structure (Figs. 1 and 2). No endometrial cellular alterations have been reported in any ruminant, no decidual reaction(s) results from the changes in uterine epithelium from cellular to syncytial. Although the sheep-goat and cow-deer types have significantly different definitive synepitheliochorial placental structure,[7] at implantation BNC migration and fusion produces a similar conversion of the

Ruminant Implantation

1. Immobilization by papillae, and elongation

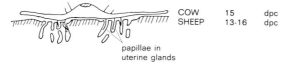

2. Cellular apposition and subsequent interdigitation of microvilli

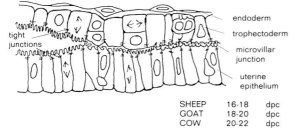

3. Binucleate cell development and migration

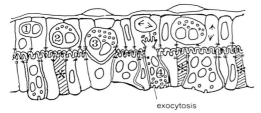

The uterine epithelium is greatly modified by migration and fusion (1-4) of fetal binucleate cells with some uterine epithelial cells and the death of others, *

Figure 1. (Above Left) Diagrams of the cellular changes at ruminant implantation.

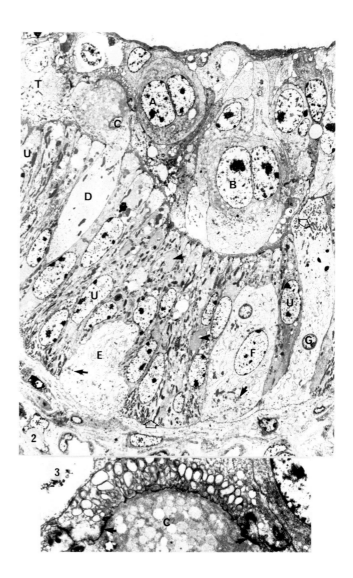

Figure 2. (Top Right) Electron micrograph of 20 dpc cow blastocyst apposed to uterine epithelium. The young (A) binucleate cell (BNC) is deep in the trophectoderm (T), the mature (B) BNC has migrated up to the microvillar junction. C is a BNC which has fused with a uterine epithelial cell (D), its granules are still on the fetal side but the BNC has almost completely migrated through its trophectoderm tight junction and is shedding excess plasma membrane from its fetal side (see higher magnification, Fig. 3). The cell profiles E, F, and G are considered to be of trinucleate cells. E and F contain BNC derived granules (arrows), many individual strands of rough endoplasmic reticulum (E) and small, apically clustered mitochondria (open arrow in G). The uterine epithelial cells (U) do not contain any similar granules, have aggregates of smooth endoplasmic reticulum (arrowheads) and show basal aggregates of elongate mitochondria (open arrow). There are no visible "decidual" changes in the endometrial stromal fibroblasts (*). 20 dpc Glutaraldehyde-Osmium-Araldite-Lead and Uranyl acetate stain X1900.

Figure 3. (Bottom Right). Detail from Fig. 2 showing the removal by vesiculation of residual trinucleate cell (C, Fig. 2) plasma membrane between the tight junction (arrows) through which the originally binucleate cell migrated. 20 dpc, G/O/A/L+U, X7100.

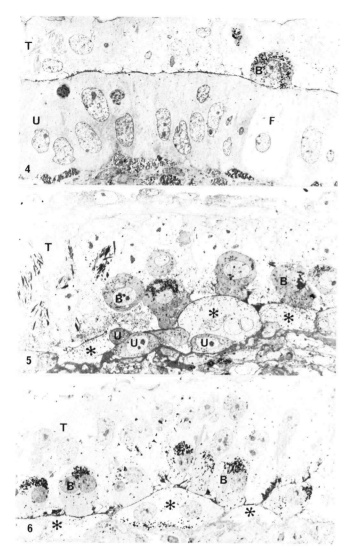

Figures 4, 5, and 6. *Electron micrographs of sheep implantation to illustrate the sequence of cellular changes mediated by the binucleate cells (B) in the trophectoderm (T) which convert the columnar uterine epithelial cells (U) into multinucleated plaques (*). Cells marked with an asterisk are equivalent to those shown by serial semi-thin sectioning to contain 3, 5, or 7 nuclei. Note the BNC-derived granules in some of the plaques. The pale cell marked F in Fig. 4 is a trinucleate cell very recently formed from fusion of the fully granulated BNC (B) with a uterine epithelial cell. Note the large number of BNC (e.g., B) at the microvillar junction in Figs. 5 and 6, easily identified by their granules and cytoplasmic densities which are emphasized by this method of section preparation. Glutaraldehyde-Araldite-Phosphotungstic Acid. 4, 16 dpc X1200; 5, 17 dpc, X1100; 6, 19 dpc, X1200 (Figs. 5 and 6 from Wooding, 1984).*

caruncular epithelium from unicellular to a mixture of uninucleate cells plus fetomaternal tri- and multinucleate (syncytial) plaques[11,12] (Figs. 4, 5, 6). Previous authors have referred to the cells with more than one nucleus as fetal or maternal "giant cells."[13] This imprecise terminology obscures the possible interrelationships between these cells and suggests a misleading analogy with rodent giant cells, which are uninucleate and polyploid.[14] In our developmental investigations, it was found more useful to define cell populations by specifying the number of nuclei. The evidence for the BNC migration and fusion interpretation of the cellular changes observed, rather than the simpler hypothesis of fusion between uterine epithelial cells, is based upon the following morphometrical,[11] ultrastructural,[11,12] histochemical,[11,12] and immunocytochemical[15] evidence.

In the pseudopregnant and pregnant rabbit, lateral fusion of uterine epithelial cells has been clearly documented.[16] The process is easily recognized by the presence of residual apical junctional complexes. Such structures have never been observed in ruminant trinucleate cells or multinucleated plaques (MNP).

At the earliest stage of implantation in sheep and goat, evidence from light microscope serial semi-thin section counting of the number of nuclei within each cellular boundary in the uterine epithelium indicates that possible fusions are restricted. All cells observed had one or three or five or more nuclei.[11] A BNC can fuse with the apex of a single uterine epithelial cell to form a trinucleate cell (TNC) and further BNC can fuse apically to extend this minisyncytium to five or seven nuclei or beyond. The fact that no evidence was found for any minisyncytia with two or four nuclei[11] indicates that syncytia in the uterine epithelium do not result from a random lateral fusion of uterine epithelial cells since that would produce a continuous range of nuclear numbers per minisyncytium. There is no technical problem in recognizing cells with two nuclei, since the same study clearly confirmed that the trophectoderm consisted of uninucleate cells and BNC.[11]

Ultrastructural examination of perfusion fixed material in the initial stages of implantation in cow,[12] sheep,[11] and goat shows that BNC differentiate, that is, develop a full complement of their characteristic granules isolated within the trophectodermal epithelium, touching neither the basement membrane nor the tight junction (Figs. 1, 11). Only mature fully granulated BNC were found at all stages of apparent migration through that tight junction while maintaining its structure (Fig. 1).

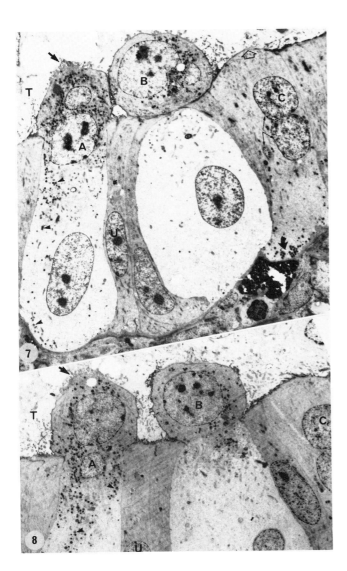

Figure 7 and 8. *Two different sections through the same three recently formed sheep trinucleate cells A, B, C. Note the vesiculation of residual membrane (arrows) at the fetal side of A. The BNC-derived granules stream down (arrowheads) into the maternal half of TNC (A) but are only present at the base of (C) (curved arrow). B shows clear fusion in Fig. 8 but only two nuclear profiles; the three nuclei are visible on Fig. 7 but the fusion is not apparent. C has three nuclei (thin arrows) and has lost all its residual membrane on the fetal side, but there is a tight junction remanent (open arrow) interrupting the dense phosphotungstic acid stained microvillar junction. T, trophectoderm; U uterine epithelium. Fig. 7, 16 dpc, G/Ar/PTA/Lead, X2500; Fig. 8, 16 dpc, G/Ar/PTA only, X3000.*

The front of the BNC which first penetrates the junction is usually a smooth pseudopodium (Fig. 2). The farther this BNC pseudopodium protrudes through the tight junction band, the flatter the BNC-uterine epithelial cell apposition becomes, until eventually the uterine epithelial microvilli are displaced entirely leaving the two cell plasmalemmas in close apposition. Fusion of these closely apposed membranes would produce a trinucleate cell whose BNC synthesized granules could translocate to the base of the uterine epithelium for exocytosis (Fig. 7). We have not yet captured the moment of membrane fusion in conventionally fixed material, but uterine epithelial cells undergoing fusion demonstrate the fact by becoming much less dense and usually considerably larger than their neighbors (Figs. 2, 4, 7). The TNC produced by such fusion is attached to both the trophectoderm and uterine epithelium tight junction seals emphasizing its dual origin. As the bulk of what was the BNC cytoplasm flows into the uterine epithelial cell, the excess plasma membrane on the fetal side of the trophectodermal tight junction is removed by vesiculation and phagocytosis by the trophectoderm, a dramatically visible process in the cow (Figs. 2, 3). As a result of this membrane loss the trinucleate cell is now separated from the trophectoderm by a patch of tight junction which interrupts the microvillar junction (Fig. 7) and is a good marker for completed BNC migration since there are no junctions between maternal and fetal cells elsewhere. Eventually this tight junction remanent is resorbed and the microvillar junction reforms leaving no trace of any BNC passage (Fig. 9).

Many BNC are found at the microvillar junction (Figs. 2,5,6,7) and many TNC and multinucleate plaques (MNP) are present in what was the uterine epithelium[11,12] but examples of cells actually fusing are very difficult to find, suggesting that the process occurs abruptly rather than rarely. Further evidence that fusion is normal and frequent can be derived by close examination of ultrastructure.

The TNC and MNP in the uterine epithelium have mitochondria, Golgi bodies, and endoplasmic reticulum much more like those in the BNC than the uninucleate uterine epithelial cells (Fig. 2). TNC and MNP often, but not always, include large numbers of granules of characteristic ultrastructure close to the basement membrane—very similar to those in the BNC but never found in uninucleate uterine epithelial cells (UUEC). All these granules can be selectively stained with phosphotungstic acid at low pH in non-osmicated material indicating a glycoprotein content (Figs. 4-10). The Golgi cisternae which produce the granules in the BNC also stain, but never the Golgi in the TNC/MNP/UUEC.[11,12] The PTA stain is only

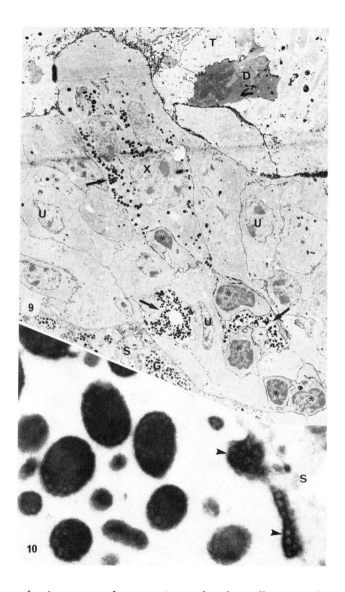

Figure 9. Sheep trinucleate cell (X7), 19 dpc, which has five intraepithelial lymphocytes (*) closely associated with its bottom end. BNC-derived granules (arrows) are streaming down the TNC to exocytose (see Fig. 10) to the maternal stroma (S) and to the lymphocyte surface. The stroma contains melanocytes whose granules (G) can be easily distinguished from those derived from the BNC. The three groups of binucleate cell granules (arrows) are probably all in the same TNC, illustrating the ability of such cells to flow around others. The trophectoderm (T) frequently includes dead cells (D), probably originating from uterine epithelial cells (U). 19 dpc, G/Glycolmethacrylate/PTA X2500.

Figure 10. Detail of BNC-derived granules at the base of a TNC. Note the similarity in microstructure of the granules and the densely stained areas (arrowheads) continuous with the stroma (S) which are 19 dpc, G/GMA/PTA X39,000.

selective, any glycoprotein molecule will stain, but immunocytochemistry on ultra-thin frozen sections has recently demonstrated[15] a specific protein, ovine placental lactogen (OPL), also restricted to the BNC Golgi but present in all BNC, TNC and MNP granules (Figs. 11, 12, 13). The simplest explanation is that the OPL-containing granules are only synthesized in the BNC in the fetal trophectoderm and are present in the TNC/MNP as a result of their formation by migration and fusion of BNC with UUEC.

Once the TNC has formed, the granules initially located at the fetal end of the BNC stream down the TNC past the nuclei (Fig. 7) and are exocytosed at the basolateral plasmalemma of the original UUEC,[11] thus releasing their contents to the maternal compartment (Fig. 10).

During early implantation in the sheep (17-24 dpc) few multinucleated plaques contain more than 5 nuclei.[11] Since no nuclear division has ever been observed in the syncytium these must originate from fusion. If this is restricted to the apex of the cells the nuclear contribution and presumably cell characteristics will be predominantly fetal, but it is not possible as yet to verify this. The basal plasmalemma of the original uterine epithelium is considerably modified, the MNP have many microvilli and large cellular processes penetrating the basement membrane and extending into the uterine stroma.[11]

The first TNC formed at implantation frequently appear to be associated with intraepithelial lymphocytes.[11] Groups of lymphocytes are often found at the fetomaternal interface during this time (Fig. 9). It is tempting to suggest an analogy with the lymphocytes recruited into the decidua in early pregnancy by mice and human conceptuses.[17] However, these ruminant lymphocytes need to be better characterized before any similar functions can be attributed to them. During implantation there is evidence in the uterine epithelium for both cell division (Fig. 10) and cell death (Fig. 9) with the latter predominating.[11] Since there is little increase in area of the uterine epithelium at this time the cell death could be a result of the considerable influx of BNC and consequent crowding out of the uninucleate uterine epithelial cells. The TNC and MNP formed certainly seem capable of flowing round and under to isolate such cells. There is no evidence, however, that they phagocy-

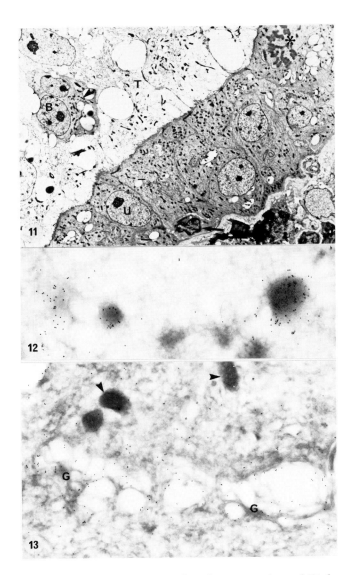

Figures 11, 12 and 13. *Ultra-thin cryosections of 17 dpc sheep blastocyst trophectoderm (T) apposed to uterine epithelium (U). A BNC (B) with a lymphocyte (arrow) and a dividing cell (*) in the uterine epithelium are clearly visible in Fig. 11. Fig. 12 shows BNC granules and Fig. 13 a BNC Golgi body (G) which are both marked with gold label after immunocytochemical processing using anti-ovine placental lactogen antibodies. Arrowheads, mitochondria. 17 dpc; G/Frozen sections/immunocytochemistry/Uranylacetate, Fig. 11 X2000; Fig. 12 X34000; Fig. 13 X20000. From Morgan and Wooding (1987).*

tose the residues. The uninucleate trophectodermal cells seem to play that role[11] (Fig. 9).

The reason for formation of the syncytial plaques is not obvious. They can form no more significant immunological or biophysical barrier than a cellular epithelium since they are noncontinuous, and in the cow, essentially transient. Rapid delivery of the BNC granule content to the maternal compartment seems to be their most consistent function. So far, only the placental lactogens have been definitely identified in the BNC granules at this early stage of pregnancy,[15] but it is clear that several other constituents are present. These may play an important role in modulating the maternal physiological and immune responses and/or providing the immunological camouflage for the fetal tissue, necessary for establishing and maintaining pregnancy.

The end of implantation may be defined by the start of villus formation on the flat caruncles.[11,12] (ewe, 24 dpc; cow, 30 dpc). This process produces a continuous and eventually enormous (approx. 50,000X) increase in the area of the fetomaternal junction during pregnancy. In the sheep and goat the syncytial plaques are maintained and extended by continuous BNC migration. In the cow and deer, residual uninucleate uterine epithelial cells displace the plaques, although these rapidly dividing uninucleate cells are very different ultrastructurally from the original uterine epithelial cells.[12] BNC formation and migration continues unabated, but only transient TNC are formed in the cellular uterine epithelium.

Binucleate cells form and migrate throughout pregnancy in all ruminants so far examined.[7] They are not solely concerned with implantation. There is increasing evidence for changes in their granule content at differing stages of development[15] and they have been shown to be capable of synthesizing steroids and prostaglandins later in pregnancy (see refs. in 15). These remarkably versatile cells appear to be of primary importance in implantation and placental growth in ruminants, but as yet little is known about control of their growth and differentiation.

References

1. Rowson LEA, Moor RM. Development of the sheep conceptus during the first 14 days. *J Anat* 1966; 100:777-785.
2. Lee SY, Mossman HW, Mossman AS, Delpino G. Evidence for a specific implantation site in ruminant. *Amer J Anat* 1977; 150:631-640.
3. Wooding FBP, Staples LD, Peacock M. Structure of trophoblast papillae on the sheep conceptus at implantation. *J Anat* 1982; 134:507-516.

4. Guillomot M, Guay P. Ultrastructural features of the cell surfaces of uterine and trophoblastic epithelium during embryonic attachment in the cow. *Anat Rec* 1982; 204:315-322.
5. Godkin JD, Bazer FW, Thatcher WW, Roberts RM. Proteins released by cultured day 15-16 conceptuses prolong luteal maintenance when introduced into the uterine lumen of cyclic ewes. *J Reprod Fertil* 1984; 71:57-64.
6. Heap RB, Fleet IR, Hamon M. $PGF_2\alpha$ is transferred from the uterus to the ovary in the sheep by lymphatic and blood vascular pathways. *J Reprod Fertil* 1985; 74:645-656.
7. Wooding FBP, Flint APF. Placentation In: Lamming GE, ed. *Marshalls physiology of reproduction*, Fourth Edition, Vol III, London: Churchill-Livingstone, in press, 1989.
8. Guillomot M, Fléchon E, Wintenberger-Torres S. Cytochemical studies of uterus and trophoblastic surface coats during blastocyst attachment in the ewe. *J Reprod Fertil* 1982; 65:1-8.
9. Leiser R, Wille KH. Alkaline phosphatase in the bovine endometrium and trophoblast during the early phase of implantation. *Anat Embryol* 1975; 148:145-157.
10. Leiser R. Kontaktaufnahme zwischen Trophoblast und Uterus epithel wahrend der fruhen Implantation beim Rind. *Anat Histol Embryol* 1975; 4:63-86.
11. Wooding FBP. Role of binucleate cells in fetomaternal cell fusion at implantation in the sheep. *Amer J Anat* 1984; 170:233-250.
12. Wathes DC, Wooding FBP. An electronmicroscope study of implantation in the cow. *Amer J Anat* 1980; 159:285-306.
13. King GJ, Atkinson BA, Robertson HA. Development of the bovine placentome from days 20 to 29 of gestation. *J Reprod Fertil* 1980; 59:95-100.
14. Kaufman MH. Origin, properties and fate of trophoblast in the mouse. In: Loke C, Whyte A eds. *Biology of trophoblast*. Amsterdam: Elsevier, 1983.
15. Morgan G, Wooding FBP, Brandon MR. Immunogold localisation of placental lactogen and the SBU3 antigen by ultracryomicrotomy at implantation in the sheep. *J Cell Science* 1987; 88:503-512.
16. Davies J, Hoffman LH. Studies on the progestational endometrium of the rabbit. II Electronmicroscopy, day 0 to day 15 of gonadotrophin induced pseudopregnancy. *Amer J Anat* 1975; 142:355-366.
17. Clark DA. Maternofetal relationships. *Immunology Letters* 1985; 9:239-247.

SECTION IV: DECIDUALIZATION, IMMUNOLOGICAL CONSIDERATIONS

MORPHOLOGY OF THE DECIDUA

Paulo A. Abrahamsohn

Department of Histology and Embryology
Institute of Biomedical Sciences
University of Sao Paulo, Brazil

SINCE the morphological description of the decidua presented by Krehbiel,[1] many papers and reviews have appeared dealing with light microscopical, histochemical, and ultrastructural aspects of the decidua. The morphology of the decidua has mainly been studied in rats and mice, and to a lesser extent in hamsters, guinea pigs, humans, and nonhuman primates.[2-12] Therefore, most of this chapter will deal with the first two mentioned species. Emphasis will be given to newer developments on the subject.

GENERAL MORPHOLOGY OF THE DECIDUA

The decidua that develops in the antimesometrial wall of the uterus differs from the mesometrial decidua in its temporal development, cellular arrangement, and some morphological features. Their fate is also different: the antimesometrial decidua develops rapidly and regresses simultaneously with the growth of the embryo, whereas the mesometrial decidua grows more slowly, gradually providing the groundwork for the development of the hemochorial placenta. Several regions are seen in the fully decidualized endometrium of rodents. The following description is primarily based on the work of Welsh and Enders.[12]

1. In the *antimesometrial decidua*, the layer of decidual cells closest to the lateral walls of the embryo consists of relatively small, mostly flattened decidual cells. Many of these cells show signs of degeneration. The group of decidual cells that surrounds the antimesometrial pole of the embryo is called the *decidual crypt*. These cells are less closely packed than mature decidual cells and have longer processes. Red blood cells are often present in the extracellular spaces as well as in the cytoplasm of decidual cells. Many of these cells are degenerating. A wide layer of large, closely packed decidual cells (fully transformed or mature decidual cells) surrounds the flattened cells and the cells of the decidual crypt. These cells have round nuclei and prominent nucleoli. They are often binucleate (rat) or multinucleate (mouse). Their cytoplasms have numerous ribosomes, well-developed endoplasmic reticulae and Golgi complexes, and lysosome-like bodies. Intermediate filaments are a prominent feature of rodent decidual cells. The intermediate filament protein *desmin* is expressed by these cells.[13] Surrounding the region of mature decidual cells exists a layer of cells exhibiting intermediate features of mature decidual cells and of fibroblast-like cells. These cells (predecidual cells) are smaller than the mature cells and have longer processes that touch processes of other cells; the extracellular spaces are larger than in the mature cell region. Since there is a gradient of transformation of predecidual cells into mature cells, the limits between both layers are ill-defined. At the periphery of the predecidual cells, flattened and closely packed cells form a layer that is very distinct in the rat (fibrinoid capsule) but not in the mouse.

2. The *mesometrial decidua* consists of decidual cells and granular cells. The decidual cells are smaller than the mature antimesometrial cells and their cytoplasms have fewer organelles. They are often binucleate. A marked feature of these cells is the processes that span the extracellular spaces, giving a spiny appearance. These decidual cells are found up to the neighborhood of the myometrium. The granular cells are intermingled with decidual cells but differ from the latter with respect to the following: they have a clear cytoplasm, electron-dense granules, and do not establish intercellular junctions.[12] The granular cells appear in the decidua at early stages of pregnancy and gradually accumulate in the mesometrial triangle.[14] In contrast to the decidual cells that originate from endometrial fibroblastic cells, small endometrial cells, similar to lymphocytes, are thought to be precursors of the granular cells.[15] Experiments using irradiated mice reconstituted with rat bone marrow indicate that granular cell precursors originate from the bone marrow.[16]

3. The *glycogen region* (glycogen wings) is a funnel-shaped region situated between the antimesometrial decidua and the mesometrial decidua. In addition to containing much glycogen, the cells of this region have well-developed granular endoplasmic reticulae and Golgi complexes. Fewer lysosome-like bodies and intermediate filaments exist as compared to mature antimesometrial decidual cells. The cells of the glycogen region are closely packed and often binucleate.

4. The *undifferentiated stroma* (nondecidualized stroma, basal zone) is a layer of fibroblast-like cells and intercellular matrix, situated between the antimesometrial decidua and the myometrium. At the beginning of decidualization this region also extends into the mesometrial endometrium.

CELL SURFACE

Cell processes and intercellular junctions are the most prominent features of the decidual cell surface of rodents. Finger-like or lamellar processes frequently interdigitate with processes of adjacent cells or of the same cell, often establishing junctions. The processes emitted by mature rat decidual cells seem to be longer and more interdigitated than those of the mouse decidua. In the rat decidua, lamellar processes may interdigitate intensively, forming series of parallel stacks, especially in the antimesometrial decidua and glycogen area, whereas in the mouse these stacks are rarely seen.[12,17,18] Larger spaces exist between human decidual cells as compared to those present between mature rodent decidual cells. Human decidual cells characteristically have small club-shaped processes that contain membrane-bound electron-dense granules.[7] The junctions in rodents occur between cell bodies, between processes, and between processes and cell bodies. On the 5th day of pregnancy (d.o.p.) in the mouse, small surface areas participate in intercellular junctions; from day 6 on, the junctions occupy large areas of the cell surface. Two main types of intercellular junctions are found in rodent decidual cells: gap and adherens. Additionally, tight junctions are present in the rat primary decidual zone.[19] Gap junctions are highly developed in the mature decidual cell region, both in number and size. The length of the gap junctions seen in cross-sections of mouse decidual cell membranes may reach 2 μm. Many gap junctions of the rodent decidua have a peculiar arrangement: tips of bulb-ended processes establish gap junctions at the surface of recesses of adjacent cells. Cross-sections of the bulbs appear as circles. Hence these junctions have been termed annular gap junctions. Gap junctions established between parts of the same cell are occasionally seen. The human decidual cells have few intercellular junctions but many gap junctions form between parts of the same cell.[7] Gap junctions are known as sites of cell communication and could play an important role in the process of decidualization by transmitting appropriate messages between stromal cells.[20] They could provide means to coordinate decidual cell transformation, division, polyploidization, and perhaps cell death. Possibly in this regard, small gap junctions can be found between mouse endometrial stromal cells before overt decidualization, by 4 d.o.p. The adherens-type junctions have been variously named by different authors. This junction shows a regular intercellular space of about 20 nm between the membranes. A delicate electron-dense mesh appears in the subplasmalemmal cytoplasm of the junction. Its morphology is very similar to the zonula adherens present in the lateral membranes of many epithelial cells. However, since the surface of the decidual cell is quite irregular it is unlikely that this junction is arranged as a belt along the cell surface. Thus, because these junctions are probably discontinuous, they are most likely fasciae adherens. A definition of this junction must await the demonstration of proteins associated with it, such as vinculin, talin and the 135-kDa protein.[21] Very small adherens junctions exist in mouse decidual cells during early stages of decidualization, 5 d.o.p. These junctions resemble the focal contacts established by cells during embryonic development as well as during *(in vitro)* reaggregation or sorting out.[22] Adherens junctions become prominent on the 7th and following days of pregnancy in the mouse. At these stages they frequently alternate with small gap junctions along extensive areas of the cell surface, leaving small junction-free zones that seem to form intercellular channels into which small microvilli protrude. In the rat primary decidual zone, tight junctions are adjacent to expanded extracellular spaces that contain cell processes.[18] In the mouse, the neck of most bulb-ended processes forming gap junctions with adjacent cells contains an adherens junction as if to hold both cells together. An obvious role of the adherens junction is to promote adhesion between decidual cells. As these junctions are thought to transmit active forces between cells, they may permit the contraction and relaxation of a whole tissue or of parts of it.[22] Accumulation of these junctions after 7 d.o.p. may reflect an increasing pressure exerted by the conceptus against the decidua. An ultrastructural study on the permeability of intravenously injected horseradish peroxidase (HRP) and HRP-labeled immunoglobulin G (IgG) across the rat primary decidual zone, supplemented with en bloc tracing with lanthanum nitrate, suggested that besides the barrier rendered by the endothelial cell junctions, a second barrier is present in the primary decidua.[19] This barrier is probably formed by tight junctions that, albeit discontinuously, join the cells of this region.[18,19] The rat primary decidual zone may be regarded as a temporary barrier surrounding the embryo, protecting it from exposure to maternal IgG, microorganisms, and immunocompetent cells.[19,23]

CELL TYPES IN THE DECIDUA

Morphological analysis reveals that the main cell types present in the decidua are decidual cells, granular cells, and endothelial cells. Some morphological differences exist among decidual cells within each decidual region (mainly due to progressive degrees of cell transformation) as well as among cells of the several regions of the decidua. One may wonder whether these differences conceal the existence of different cell types in the decidua, not distinguishable by morphological criteria alone (see below). Leukocytes, commonly present in the connective tissues, are rarely found among fully transformed decidual cells, but they, as well as macrophages and plasma cells, are present between predecidual cells and in the nondecidualized stroma.[5,10] Lymphocytes are found in the human decidua.[9] The endometrium of implantation sites of Rhesus monkeys analyzed up to 35 d.o.p. has leukocytes, macrophages, and granular cells.[11] Cell surface marker labeling permits the identification of cells present in suspensions of mouse endometrial stromal cells. As about 50% of mouse decidual or deciduomal cells express Thy-1 antigen, this was thought to denote their fibroblastic origin.[24,25]

Receptors for Fc (characteristic of phagocytic cells) were found in 10-20% of cells obtained from decidual tissue or from deciduomata.[25] Both Thy-1 and Fc receptors are thus expressed independently of the presence of an embryo.[25] Supernatants of cultures prepared from mouse decidual tissue exhibit immunosuppressor activity.[26] Two major cell populations could be observed in these cultures: large flat, spindle-shaped or stellate cells (probably decidual cells) and small round cells (probably an infiltrate).[26] The *in vitro* assay of immunosuppressor activity in mouse endometrial stromal cells was found to be associated with "large" cells in early stages of pregnancy or pseudopregnancy with small lymphocytes during the second half of pregnancy.[27]

THE DYNAMIC NATURE OF THE DECIDUA

During early stages of embryo-implantation in rodents, the first decidual cells appear in the subepithelial stroma, surrounding the embryo antimesometrially. In the mouse these decidual cells might be termed immature decidual cells since they have few cisternae or endoplasmic reticulae and Golgi complexes but many free ribosomes.[10] The growth of the decidua results mainly from cell division (especially of predecidual cells) and enlargement of stromal cells as they transform into decidual cells. As the embryo grows, the decidual cells situated close to the embryo die, while newly transformed decidual cells are added at the periphery of already existing decidual cells. The antimesometrial decidua grows rapidly following embryo-implantation and attains its maximum development around days 10 and 11 in the rat[12] and around days 8 and 9 in the mouse. After these stages, the balance between death and addition of new decidual cells is probably shifted in favor of the regression of the antimesometrial decidua. On day 14 in the rat and on day 11 in the mouse the antimesometrial decidua has turned into a mass of dead cells which is sloughed off into the new (antimesometrial) uterine lumen.[12] The new lumen arises out of the gradual growth of the luminal epithelium of adjacent interimplantation sites, within the nondecidualized stroma and around the antimesometrial decidua. The epithelium begins growing one or two days after implantation and expands until the fronts of the lumina merge sometime around day 14 in the rat; around day 12 or 14 in the mouse.[28,29]

The degenerating antimesometrial decidual cells accumulate clumps of heterochromatin in the nucleus, and have heterophagosomes, and dilated perinuclear and endoplasmic reticulum cisternae.[12,30] Terminally deteriorated cells round up and become fragmented. The debris of dead cells situated close to the embryo are phagocytosed by trophoblastic giant cells or enter the blood spaces formed by the trophoblastic giant cells and are probably carried to other parts of the body.[30]

In the mouse, early signs of decidualization of the mesometrial decidua are apparent by 5 d.o.p.: stromal cells are polygonal and have round nuclei with prominent nucleoli. Their arrangement is different from that of interimplantation sites because the cells have long processes that, touching processes of other cells, form a net with large extracellular spaces. These cells gradually transform into spiny mesometrial decidual cells.

The regression of decidual cells at the trophoblast-decidua interface and the addition of newly decidualized cells at the periphery make the decidua a difficult tissue to analyze, especially in studies where different gestational ages are to be compared. This happens because cells that are close to the embryo at one stage may have disappeared at subsequent stages. On the other hand, predecidual cells, which are situated far from the embryo, become decidual cells and move closer to the embryo at later stages.

BLOOD VESSELS

The decidua has been held responsible for nutrition of the embryo before the establishment of the definitive hemochorial placenta. It is currently thought that lipids and glycogen are transferred from decidual cells to the embryo;[1] however, no experimental evidence has been provided to support this concept. Initially, the nutrition of the embryo is probably supplied by materials originating from decidual blood vessels, even considering that the traffic of molecules in the intercellular spaces of the decidua is not unrestricted.[19,22] Nutrients present in the extracellular spaces have access to the parietal endoderm after crossing the trophoblastic cells (or pores of these cells) as well as Reichert's membrane.[31,32] A few days after embryo-implantation in rodents, the blood spaces of the trophoblastic giant cells probably provide most of the nutrients in this stage of pregnancy.

During the beginning of decidualization in rodents, endometrial blood vessels of implantation sites leak plasma into the extracellular spaces; when dyes that bind albumin (Pontamine blue, Evans blue) are injected intravenously, they leak and delineate implantation sites.[33] Fenestrated post-capillary venules situated at the periphery of the decidua are probably the sites of leakage.[34] Fenestrated capillaries are present in the pregnant rat endometrium.[12,17] Scanning electron microscopy studies of castings of endometrial blood vessels show that the spacing between the blood vessels of implantation sites increases soon after embryo-implantation and that the vessels spread out from the embryo.[35,36]

Endothelial cells in implantation sites undergo cell division and show morphological features of metabolic activation.[5,12,17,34,36] Areas of close contact between decidual cells and endothelial cells are present in the rat.[17,31] In the neighborhood of the embryo, decidual cells may interpose between endothelial cells and between trophoblastic cells that form blood spaces.[12,31] No capillaries, or very few of them, are found in the primary decidual zone.[1,5,18,36] Castings of blood vessels show that the antimesometrial capillaries approaching the embryos are blind-ended.[35,36] This is probably due to a narrowing of their lumina just outside the primary zone, preventing the access of blood to this region and possibly influencing the sloughing of the uterine epithelium during embryonic invasion.[5,35,36] The shutdown of the capillaries occurs probably around the primary decidual zone. The mesometrial blood capillaries, especially those in the glycogen region, are large and resemble sinusoids; their endothelial cells are thick and their nuclei bulge into the lumen.[12] Many of these blood vessels later form the maternal blood channels of the placenta.[1,37]

DECIDUAL CELL MATRIX

During the early invasion of the stroma by the rat embryo, decidual cell processes penetrate through perforations of the basal lamina of the implantation crypt.[18,38] It is suggested that the perforations result from the activity of decidual cells that may thus be instrumental for the breakdown of the basal lamina, necessary for trophoblastic invasion.[18,28]

Small electron-dense plaques are attached to the surface of rodent decidual cells in places where a cytoplasmic plaque is attached to the plasmalemma. In mice these plaques are found mainly in immature decidual cells (5 d.o.p.) and in predecidual cells. When mouse endometrium is fixed with a fixative containing ruthenium red, granules of the stain accumulate in the cell surface plaques indicating that heparan sulfate might be present. These plaques are similar to the fibronexus or to focal adhesions present in points where the surface of (in vitro growth) fibroblasts touch their substrate.[39] The plasmalemma of focal adhesions is supposed to have intramembrane proteins that connect extracellular components to cytoskeletal molecules. As these structures predominate in cells that are not highly migratory, it is thought that they may provide stable attachment of cells to extracellular matrix components.[39] An

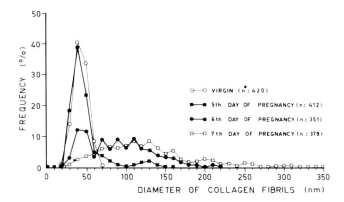

Figure 1. *Frequency of diameters of collagen fibrils of the endometrial stroma of virgin mice and of the region of fully-transformed antimesometrial decidual cells of pregnant mice. n*: number of measured fibrils (unpublished data from M.C. Alberto-Rincon and T.M.T. Zorn).*

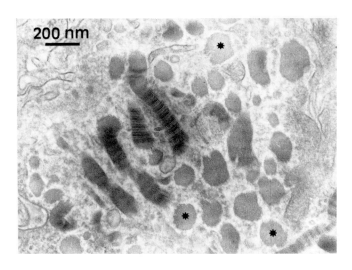

Figure 2. *Collagen fibrils of the region of fully transformed antimesometrial decidual cells of 7-day pregnant mice. Cross-sectioned fibrils (*) have irregular profiles (electron micrograph from M.C. Alberto-Rincon and T.M.T. Zorn).*

immunocytochemical study on the distribution of fibronectin during decidualization in the rat showed that while the stromal cells are spindle-shaped, fibronectin is widely distributed in a fibrillar arrangement. However, when the cells round up, fibronectin becomes present as small patches on the cell surfaces and finally disappears, except around blood vessels and in basement membranes.[40] Other studies showed that fibronectin, as well as laminin, entactin, type-IV collagen and heparan sulfate, are produced by rodent decidual cells and are detected around the cells.[13,41] Human decidual cells, as seen under the electron microscope, are surrounded by a thin sheet of amorphous material, similar to a basal lamina.[7,42] Light microscope studies indicated that fibronectin, laminin, heparan sulfate and collagen types IV and V are associated with this lamina.[42-45] The accumulation of these molecules around human decidual cells seems to parallel the progressive transformation of stromal cells into decidual cells.[42] Collagen types I and III are distributed in the matrix of the human decidua.[44] Decidual cells of the Rhesus monkey, at least until day 35 of pregnancy, are not bordered by a basal lamina-like material and have fewer processes (with fewer membrane-bound granules) than in humans.[11]

In virgin mouse endometrium fixed with glutaraldehyde-containing stains that preserve proteoglycans (alcian blue, safranine O), the extracellular space becomes homogeneously electron dense. In similarly fixed endometria, on the 7th day of pregnancy, areas of expanded extracellular spaces exhibit nets of granules and bottle-brush structures that have a central filamentous core and spiny lateral projections. This net is associated with the cell surface and collagen fibrils. In the mature decidual cell region there is much less material in the extracellular spaces; electron dense material is usually associated with small bundles of collagen fibrils. Patches of an electron dense amorphous material of unknown composition have been observed in the matrix of rat decidual cells.[12,18] The morphology and distribution of this material seem to be different from the proteoglycans studied in the mouse.

There is evidence of an active influence of decidual cells on their matrix. Human decidual explants were shown to produce collagen types I, III, IV and V *in vitro*.[44] Basement membrane components are produced by human and rodent.[13,41,44] Both in the rat[17,18,31,38] and in the mouse, collagen fibrils are embraced by flanges of decidual cells, as if the cells anchor to collagen fibrils: this may be an important provision for the structural stability of the decidua. Decidual cell processes may limit extracellular compartments where collagen bundles may be assembled and organized.[18] Another finding that may indicate an influence of decidual cells on the cell matrix is the arrangement of collagen fibrils along a mesometrial-antimesometrial axis in the primary decidual zone of rats and mice.[18,31,38] Collagen fibrils were found within vacuoles in the cytoplasm of mouse decidual cells (7 d.o.p.). Many vacuoles showed acid phosphatase activity. These features are similar to those observed in other tissues, such as gingiva and periodontal ligament, and indicate that decidual cells may phagocytose collagen.

The diameters of collagen fibrils in the mouse decidua are heterogeneous.[46,47] The fibrils of virgin endometria as well as of the nondecidualized stroma and interimplantation sites are thin. Their diameters are somewhat increased in the predecidual cell region and much more so in the region of mature decidual cells. In this region the fibril diameter increases gradually from days 5 to 7 (Fig. 1). It appears that the fibrils present in the mature decidual cell region belong to one population and that the thicker fibrils result from the growth or aggregation of thinner fibrils. The outline of the cross-sectional view of fibrils larger than about 70 nm is irregular (Fig. 2). Thick collagen fibrils are also found in the mouse deciduoma.

Acknowledgment

I wish to thank Telma M.T. Zorn, Estela M.A.F. Bevilacqua, A. Tania Bijovsky, D. Loch, and Maria C. Alberto-Rincon for their unpublished results on the mouse decidua. Dr. Allen C. Enders kindly read a preliminary version of the manuscript. Supported by FAPESP, CNPq, and FINEP.

References

1. Krehbiel RH. Cytological studies of the decidual reaction in the rat during early pregnancy in the production of deciduomata. *Physiological Zoology* 1937: 10:212-233.
2. De Feo VJ. Decidualization. In: Wynn RM, ed. *Cellular biology of the uterus.* Amsterdam: North Holland, 1967:192-291.
3. Finn CA. The implantation reaction. In: Wynn RM, ed. *Biology of the uterus.* 2nd edition, New York: Plenum Press, 1977:245-308.
4. Weitlauf HM. Biology of implantation. In: Knobil E, Neill JD, Ewing LL, Markert CL, Greenwald GS, Pfaff DW, ed. *Physiology of reproduction.* Raven Press, 1988.
5. Enders AC, Schlafke S. A morphological analysis of the early implantation stages in the rat. *Am J Anat* 1967; 120:185-226.
6. Orsini MW, Wynn RM, Harris JA, Bulmash JM. Comparative ultrastructure of the decidua in pregnancy and pseudopregnancy. *Amer J Obstet Gynecol* 1970; 106:14-25.
7. Lawn AM, Wilson EW, Finn CA. The ultrastructure of human decidual and predecidual cells. *J Reprod Fertil* 1971; 26:85-90.
8. Wynn RM. Cytotrophoblastic specializations: an ultrastructural study of the human placenta. *Am J Obstet Gynecol* 1972; 114:339-355.
9. Liebig W, Stegner HE. Die Dezidualization der endometrialen Stromazelle. *Arch Gynak* 1977; 223:19-31.
10. Abrahamsohn PA. Ultrastructural study of the mouse antimesometrial decidua. *Anat Embryol* 1983; 166:263-274.
11. Enders AC, Welsh AO, Schlafke S. Implantation in the Rhesus monkey: endometrial responses. *Am J Anat* 1985; 173:147-169.
12. Welsh AO, Enders AC. Light and electron microscopic examination of the mature decidual cells of the rat with emphasis on the antimesometrial decidua and its degeneration. *Am J Anat* 1985; 172:1-29.
13. Glasser SR, Lampelo S, Munir MI, Julian JA. Expression of desmin, laminin and fibronectin during *in situ* differentiation (decidualization) of rat uterine stromal cells. *Differentiation* 1987; 35:132-142.
14. Stewart I, Peel S. The differentiation of the decidua and the distribution of metrial gland cells in the pregnant mouse uterus. *Cell Tissue Res* 1978; 187:167-179.
15. Peel S, Bulmer D. The fine structure of the rat metrial gland in relation to the origin of the granulated cells. *J Anat* 1977; 123:687-696.
16. Peel S, Stewart IJ, Bulmer D. Experimental evidence for the bone marrow origin of granulated metrial gland cells of the mouse uterus. *Cell Tissue Res* 1983; 233:647-656.
17. O'Shea JD, Kleinfeld RG, Morrow HA. Ultrastructure of decidualization in the pseudopregnant rat. *Am J Anat* 1983; 166:271-298.
18. Parr MB, Tung HN, Parr EL. The ultrastructure of the rat primary decidual zone. *Am J Anat* 1986; 176:423-436.
19. Tung HN, Parr MB, Parr EL. The permeability of the primary decidual zone in the rat uterus: an ultrastructural tracer and freeze-fracture study. *Biol Reprod* 1986; 35:1045-1058.
20. Finn CA, Lawn AM. Specialized junctions between decidual cells in the uterus of the pregnant mouse. *J Ultrastruct Res* 1967; 20:321-327.
21. Geiger B, Volk T, Volberg T. Molecular heterogeneity of adherens junctions. *J Cell Biol* 1985; 101:1523-1531.
22. Staehelin AL. Structure and function of intercellular junctions. *Int Rev Cytol.* 1974; 39:191-283.
23. Parr MB, Parr EL. Permeability of the primary decidual zone in the rat uterus: studies using fluorescein-labeled proteins and dextrans. *Biol Reprod.* 1986; 34:393-403.
24. Bernard O, Scheid MP, Ripoche MA, Bennet D. Immunological studies of mouse decidual cells. *J Exp Med.* 1978; 148:580-591.

25. Rachman F, Bernard O, Scheid MP. Immunological studies of mouse decidual cell. II Studies of cells in artificially induced decidua. *J Reprod Immunol* 1981; 3:41-48.
26. Badet MT, Bell SC, Billington WD. Immunoregulatory activity of supernatants from short-term cultures of mouse decidual tissue. *J Reprod Fertil* 1983; 68:351-358.
27. Brierley J, Clark DA. Characterization of hormone-dependent suppressor cells in the uterus of mated and pseudopregnant mice. *J Reprod Immunol* 1987; 10:201-217.
28. Welsh AO, Enders AC. Occlusion and reformation of the rat uterine lumen during pregnancy. *Am J Anat* 1983; 167:463-477.
29. Peel S, Bulmer D. A study of proliferative activity of the uterine epithelium of the pregnant rat in relation to the morphogenesis of the new lumen. *J Reprod Fertil* 1975; 42:189-193.
30. Katz S, Abrahamsohn PA. Involution of the antimesometrial decidua in the mouse. *Anat Embryol* 1987; 176:251-258.
31. Welsh AO, Enders AC. Trophoblast-decidual cell interactions and establishment of maternal blood circulation in the parietal yolk sac placenta of the rat. *Anat Rec* 1987; 217:203-219.
32. Bevilacqua EMAF, Abrahamsohn PA. Ultrastructure of trophoblast giant cell transformation during the invasive stage of implantation of the mouse embryo. *J Morph*, in press.
33. Psychoyos A. La réaction déciduale est précédée de modifications précoces de la perméabilité capillaire de l'utérus. *C R Soc Biol* 1960; 154:1384-1387.
34. Abrahamsohn PA, Lundkvist O, Nilsson O. Ultrastructure of the endometrial blood vessels during implantation of the rat blastocyst. *Cell Tissue Res* 1983; 229:269-280.
35. Rogers PAW, Murphy CR, Gannon BJ. Changes in the spatial organization of the uterine vasculature during implantation in the rat. *J Reprod Fertil* 1982; 65:211-214.
36. Christofferson RH, Nilsson BO. Morphology of the endometrial microvasculature during early placentation in the rat. *Cell Tissue Res* 1988; 253:209-220.
37. Christofferson RH. Angiogenesis as induced by trophoblast and cancer cells. *Doctoral Thesis*. University of Uppsala, 1988.
38. Schlafke S, Welsh AO, Enders AC. Penetration of the basal lamina of the uterine luminal epithelium during implantation in the rat. *Anat Rec* 1985; 212:47-56.
39. Woods A, Couchman JR. Focal adhesions and cell-matrix interactions. *Collagen Rel Res* 1988; 8:155-182.
40. Grinnell F, Head JR, Hoffpauir J. Fibronectin and cell shape *in vivo* : studies on the endometrium during pregnancy. *J Cell Biol* 1982; 94:597-606.
41. Wewer UM, Damjanov A, Weiss J, Liotta LA, Damjanov I. Mouse endometrial stromal cells produce basement-membrane components. *Differentiation* 1986; 32:49-58.
42. Wewer UM, Faber M, Liotta LA, Albrechtsen R. Immunochemical and ultrastructural assessment of the nature of the pericellular basement membrane of human decidual cells. *Lab Invest* 1985; 53:624-633.
43. Aplin JD, Campbell S. An immunofluorescence study of extracellular matrix associated with cytotrophoblast of the chorion laeve. *Placenta* 1985; 6:469-479.
44. Kisalus LL, Herr JC, Little CD. Immunolocalization of extracellular matrix proteins and collagen synthesis in first-trimester human decidua. *Anat Rec* 1987; 218:402-415.
45. Charpin C, Kopp F, Pourreau-Schneider N, et al. Laminin distribution in human decidua and immature placenta. An immunoelectron microscopic study (avidin-biotin-peroxidase complex method). *Am J Obstet Gynecol* 1985; 151:822-827.
46. Zorn TMT, Bevilacqua EMAF, Abrahamsohn PA. Collagen remodeling during decidualization in the mouse. *Cell Tissue Res* 1986; 244:443-448.
47. Alberto-Rincon MC, Zorn TMT, Abrahamsohn PA, Bevilacqua EMAF. Distribution of collagen fibrils in the endometrium during the sixth day of pregnancy. *Proc 11th Meeting Braz Soc Electron Microscopy.* 1987:121-122.

MEDIATORS INVOLVED IN DECIDUALIZATION

T.G. Kennedy, P.M. Squires, G.M. Yee

MRC Group in Reproductive Biology
Departments of Obstetrics & Gynaecology and of Physiology
The University of Western Ontario
London, Ontario N6A 5A5 Canada

THERE are considerable differences among species in the process of blastocyst implantation, particularly in the extent of trophoblastic invasion of the endometrium.[1,2] In many species, the endometrium undergoes decidual transformation in response to an implanting embryo, ultimately giving rise to the maternal component of the placenta.[2] Although decidualization, which involves proliferation and differentiation of endometrial stromal cells, is a conspicuous part of the process of implantation, the function of this specialized tissue is uncertain.[3] Decidualization can also be obtained in some species, particularly rodents, in response to artificial stimuli. Because the basic processes involved in decidualization in response to blastocysts and artificial stimuli appear to be the same, artificially induced decidualization has become widely accepted as a mode for the maternal component of implantation.[3]

In all species that have been investigated, the earliest macroscopically identifiable sign of blastocyst implantation is an increase in endometrial vascular permeability which is confined to areas adjacent to the blastocysts.[2] The increase in permeability is usually taken as indicative of the initiation of implantation, and is thought to be essential for successful implantation.[2] In species in which artificial stimuli induce decidualization, an increase in endometrial vascular permeability precedes the differentiation of decidual cells.[2]

The localized nature of the endometrial vascular permeability response and subsequent decidualization at implantation suggests that these responses are mediated by localized factors. The primary signal from the blastocyst may be chemical or physical in nature; if the latter, it must be transduced within the endometrium to a chemical signal to bring about the endometrial responses. This review will restrict itself to the compounds which have received the most attention as proposed mediators of implantation and/or artificially induced decidualization, namely, histamine, estrogen, prostaglandins (PGs), leukotrienes (LTs), and platelet-activating factor (PAF). These mediators are by no means mutually exclusive, and it is possible that the mediators of the vascular responses differ from those involved in the subsequent proliferation and differentiation of stromal cells.

HISTAMINE

A role for histamine in decidualization was first proposed by Shelesnyak.[4] Assuming that a factor common to all artificial deciduogenic stimuli was some degree of tissue damage and arguing by analogy with the inflammatory response, he suggested that uterine trauma caused the release from mast cells of histamine, and that this substance was the prime inducer of decidualization.

Evidence, acquired mainly in the rat, for this proposal included the observations that intrauterine injections of antihistaminic drugs blocked the artificially induced decidual response,[4,5] and that systemic administration of histamine or drugs which cause its release could induce decidualization in uteri without physical or surgical contact.[6] In addition, a decline in uterine histamine content was associated with implantation[7] and decidual growth,[8] correlated with a decline in the uterine mast cell population. The uterine retention of labeled histamine associated with decidualization has also been reported suggesting the presence of endometrial receptors for histamine.[9]

Other studies, however, do not support Shelesnyak's proposal. Various workers have reported that antihistamines given systemically to mice[10] or into the uterine lumen of rats[11,12] did not block decidualization, while others found that intrauterine injections of antihistamines decreased the size of the decidual cell reaction, as indicated by uterine weight, without blocking its induction as indicated by the proportion of uteri responding.[13,14] Intrauterine administration of histamine was no more effective than its vehicle in inducing decidualization in mice[15] and rats.[12,16-18] In addition, decidualization induced by the intrauterine injection of the putative histamine releaser 48/80[6] was not inhibited by prior depletion of uterine histamine,[11,15] thus raising questions about the specificity of the effect of 48/80.

Because of the conflicting evidence reviewed extensively by De Feo,[19] the concept of histamine as a prime inducer of decidualization lost favor. However, interest was renewed with the identification of two populations of histamine receptors, H_1 and H_2. The localized increase in endometrial vascular permeability which defines the initiation of blastocyst implantation was found to be inhibited by a combination of histamine H_1 and H_2 receptor antagonists in rats[20] and rabbits.[21] However, when the H_2 antagonist, burimamide, used in the investigation in rats, was replaced with the more specific and potent metiamide, inhibitory activity of the combination was lost.[22] Furthermore, Brandon[23] noted that histamine antagonists have detrimental effects on blastocysts, apparently delaying loss of the zona pellucida. Thus the use of histamine receptor antagonists during pregnancy had not clarified the role of histamine in decidualization because the blastocysts, as a consequence of exposure to the antagonists, may not have signaled their presence. It is interesting to note, however, that rabbit endometrial cells have histamine H_1 receptors[24] and are therefore presumably able to respond to histamine. Furthermore, the H_2 antagonist burimamide, which was effective in rats when combined with a H_1 antagonist,[20] has now been shown to have partial antagonist activity at the recently identified histamine H_3 receptor subtype which is thought to be important in the control of the circulation.[25] The possible involvement of the H_3 receptor in decidualization remains to be investigated.

There is some evidence that histamine of embryonic origin may be involved in decidualization. In rabbits, intrauterine administration of the inhibitor of histamine release, disodium cromoglycate, inhibited implantation;[26] the authors suggested that the blastocysts took up the drug and released it during invasion of the endometrium. Rabbit blastocysts have histidine decarboxylase activity and thus presumably are able to synthesize histamine from histidine.[27] Intrauterine injection of a histidine decarboxylase inhibitor blocked implantation in rabbits, suggesting that histamine of embryonic origin acts as a signal for the initiation of decidualization.[27] However, in mice, inhibitors of histidine decarboxylase block embryonic development;[28] if this also occurs in rabbits, then the effect of intrauterine inhibitors of this enzyme on implantation is difficult to interpret.

There is evidence of interactions between histamine and PGs within the uterus; this will be presented in a later section.

ESTROGEN

The proposal that blastocyst-produced estrogen initiates implantation is an attractive hypothesis because it has the potential of explaining why some species require both estrogen and progesterone of maternal origin for implantation while others require only progesterone. Perhaps all species require both hormones, with the only difference between species being the relative importance of maternal and embryonic sources of estrogen.[29]

A non-maternal source of steroids during pregnancy was first suggested by the observation that day 6 rabbit blastocysts could not only synthesize cholesterol and pregnenolone from acetate, but also metabolize several steroids.[30] Subsequently, histochemical methods were used to demonstrate that 3β-hydroxysteroid dehydrogenase[31-33] and 17β-hydroxysteroid dehydrogenase[34] enzyme activities appeared in rat embryos at the late morula stage, and increased to maxima in the blastocyst at the time of implantation. A similar pattern of enzyme activities was reported for rabbit pre-implantation embryos.[35] With the observation that intrauterine instillation of a nonsteroidal antiestrogen interfered with implantation in the rabbit, Dickmann et al.[29] proposed that pre-implantation embryos can produce steroids which are prime regulators of implantation and decidualization.

Not all attempts to demonstrate steroidogenesis by preimplantation embryos, particularly in rodents, have been successful, and the specificity of the histochemical techniques used by Dickmann and his colleagues has been queried.[36]

Consequently, the Dickmann hypothesis remains controversial. Evidence for and against steroidogenesis by embryos is beyond the scope of this contribution (for reviews see refs. 3 and 37).

There is evidence that estrogen may act as a local signal to initiate the early vascular events of decidualization and implantation. When 2-4 cell rat embryos were briefly cultured in the presence or absence of estradiol before being transferred to the uteri of day 5 pseudopregnant hosts, only estrogen-exposed embryos were able to induce local increased endometrial vascular permeability responses.[38] The endometrium can synthesize estrogens from steroid precursors, and this synthesis is augmented by the presence of embryos.[39] Thus it is possible that the embryo, by some unknown mechanism, stimulates the adjacent endometrium to produce estrogens which then modify vascular permeability.

More recently, attention has been focused on the catechol estrogens which are formed by aromatic hydroxylation of primary estrogens at either the C-2 or C-4 positions.[40] Human endometrial and rat uterine homogenates can form catechol estrogens.[41,42] Implantation can be induced in ovariectomized pregnant mice by the systemic administration of 4-hydroxy- or 2-hydroxy-estradiol, although extremely high doses of the latter are required.[43] Similarly, in the delayed implanting rat, local increases in endometrial vascular permeability, indicative of the initiation of implantation, are induced by systemically administered catechol estrogens, but their potency is less than that of estradiol,[44] possibly as a consequence of their rapid metabolic clearance. Studies employing fluorinated estrogens, which are potent estrogens with reduced catechol-forming capacity, have suggested that the formation of catechol estrogens is obligatory for the initiation of implantation and decidualization. Dey et al.[45] failed to initiate implantation in ovariectomized pregnant rats with 2-fluoro-estradiol, but could induce it with 4-fluoro-estradiol, a surprising result given the greater potency of 4-hydroxy-estradiol in inducing implantation.[43,44] These data have been interpreted to indicate that the vasoactive component of estrogen action in decidualization requires the conversion of estrogen to a catechol estrogen.[46] However, all of these studies have involved systemic administration of estrogens, and it is clear that the local effects of catechol estrogens on the uterus must be investigated before a role for these compounds in decidualization can be assigned.

Interactions between histamine and estrogens may occur; histamine combined with 2-fluoro-estradiol induces implantation in ovariectomized pregnant rats, whereas either alone is ineffective.[45,46] Interactions between estrogens and prostaglandins will be presented later.

PROSTAGLANDINS

There is now considerable evidence that PGs have an obligatory role in endometrial vascular permeability changes and decidualization in a number of species.

In pregnant animals, indomethacin, an inhibitor of PG synthesis,[47] delays or inhibits the localized increase in endometrial vascular permeability in rats,[48,49] mice,[50] hamsters,[51] and rabbits[52] and implantation in rats,[53,54] mice,[55-57] and rabbits[58,59] and the establishment of pregnancy in pigs.[60] To date, two exceptions have been reported, both involving species with central implantation. In ferrets, indomethacin administration did not affect the increase in endometrial vascular permeability, but did cause a reduction in the number and size of uterine swellings and delayed or inhibited attachment of the trophoblast to the uterine luminal epithelium in some animals.[61] Unfortunately, no measurements of PGs were made in this study and consequently the extent to which PG synthesis was inhibited by the treatment with indomethacin is unknown. In addition, the effect of the treatment with indomethacin on the outcome of pregnancy was not determined. The second exception reported that the treatment of ewes, from days 7 to 22 after mating, with either indomethacin or acetylsalicylic acid at doses which substantially reduced endometrial PG concentrations had no apparent effect on the establishment of pregnancy.[62] Perhaps PGs are involved only in those species with invasive implantation, and not in those with central implantation, although the results obtained in pigs[60] do not support this generalization if indeed the effect of indomethacin in that study was on blastocyst attachment.

Additional evidence for the involvement of PGs in implantation has come from the observation that the concentrations of PGs are elevated in the areas of increased endometrial vascular permeability.[48,51,63,64] Furthermore, exogenous PGs can reverse, at least partially, the effects of indomethacin on implantation,[56,57,65] and when combined with histamine, produce a complete reversal.[56]

In species in which stimulation of the sensitized uterus results in decidualization, the extent of the decidual response is reduced by indomethacin administration,[66-73] as also is the endometrial vascular permeability increase which precedes decidualization.[74] The increase in endometrial alkaline phosphatase activity, an early event in decidualization, is also reduced by indomethacin treatment.[75] Uterine concentrations of the PGs are elevated by artificial deciduogenic stimuli[72,74,76-79] before there are detectable changes in permeability, a time-course consistent with the notion that PG levels are elevated as a cause, rather than a consequence, of the changes in permeability. PGs administered into the uterine lumen of animals in which endogenous PG production has been inhibited increase endometrial vascular permeability,[70,74,76] endometrial alkaline phosphatase activity,[75] and restore decidualization.[70,71,78,80] These observations that the inhibitory effects of indomethacin can be overridden by exogenous PGs strongly suggest that PGs are involved as physiological mediators of the responses, although it remains possible that concentrations of PGs within the endometrium after exogenous administration are supraphysiological and consequently the responses are pharmacological.

PGs are probably involved not only in the endometrial vascular changes, but also during proliferation and differentiation of decidual cells. Administration of indomethacin 12 hrs[67] or up to 48 hrs[71] after the application of a deciduogenic stimulus suppressed the extent of decidualization in rats. Since the endometrial vascular permeability response to the deciduogenic stimulus occurs by 12 hrs,[74,81] these observations suggest that PGs are involved in the later stages of the decidual cell reaction.

The identity of the PGs involved in implantation and decidualization is uncertain. No single PG has been identified unequivocally as the mediator based on PG measurements. The concentration of PGs of the E, F, and I series are elevated at implantation sites[48,63,64,82] and in the uterus following the application of an artificial deciduogenic stimulus.[72,74,76,77,83] In the rat, a deciduogenic stimulus does not increase the uterine concentrations of 6-oxo-PGE_1.[84] The uterine responses to exogenously administered PGs have been no more enlightening. Indirect evidence that $PGF_2\alpha$ may be involved comes from reports that this PG can induce implantation in rats and mice when given systemically;[56,65] PGE_2 has not been studied in this context. However, when administered into the uterine lumen, $PGF_2\alpha$ is less effective than PGE_2 at inducing implantation in mice.[57] PGE_2 and $PGF_2\alpha$ have in most circumstances been found to be equipotent at increasing endometrial vascular permeability and producing decidualization when infused into the uterine lumen of rats treated with indomethacin to inhibit endogenous PG production.[70,71] Under the same conditions, 6-oxo-PGE_1, but not PGI_2 or a stable analogue of PGI_2, produced decidualization.[78,84] Collectively, these data suggest that, at least for the rat, PGE_2 and $PGF_2\alpha$ are the PGs most likely involved since they alone meet the criteria of being found within the uterus in elevated concentrations at the appropriate times, and produce appropriate responses when given exogenously. However, the activity of $PGF_2\alpha$ is perplexing because, while endometrial binding sites, presumably representing receptors, have been reported for the E-series PGs in rats, pigs and humans,[85-88] no equivalent sites for $PGF_2\alpha$ have been found.[87,89] When analogues of PGE_2 and $PGF_2\alpha$ were infused into the uterine lumen of indomethacin-treated rats, decidualization was only obtained in response to the E-analogue.[90] These results have been interpreted as suggesting that PGE_2 mediates the endometrial responses, and that decidualization in response to $PGF_2\alpha$ may involve its conversion within the uterus to PGE_2; presumably the $PGF_2\alpha$ analogue was ineffective because it could not be converted to a corresponding PGE_2 analogue. In support of this proposal are observations that, whenever differences have been detected, in general, PGE_2 is more effective than $PGF_2\alpha$ at bringing about implantation and decidualization.[57,91,92]

Interactions between estrogens and PGs may occur within the uterus. Estrogens stimulate uterine PG production, probably by a mechanism which does not involve "classical" steroid-receptor interactions[93] in that it is not inhibited by estrogen receptor antagonists nor by inhibitors of RNA and protein synthesis. It is possible that conversion of estrogens to catechol estrogens is the mechanism by which estrogen stimulates uterine PG production. 2-Hydroxy-estradiol is more effective than estradiol in stimulating PGE_2 and $PGF_2\alpha$ production by homogenates of rat and human endometrium;[42,94] 4-hydroxy-estradiol had similar effects but also increased levels of 6-oxo-$PGF_1\alpha$, the hydrolysis product of PGI_2. In rabbits, endometrial PG release was augmented by catechol estrogens, but not by estradiol.[95]

LEUKOTRIENES

Recently, evidence supporting a possible role for leukotrienes (LTs) in decidualization has surfaced; interest in these compounds arose in part because of their vasoactive properties.

Indirect evidence has come from demonstrations that rabbit blastocysts and endometrium have an active 5-lipoxygenase pathway, as indicated by the synthesis of 5(S)-hydroxy-6,8,11,14-eicosatetraenoic acid.[96,97] Subsequently, the pregnant rat uterus was shown to produce LTB_4 and LTC_4, with a peak in synthesis around noon on day 4.[98] As well, human endometrium is capable of metabolism and release of leukotrienes throughout the menstrual cycle.[99] In addition, specific LTC_4 binding sites have been found in non-pregnant human and bovine endometrium,[100,101] suggesting that LTC_4 may have effects within the endometrium.

More direct evidence for the involvement of LTs in decidualization have come from studies in which compounds were infused into the uterine lumen of rats. LTC_4 produces decidualization which is augmented when combined with PGE_2. Infusion of FPL 55712, an antagonist of LTC_4, or inhibitors of LT synthesis such as nordihydroguairetic acid (NDGA) inhibits decidualization;[102,103] these inhibitions can be overridden in part by the simultaneous infusion of LTC_4 but best by a combination of LTC_4 and PGE_2. Based on measurements of production of PGs and LTs, NDGA apparently inhibits the synthesis of both classes of compounds. Hence the requirement for infusion of both PGE_2 and LTC_4 to restore the response. These data suggest that PGs and LTs are required for decidualization. As yet, the involvement of LTs in the early endometrial vascular response has not been investigated.

PLATELET ACTIVATING FACTOR

PAF has been implicated in a variety of physiological processes and is a potent vasoactive compound.[104] There are suggestions that it may be involved in implantation and decidualization. Mouse and human embryos produce PAF which induces a mild thrombocytopenia during the first days of pregnancy.[105,106] PAF may be the first signal produced by the embryo for maternal recognition of pregnancy.[107]

Because PAF antagonists inhibit implantation,[107,108] it has been suggested that PAF is the primary embryonic signal which, as a consequence of its vasoactive properties,[104,109,110] initiates implantation. Evidence for this proposal comes from the observation that BN 52021, a specific PAF antagonist, inhibits decidualization; this inhibition can be overridden by the simultaneous instillation of PAF into the uterus.[111] PAF need not necessarily be of embryonic origin since both the rabbit and rat uterus are apparently capable of its synthesis.[112,113]

PAF may have direct effects on the endometrial microvasculature, or alternatively, it may act indirectly by stimulating the synthesis of PGs. Smith and Kelly[114] have reported that PAF causes a dose-dependent increase in the synthesis of PGE_2 by a glandular, but not a stromal, fraction from human endometrium. The effects of PAF in some other responses are thought to be mediated, at least in part, by PG synthesis.[115,116]

SUMMARY

The experimental evidence that histamine, estrogen, PGs, LTs and PAF may act as mediators in blastocyst implantation and decidualization is reviewed. It is not possible to exclude any of these compounds with certainty. There is evidence that these compounds may interact within the endometrium.

References

1. Amoroso EC. Placentation. In: Parkes AS, ed. *Marshall's physiology of reproduction.* Vol. II London: Longmans, Green and Co., 1952:127-311.
2. Psychoyos A. Endocrine control of egg implantation. In: Greep RO, Astwood EB, Geiger SR, eds. *Handbook of physiology.* Sect. 7, Vol. II, Pt. 2. Bethesda: American Physiological Society, 1973:187-215.
3. Weitlauf HM. Biology of implantation. In: Knobil E, Neill JD, eds. *The physiology of reproduction.* Vol. 1. New York: Raven Press, 1988:231-262.
4. Shelesnyak MC. Inhibition of decidual cell formation in the pseudopregnant rat by histamine antagonist. *Am J Physiol* 1952; 170:522-527.
5. Shelesnyak MC. Comparative effectiveness of antihistamines in suppression of the decidual cell reaction in the pseudopregnant rat. *Endocrinology* 1954; 54:396-401.
6. Kraicer P, Shelesnyak MC. The induction of deciduomata in the pseudopregnant rat by systemic administration of histamine and histamine releasers. *J Endocrinol* 1958; 17:324-328.
7. Shelesnyak MC. Fall in uterine histamine associated with ovum implantation in pregnant rats. *Proc Soc Exp Biol Med* 1959; 100:380-381.
8. Cecil HC, Wrenn TR, Bitman J. Uterine histamine in rat deciduomata. *Endocrinology* 1962; 71:960-963.
9. Marcus GJ, Shelesnyak MC. Studies on the mechanism of nidation. XXV. A receptor theory for induction of decidualization. *Endocrinology* 1967; 80:1032-1037.
10. Goldstein A, Hazel MM. Failure of an antihistamine drug to prevent pregnancy in the mouse. *Endocrinology* 1955; 56:215-216.
11. De Feo VJ. Comparative effectiveness of several methods for the production of deciduomata in the rat. *Anat Rec* 1962; 142:226.
12. De Feo VJ. Determination of the sensitive period for the induction of deciduomata in the rat by different inducing procedures. *Endocrinology* 1963; 73:488-497.
13. Finn CA, Keen PM. Influence of systemic antihistamines on formation of deciduomata. *J Endocrinol* 1962; 24:381-382.

14. Lobel BL, Tic L, Shelesnyak MC. Studies on the mechanism of nidation. XVII. Histochemical analysis of decidualization in the rat. *Acta Endocrinol* 1965; 50:560-583.
15. Humphrey KW, Martin L. Attempted induction of deciduomata in mice with mast-cell, capillary permeability and tissue inflammatory factors. *J Endocrinol* 1968; 42:129-141.
16. Banik UK, Ketchel MM. Inability of histamine to induce deciduomata in pregnant and pseudopregnant rats. *J Reprod Fertil* 1964; 7:259-261.
17. De Feo VJ. Intraluminal histamine and massive deciduomata formation? *Anat Rec* 1961; 139:298.
18. Wrenn TR, Bitman J, Cecil HC, Gilliam DR. Uterine deciduomata: Role of histamine. *J Endocrinol* 1964; 28:149-152.
19. De Feo VJ. Decidualization. In: Wynn RM, ed. *Cellular biology of the uterus*. Amsterdam: Appleton-Century-Crofts, 1967:191-290.
20. Brandon JM, Wallis RM. Effect of mepyramine, a histamine H_1-, and burimamide, a histamine H_2-receptor antagonist, on ovum implantation in the rat. *J Reprod Fertil* 1977; 50:251-254.
21. Hoos PC, Hoffman LH. Effect of histamine receptor antagonists and indomethacin on implantation in the rabbit. *Biol Reprod* 1983; 29:833-840.
22. Brandon JM, Raval PJ. Interaction of estrogen and histamine during ovum implantation in the rat. *Eur J Pharmacol* 1979; 57:171-177.
23. Brandon JM. Some recent work on the role of histamine in ovum implantation. *Progr Reprod Biol* 1980; 7:244-252.
24. Dey SK, Villanueva C, Abdou NI. Histamine receptors on rabbit blastocyst and endometrial cell membranes. *Nature* 1979; 278:648-649.
25. Ishikawa S, Sperelakis N. A novel class (H_3) of histamine receptors on perivascular nerve terminals. *Nature* 1987; 327:158-160.
26. Dey SK, Villanueva C, Chien SM, Crist RD. The role of histamine in implantation in the rabbit. *J Reprod Fertil* 1978; 53:23-26.
27. Dey SK, Johnson DC, Santos JG. Is histamine production by the blastocyst required for implantation in the rabbit? *Biol Reprod* 1979; 21:1169-1173.
28. Dey SK, Johnson DC. Histamine formation by mouse preimplantation embryos. *J Reprod Fertil* 1980; 60:457-460.
29. Dickmann Z, Dey SK, Sengupta J. A new concept: control of early pregnancy by steroid hormones originating in the preimplantation embryo. *Vit Horm* 1976; 34:215-242.
30. Huff RL, Eik-Nes KB. Metabolism *in vitro* of acetate and certain steroids by six-day-old rabbit blastocysts. *J Reprod Fertil* 1966; 11:57-63.
31. Dickmann Z, Dey SK. Two theories: The preimplantation embryo is a source of steroid hormones controlling (1) morula-blastocyst transformation, and (2) implantation. *J Reprod Fertil* 1973; 35:615-617.
32. Dickmann Z, Dey SK. Evidence that Δ^5-3β-hydroxysteroid dehydrogenase activity in rat blastocysts is autonomous. *J Endocrinol* 1974; 61:513-514.
33. Dey SK, Dickmann Z. Δ^5-3β-Hydroxysteroid dehydrogenase activity in rat embryos on days 1 through 7 of pregnancy. *Endocrinology* 1974; 95:321-322.
34. Dey SK, Dickmann Z. Estradiol-17β-hydroxysteroid dehydrogenase activity in preimplantation rat embryos. *Steroids* 1974; 24:57-63.
35. Dickmann Z, Dey SK, Sengupta J. Steroidogenesis in rabbit preimplantation embryos. *Proc Natl Acad Sci USA* 1975; 72:298-300.
36. Bleau G. Failure to detect Δ^5-3β-hydroxysteroid oxidoreductase activity in the preimplantation rabbit embryo. *Steroids* 1981; 37:121-132.
37. Bullock DW. Steroids from the pre-implantation blastocyst. In: Johnson MH, ed. *Development in mammals. Vol. 2*. Amsterdam: Elsevier/North-Holland, 1977:199-208.
38. Dickmann Z, Sen Gupta J, Dey SK. Does 'blastocyst estrogen' initiate implantation? *Science* 1977; 195:687-688.
39. Wise T, Heap RB. Effects of the embryo upon endometrial estrogen synthesis in the rabbit. *Biol Reprod* 1983; 28:1097-1106.
40. MacLusky NJ, Naftolin F, Krey LC, Franks S. The catechol estrogens. *J Steroid Biochem* 1981; 15:111-124.
41. Reddy VR, Hanjani P, Ragan R. Synthesis of catechol estrogens by human uterus and leiomyoma. *Steroids* 1981; 37:195-203.
42. Kelly RW, Abel MH. Catechol estrogens stimulate and direct prostaglandin synthesis. *Prostaglandins* 1980; 20:613-626.
43. Hoversland RC, Dey SK, Johnson DC. Catechol estradiol induced implantation in the mouse. *Life Sci* 1982; 30:1801-1804.
44. Kantor BS, Dey SK, Johnson DC. Catechol estrogen induced initiation of implantation in the delayed implanting rat. *Acta Endocrinol* 1985; 109:418-422.
45. Dey SK, Johnson DC, Pakrasi PL, Liehr JG. Estrogens with reduced catechol-forming capacity fail to induce implantation in the rat. *Proc Soc Exp Biol Med* 1986; 181:215-218.
46. Dey SK, Johnson DC. Embryonic signals in pregnancy. *Ann NY Acad Sci* 1987; 476:49-62.

47. Vane JR. Inhibition of prostaglandin synthesis as a mechanism of action of aspirin-like drugs. *Nature [New Biol]* 1971; 231:232-235.
48. Kennedy TG. Evidence for a role for prostaglandins in the initiation of blastocyst implantation in the rat. *Biol Reprod* 1977; 16:286-291.
49. Phillips CA, Poyser NL. Studies on the involvement of prostaglandins in implantation in the rat. *J Reprod Fertil* 1981; 62:73-81.
50. Lundkvist O, Nilsson BO. Ultrastructural changes of the trophoblast-epithelial complex in mice subjected to implantation blocking treatment with indomethacin. *Biol Reprod* 1980; 22:719-726.
51. Evans CA, Kennedy TG. The importance of prostaglandin synthesis for the initiation of blastocyst implantation in the hamster. *J Reprod Fertil* 1978; 54:255-261.
52. Hoffman LM, DiPietro, McKenna TJ. Effects of indomethacin on uterine capillary permeability and blastocyst development in rabbits. *Prostaglandins* 1978; 15:823-828.
53. Gavin MA, Dominguez Fernandez-Tejerina JC, Montanes de las Heras MF, Vijil Maeso E. Efectos de un inhibidor de la biosintesis de las prostaglandinas (indometacina) sobre la implantacion en le rats. *Reproduccion* 1974; 1:177-183.
54. Garg SK, Chaudhury RR. Evidence for a possible role of prostaglandins in implantation in rats. *Arch Int Pharmacodyn* 1983; 262:299-307.
55. Lau IF, Saksena SK, Chang MC. Pregnancy blockade by indomethacin, an inhibitor of prostaglandin synthesis: its reversal by prostaglandins and progesterone in mice. *Prostaglandins* 1973; 4:795-803.
56. Saksena SK, Lau IF, Chang MC. Relationship between oestrogen, prostaglandin $F_2\alpha$ and histamine in delayed implantation in the mouse. *Acta Endocrinol* 1976; 81:801-807.
57. Holmes PR, Gordashko BJ. Evidence of prostaglandin involvement in blastocyst implantation. *J Embryol Exp Morphol* 1980; 55:109-122.
58. El-Banna AA. The degenerative effect on rabbit implantation sites by indomethacin. I. Timing of indomethacin action, possible effect on uterine proteins and the effect of replacement doses of $PGF_2\alpha$. *Prostaglandins* 1980; 20:587-599.
59. Cao ZD, Jones MA, Harper MJK. Progesterone and estradiol receptor concentration and translocation in uterine tissue of rabbits treated with indomethacin. *J Endocrinol* 1985; 107:197-203.
60. Kraeling RR, Rampacek GB, Fiorello NA. Inhibition of pregnancy with indomethacin in mature gilts and prepubertal gilts induced to ovulate. *Biol Reprod* 1985; 32:105-110.
61. Mead RA, Bremner S, Murphy BD. Changes in endometrial vascular permeability during the periimplantation period in the ferret (*Mustela putorius*). *J Reprod Fertil* 1988; 82:293-298.
62. Lacroix MC, Kann G. Comparative studies of prostaglandin $F_2\alpha$ and E_2 in late cyclic and early pregnant sheep: *in vitro* synthesis by endometrium and conceptus effect of *in vivo* indomethacin treatment on establishment of pregnancy. *Prostaglandins* 1982; 23:507-526.
63. Kennedy TG, Zamecnik J. The concentration of 6-keto-prostaglandin $F_1\alpha$ is markedly elevated at the site of blastocyst implantation in the rat. *Prostaglandins* 1978; 16:599-605.
64. Sharma SC. Temporal changes in PGE, $PGF\alpha$, estradiol 17β and progesterone in uterine venous plasma and endometrium of rabbits during early pregnancy. *INSERM Symp* 1979; 91:243-264.
65. Oettel M, Koch M, Kurischko A, Schubert K. A direct evidence for the involvement of prostaglandin $F_2\alpha$ in the first step of estrone-induced blastocyst implantation in the spayed rat. *Steroids* 1979; 33:108.
66. Castracane VD, Saksena SK, Shaikh AA. Effect of IUDs, prostaglandins and indomethacin on decidual cell reaction in the rat. *Prostaglandins* 1974; 6:397-404.
67. Tobert JA. A study of the possible role of prostaglandins in decidualization using a nonsurgical method for the instillation of fluids into the rat uterine lumen. *J Reprod Fertil* 1976; 47:391-393.
68. Sananes N, Baulieu EE, Le Goascogne C. Prostaglandin(s) as inductive factor of decidualization in the rat uterus. *Mol Cell Endocrinol* 1976; 6:153-158.
69. Sananes N, Baulieu EE, Le Goascogne C. A role for prostaglandins in decidualization of the rat uterus. *J Endocrinol* 1981; 89:25-33.
70. Kennedy TG, Lukash LA. Induction of decidualization in rats by the intrauterine infusion of prostaglandins. *Biol Reprod* 1982; 27:253-260.
71. Kennedy TG. Evidence for the involvement of prostaglandins throughout the decidual cell reaction in the rat. *Biol Reprod* 1985; 33:140-196.
72. Rankin JC, Ledford BE, Jonsson HT, Baggett B. Prostaglandins, indomethacin and the decidual cell reaction in the mouse uterus. *Biol Reprod* 1970; 20:399-404.
73. Buxton LE, Murdoch RN. Lectins, calcium ionophore A23187 and peanut oil as deciduogenic agents in the uterus of pseudopregnant mice: effects of tranylcypromine, indomethacin, iproniazid and propranolol. *Aust J Biol Sci* 1982; 35:63-72.
74. Kennedy TG. Prostaglandins and increased endometrial vascular permeability resulting from the application of an

artificial stimulus to the uterus of the rat sensitized for the decidual cell reaction. *Biol Reprod* 1979; 20:560-566.
75. Yee GM, Kennedy TG. Stimulatory effects of prostaglandins upon endometrial alkaline phosphatase activity during the decidual cell reaction in the rat. *Biol Reprod* 1988; 38:1129-1136.
76. Kennedy TG. Timing of uterine sensitivity for the decidual cell reaction: role of prostaglandins. *Biol Reprod* 1980; 22:519-525.
77. Kennedy TG. Estrogen and uterine sensitization for the decidual cell reaction: role of prostaglandins. *Biol Reprod* 1980; 23:955-962.
78. Kennedy TG, Barbe GJ, Evans CA. Prostaglandin I_2 and increased endometrial vascular permeability preceding the decidual cell reaction. In: Kimball FA, ed. *The endometrium*. New York: Spectrum, 1980:331-344.
79. Milligan SR, Lytton FDC. Changes in prostaglandin levels in the sensitized and non-sensitized uterus of the mouse after the intrauterine instillation of oil or saline. *J Reprod Fertil* 1983; 67:373-377.
80. Miller MM, O'Morchoe CCC. Inhibition of artificially induced decidual cell reaction by indomethacin in the mature oophorectomized rat. *Anat Rec* 1982; 204:223-230.
81. Milligan SR, Mirembe FM. Time course of the changes in uterine vascular permeability associated with the development of the decidual cell reaction in ovariectomized steroid-treated rats. *J Reprod Fertil* 1984; 70:1-6.
82. Pakrasi PL, Dey SK. Blastocyst is the source of prostaglandins in the implantation site in the rabbit. *Prostaglandins* 1982; 24:73-77.
83. Jonsson HT, Rankin JC, Ledford BE, Baggett B. Uterine prostaglandin levels following stimulation of the decidual cell reaction: effect of indomethacin and tranylcypromine. *Prostaglandins* 1979; 18:847-857.
84. Doktorcik PE, Kennedy TG. 6-Keto-prostaglandin E_1 and the decidual cell reaction in rats. *Prostaglandins* 1986; 32:679-689.
85. Kennedy TG, Martel D, Psychoyos A. Endometrial prostaglandin E_2 binding: characterization in rats sensitized for the decidual cell reaction and changes during pseudopregnancy. *Biol Reprod* 1983; 29:556-564.
86. Kennedy TG, Martel D, Psychoyos A. Endometrial prostaglandin E_2 binding during the estrous cycle and its hormonal control in ovariectomized rats. *Biol Reprod* 1983; 29:565-571.
87. Hofmann GE, Rao CV, De Leon FD, Toledo AA, Sanfillippo JS. Human endometrial prostaglandin E_2 binding sites and their profiles during the menstrual cycle and in pathologic states. *Am J Obstet Gynecol* 1985; 151:369-375.
88. Chegini N, Rao CV, Wakim N, Sanfillipo J. Prostaglandin binding to different cell types of human uterus: quantitative light microscope autoradiographic study. *Prostagl Leukotr Med* 1986; 22:129-138.
89. Martel D, Kennedy TG, Monier MN, Psychoyos A. Failure to detect specific binding sites for prostaglandin $F_2\alpha$ in membrane preparations from rat endometrium. *J Reprod Fertil* 1985; 75:265-274.
90. Kennedy TG, Doktorcik PE. Effects of analogues of prostaglandin E_2 and $F_2\alpha$ on the decidual cell reaction in the rat. *Prostaglandins* 1988; 35:207-219.
91. Hoffman LH, Strong GB, Davenport GR, Frolich JC. Deciduogenic effect of prostaglandins in the pseudopregnant rabbit. *J Reprod Fertil* 1977; 50:231-237.
92. Kennedy TG. Intrauterine infusion of prostaglandins and decidualization in rats with uteri differentially sensitized for the decidual cell reaction. *Biol Reprod* 1986; 34:327-335.
93. Castracane VD, Jordan VC. Considerations into the mechanism of estrogen-stimulated uterine prostaglandin synthesis. *Prostaglandins* 1976; 12:243-251.
94. Kelly RW, Abel MH. A comparison of the effects of 4-catechol estrogens and 2-pyrogallol estrogens on prostaglandin synthesis by the rat and human uterus. *J Steroid Biochem* 1981; 14:787-791.
95. Pakrasi PL, Dey SK. Catechol estrogens stimulate synthesis of prostaglandins in the preimplantation rabbit blastocyst and endometrium. *Biol Reprod* 1983; 29:347-354.
96. Pakrasi PL, Dey SK. Evidence for an inverse relationship between cyclooxygenase and lipoxygenase pathways in the pregnant rabbit endometrium. *Prostagl Leukotr Med* 1985; 18:347-352.
97. Pakrasi PL, Becka R, Dey SK. Cyclooxygenase and lipoxygenase pathways in the preimplantation rabbit uterus and blastocyst. *Prostaglandins* 1985; 29:481-495.
98. Malathy PV, Cheng HC, Dey SK. Production of leukotrienes and prostaglandins in the rat uterus during preimplantation period. *Prostaglandins* 1986; 32:605-614.
99. Rees MCP, DiMarzo V, Tippins JR, Morris HR, Turnbull AC. Leukotriene release by endometrium and myometrium throughout the menstrual cycle in dysmenorrhoea and menorrhagia. *J Endocrinol* 1987; 113:291-295.
100. Chegini N, Rao CV. The presence of leukotriene C_4- and prostacyclin-binding sites in nonpregnant human uterine tissue. *J Clin Endocrinol Metab* 1988; 66:76-87.

101. Chegini N, Rao CV. Quantitative light microscopic autoradiographic study on [^{3}H]leukotriene C_4 binding to nonpregnant bovine uterine tissue. *Endocrinology* 1988; 122:1732-1736.
102. Tawfik OW, Huet YM, Malathy PV, Johnson DC, Dey SK. Release of prostaglandins and leukotrienes from the rat uterus is an early estrogenic response. *Prostaglandins* 1987; 34:805-815.
103. Tawfik OW, Dey SK. Further evidence for role of leukotrienes as mediators of decidualization in the rat. *Prostaglandins* 1988; 35:379-386.
104. Braquet P, Touqui L, Shen TY, Vargaftig BB. Perspectives in platelet-activating factor research. *Pharmacol Rev* 1987; 39:97-145.
105. O'Neill C. Thrombocytopenia is an initial maternal response to fertilization in mice. *J Reprod Fertil* 1985; 73:559-566.
106. O'Neill C. Examination of the causes of early pregnancy-associated thrombocytopenia in mice. *J Reprod Fertil* 1985; 73:567-577.
107. Spinks NR, O'Neill C. Antagonists of embryo-derived platelet-activating factor prevent implantation of mouse embryos. *J Reprod Fertil* 1988; 84:89-98.
108. Acker G, Hecquet F, Etienne A, Braquet P, Mencia-Huerta JM. Role of platelet-activating factor (PAF) in the ovoimplantation in the rat: effect of the specific PAF-acether antagonist, BN 52021. *Prostaglandins* 1988; 35:233-241.
109. Humphrey DM, McManus LM, Satouchi K, Hanahan DJ, Pinckard RN. Vasoactive properties of acetyl glyceryl ether phosphorylcholine and analogues. *Lab Invest* 1982; 46:422-427.
110. Angle MJ, McManus LM, Pinckard RN. Age-dependent differential development of leukotactic and vasoactive responsiveness to acute inflammatory mediators. *Lab Invest* 1986; 55:616-621.
111. Acker GM, Braquet P, Mencia-Muerta JM. Role of platelet-activating factor (PAF) in ovoimplantation and decidualization process in the rat [Abstract]. *Prostaglandins* 1988; 35:817.
112. Angle MJ, Jones MA, McManus LM, Pindkard RN, Harper MJK. Platelet-activating factor in the rabbit uterus during early pregnancy. *J Reprod Fertil* 1988; 83:711-722.
113. Yasuda K, Satouchi K, Saito K. Platelet-activating factor in normal rat uterus. *Biochem Biophys Res Commun* 1986; 138:1231-1236.
114. Smith SK, Kelly RW. Effect of platelet-activating factor on the release of $PGF_2\alpha$ and PGE_2 by separated cells of human endometrium. *J Reprod Fertil* 1988; 82:271-276.
115. Kusner EJ, Knee CD, Krell RD. Pharmacologic analysis of 1-0-alkyl-2-acetyl-sn-glycero-3-phosphocholine-induced increases in cutaneous vascular permeability in the rat. *Agents Actions* 1987; 20:61-68.
116. Riedel A, Mest MJ. The effect of PAF (platelet-activating factor) on experimental cardiac arrhythmias and its inhibition by substances influencing arachidonic acid metabolites. *Prostagl Leukotr Med* 1987; 28:103-109.

EXPRESSION OF mRNAs AND SYNTHESIS OF PROTEINS BY RAT ANTIMESOMETRIAL AND MESOMETRIAL DECIDUA

P.G. Jayatilak, T.K. Puryear, Z. Herz, A. Fazleabas,* and G. Gibori

Department of Physiology and Biophysics and
*Department of Obstetrics and Gynecology
College of Medicine
University of Illinois
Chicago, Illinois 60680 USA

DECIDUALIZATION of the uterine endometrium, a cellular reaction to either nidation or artificial stimulation, involves a temporally and spatially coordinated differentiation of endometrial stromal cells occurring in two distinct regions of the uterus at different times.

One of the earliest events of decidualization is the transformation of stromal cells on the antimesometrial side of the uterus into large closely packed decidual cells to form the antimesometrial decidual tissue. The decidualization then proceeds laterally to the mesometrial region. Decidual cells in this region form the mesometrial decidua. Thus, the development of the two decidual zones occurs sequentially; mesometrial decidual cells appear two days after the antimesometrial decidual cells and become fully differentiated at a time when antimesometrial cells show signs of regression.[1,2] Antimesometrial and mesometrial decidual cells, which arise by proliferation and differentiation of different stem cells within these regions, differ profoundly.[1] The mesometrial cells are small, loosely packed,[2] rich in glycogen and do not achieve a ploidy greater than 4n. In contrast, the antimesometrial cells are large; their diameter may exceed 30 μm. They possess large nuclei with a high level of ploidy.[2-4] Whether the cells forming the antimesometrial and mesometrial zones secrete different proteins and if they have totally different functions remains unknown.

Rat decidual cells are the site of both secretion[5,6] and reception[7] of a protein which has the ability to bind to prolactin receptors, to stimulate steroidogenesis in the corpus luteum, and to perform various reproductive functions of prolactin.[8-12] This protein shows more similarity to human than to rat pituitary prolactin. Whereas it does not cross-react with rat prolactin antiserum, it is recognized by antibodies to human prolactin. Because of its action on the rat corpus luteum, this decidual prolactin-like hormone has been named decidual luteotropin. The recent finding that rat decidual cells possess high affinity binding sites for prolactin, which also bind the locally produced decidual luteotropin,[7] suggests a local role for this hormone. Recent evidence[13] indicates that the site of decidual luteotropin production and the location of its binding sites may be compartmentalized in the two different zones of decidual tissue. Binding sites for the hormone were localized on mesometrial cell membranes, whereas decidual luteotropin was found to be present, principally, in the antimesometrial tissue.[13] However, the presence of high concentrations of decidual luteotropin in the antimesometrial decidua does not necessarily demonstrate that this tissue synthesizes the hormone. This investigation was undertaken to determine whether mRNA for the decidual prolactin-like hormone is localized in the antimesometrial tissue, and if the antimesometrial tissue is capable of secreting this hormone.

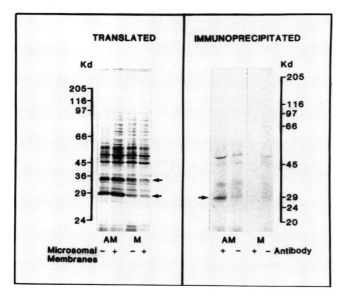

Figure 1. *(Left panel): Cell-free translation of antimesometrial (AM) and mesometrial (M) decidual RNA. Total RNA was extracted from day 9 antimesometrial and mesometrial tissue and translated in the presence or absence of canine pancreatic microsomal membranes. Translations were performed under conditions of RNA and salt concentrations previously determined to maximize the production of the 28 kDa protein. Equal amounts of TCA-precipitated proteins were run on SDS-PAGE gel, followed by fluorography. (Right panel): Immunoprecipitation of mesometrial and antimesometrial translated protein. Proteins translated in the presence or the absence of microsomal membranes were reacted with either human prolactin antiserum or control nonimmune serum, and were precipitated with Staphylococcus aureus cell suspension.*

TRANSLATION AND IMMUNOPRECIPITATION OF TRANSLATED DECIDUAL PROTEINS

Rat decidual tissue was induced by scratching the antimesometrial surface of both uterine horns on day 5 of pseudopregnancy. The day a vaginal plug was found was considered the first day of pseudopregnancy. Four days later decidual tissue was exposed and separated into mesometrial and antimesometrial tissue as described by Martel et al.[14] Total RNA was extracted from both mesometrial and antimesometrial tissues by a modification of the procedure of Cathala et al.[15] Aliquots (50 μg) of total RNA were translated in a cell-free system derived from rabbit reticulocyte lysate pretreated with micrococcal nuclease. The *in vitro* protein synthesis was performed in the presence of [^{35}S]-methionine. To detect any post- and cotranslational modifications, translation was also performed in the presence of 5 units of canine pancreatic microsomal membranes.[16] Labeled peptides that were synthesized were analyzed by SDS-PAGE.[17]

As shown in Figure 1, two proteins of molecular weight 28,000 and 35,000 were synthesized principally by the antimesometrial RNA in a cell-free system. In contrast, little of this protein was synthesized by mesometrial RNA. To determine which of these proteins is recognized by human prolactin antibodies, translated proteins were immunoprecipitated with antiserum to human prolactin. Non-immune serum served as the control. As illustrated in Figure 1, only the 28 kDa antimesometrial protein was immunoprecipitated by human prolactin antiserum. No apparent change in the molecular weight of the 28 kDa protein was observed when translation assay was performed in the presence of microsomal membranes. These results provide evidence that the cells producing 28 kDa protein belong to the antimesometrial zone of the decidual tissue. It provides no indication, however, as to whether this decidual protein is a secretory protein. It became of interest, therefore, to determine whether this protein is secreted by antimesometrial decidual tissue.

PROTEIN SECRETION BY MESOMETRIAL AND ANTIMESOMETRIAL TISSUE: RECEPTOR AFFINITY CHROMATOGRAPHY AND IMMUNOPRECIPITATION

To determine the time course of [^{35}S]-methionine incorporation into secreted proteins and levels of decidual luteotropin released into culture media, decidual tissue obtained from day 8 pseudopregnant rats was cultured in the presence of [^{35}S]-methionine and the release of radiolabeled proteins and decidual luteotropin was followed for 24 hrs. As shown in Figure 2, the secretory activity increased dramatically between 2 and 18 hrs of culture and continued for at least 24 hrs. Maximal decidual luteotropin release into the media, as measured by radioreceptor assay,[5] was also observed after 24 hrs of culture. Therefore, 24 hrs was chosen as the standard incubation time for all subsequent experiments. Approximately 7% to 8% of the radioactivity was incorporated into protein after 24 hrs of culture.

DECIDUAL PROTEIN SECRETION DURING PSEUDOPREGNANCY

To investigate the pattern of protein secretion by the antimesometrial and mesometrial decidua, antimesometrial and mesometrial tissues obtained from pseudopregnant rats between days 9-12 were cultured in the presence of

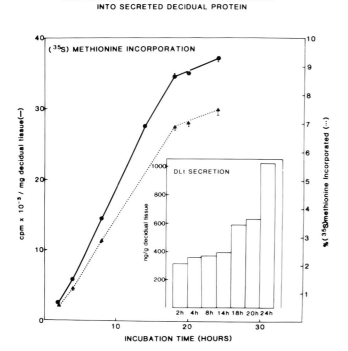

Figure 2. Time course of [^{35}S]-methionine incorporation into secreted proteins and decidual luteotropin released into culture media. Decidual tissue explants from three day-8 pseudopregnant rats were cultured in the presence of 75 µCi [^{35}S]-methionine in either triplicate or duplicate. Aliquots (250 µl) were obtained at 2, 4, 8, 15, 18, 20 and 24 hrs of culture and replaced with fresh labeled medium at each time point. The rate of incorporation of radioactive label into the secreted proteins was determined by TCA precipitation. Levels of decidual luteotropin in the media were determined by radioreceptor assay.

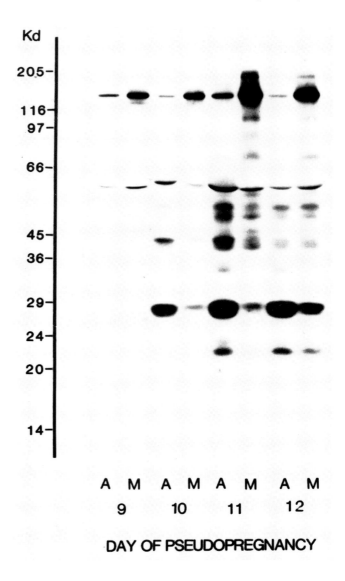

Figure 3. SDS-PAGE analysis of proteins secreted by antimesometrial and mesometrial decidual tissue throughout decidual development. Antimesometrial (A) and mesometrial (M) tissue from rats between days 9 and 12 of pseudopregnancy were incubated in the presence of 50 µCi [^{35}S]-methionine for 24 hrs. Dialyzed media samples containing 50,000 cpm were separated on 10% SDS-PAGE and the fluorograph was exposed to the film.

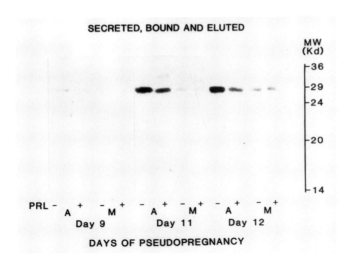

Figure 4. *Identification of the 28 kDa secreted protein by receptor affinity chromatography. Antimesometrial and mesometrial tissues were cultured independently in the presence of ^{35}S-methionine. Aliquots of dialyzed medium containing 1 µCi of activity were bound and eluted to prolactin receptors of luteal membrane in the presence (+) or absence (−) of 10 µg of ovine prolactin to assess binding specificity. Eluted proteins were run on a 12.5% SDS-PAGE and autoradiographed (Reprinted with permission from Ref. 28).*

[^{35}S]-methionine for 24 hrs. The radiolabeled secretory proteins were analyzed by SDS-PAGE. As shown in Figure 3, the pattern of synthesis and release of proteins into culture media not only differed in the mesometrial and antimesometrial zones but also differed with the advance of decidual age. One protein (approx. 180,000 Mr) was secreted in large amounts by the decidua, primarily by the mesometrial tissue. The other 28,000 Mr protein was synthesized and secreted principally by the antimesometrial tissue.

IDENTIFICATION OF A PROLACTIN-LIKE PROTEIN BY RECEPTOR AFFINITY CHROMATOGRAPHY AND IMMUNOPRECIPITATION

Proteins synthesized and secreted by antimesometrial and mesometrial tissues of different stages of decidual development were, in the first experiment, allowed to bind to prolactin receptor in the presence or absence of excess ovine prolactin. The resulting bound proteins were eluted from the receptor with MgCl$_2$, precipitated, and analyzed by SDS-PAGE. As shown in Figure 4, the 28 kDa antimesometrial protein bound to prolactin receptor from luteal membrane and was subsequently eluted by MgCl$_2$. The binding of the 28 kDa protein to the prolactin receptor was specific since it was markedly displaced by the addition of ovine prolactin.

To determine whether the secreted 28 kDa protein would cross-react with antiserum to human prolactin, 1 µCi of dialyzed media obtained from tissue incubation was immunoprecipitated with antiserum. The results shown in Figure 5 demonstrate that the [^{35}S] labeled 28 kDa protein secreted by the antimesometrium is recognized and immunoprecipitated by human prolactin antibody.

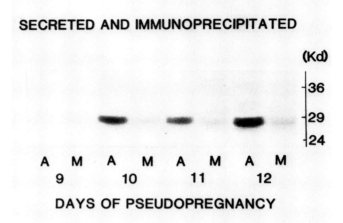

Figure 5. *Immunoprecipitation of secreted 28 kDa antimesometrial protein. One µCi of [^{35}S]-radiolabeled secreted protein, obtained from media of cultured antimesometrial (A) and mesometrial (M) tissues was incubated with antiserum to human prolactin in a final dilution of 1:100 for 24 hrs at 22°C. The antigen-antibody complexes were precipitated with 100 µl of formaldehyde-fixed Staphylococcus aureus cell suspension (10 v/v). The pellets were washed 3 times with 2 ml of buffer (Tris-HCl 50 mM, NaCl 150 mM, EDTA 5 mM, 0.02% NaN$_3$, 0.05% NP40, pH 7.6), followed by centrifugation at 3000 x g for 5 min. Pellets were resuspended in the loading buffer and separated by 12.5% SDS-PAGE and the gel was processed for fluorography. (Reprinted with permission from ref. 28).*

DISCUSSION

The results presented here demonstrate that rat decidual tissue synthesizes and selectively secretes proteins and that the secretion and individual rates of production of certain specific proteins depend on the gestational age of the decidual tissue. Further, this study demonstrates that the mesometrial tissue secretes a major 180 kDa protein whereas the antimesometrial tissue produces principally a 28 kDa protein. These proteins may represent specific markers which can serve to identify the cells of each decidual zone. The 28 kDa antimesometrial protein binds to the prolactin receptor and is immunoprecipitated by a human prolactin antibody. Cell-free translation studies indicate that the mRNA encoding this 28 kDa protein is expressed almost entirely in the antimesometrial zone. The 28 kDa protein does not appear to be a prohormone molecule, since no apparent changes in molecular weight were observed when translation studies were performed in the presence of microsomal membranes. Results obtained with [^{35}S]-methionine incorporation indicate that this protein is not only synthesized but is also abundantly secreted by the antimesometrial tissue.

Previous studies[8-12] have indicated that this molecule has luteotropic activity and was hence designated decidual luteotropin. More recent studies[13] demonstrate that the production and subsequent binding of the molecule is compartmentalized in the two zones of the rat decidua. These studies suggest the possibility that the protein may have a local effect in addition to its action on the ovary. Of the two compartments in rat decidua, the antimesometrial component forms initially and is followed by the development of the mesometrial zone. The binding site for prolactin and decidual luteotropin is localized to the mesometrial cell.[7] From a functional standpoint, this separation of site of production and site of action suggests that the decidual luteotropin may act in a paracrine manner to initially stimulate cell mitosis and subsequently control trophoblast invasion. Prolactin and prolactin-like hormones have been shown to have mitogenic properties. One possible role for decidual luteotropin during its initial stages of production could be stimulation of the development of the antimesometrial zone which is essential for blastocyst implantation. A second potential function for this prolactin-like hormone may involve regulation of the major 180 kDa protein secreted by the mesometrial tissue. A high molecular weight "decidualization associated protein" has been localized primarily in the mesometrial decidua and has been found to be similar to α_2 macroglobulin.[1,18,19] α_2 macroglobulin is thought to play a role in regulating tissue damage and its secretion by the liver is stimulated by hGH.[19,20] It appears to be of great physiological significance that 180 kDa protein is produced in the mesometrial decidual zone where the invasion of decidual cells by trophoblast cells should be prevented at a certain level, and that this mesometrial decidual zone contains the receptors for 28 kDa decidual luteotropin. Since decidual luteotropin and hGH both bind to prolactin receptor,[7,20] it is tempting to suggest that decidual luteotropin secreted by antimesometrial cells binds to prolactin receptors on mesometrial cells and up regulates the secretion of α_2 macroglobulin. α_2 macroglobulin, may, in turn, limit the damage caused by trophoblastic invasion. Further studies in this direction will establish the role(s) of 28 and 180 kDa protein in the rat decidua.

It is unclear at present, whether more than one kind of molecule similar to prolactin is produced by the rat decidua. Recently, molecules that have an amino acid sequence homologous to pituitary prolactin have been reported to be produced by the trophoblast of both the mouse[21-23] and rat.[24] These proteins do not bind to prolactin receptors and their functions are unknown. However, the finding of specific receptors for ovine placental lactogen, which have low affinity for ovine prolactin,[25-27] suggests the possibility of specific receptors for these prolactin-like molecules. Whether the decidua also produces such a molecule(s) remains to be investigated.

Acknowledgment

This work was supported by NIH grants HD 12356 and HD 22379.

References

1. Bell SC. Decidualization: regional differentiation and associated function. *Oxf Rev Reprod Biol* 1983; 5:220-271.
2. O'Shea JD, Kleinfeld RG, Morrow HA. Ultrastructure of decidualization in the pseudopregnant rat. *Am J Anat* 1983; 116:271-278.
3. McConnell KN, Sillar RG, Young BD, Green B. Ploidy and progesterone receptor distribution in flow-sorted deciduomal nuclei. *Mol Cell Endo* 1982; 25:99-104.
4. Sartor P. Déroulement des premiers stades de l'ovoimplantation chez des rattes castrées le 5e jour de la gestation avant midi. *CR Acad Sci (D) Paris* 1980; 209:481-484.
5. Jayatilak PG, Glaser LA, Basuray R, Kelly PA, Gibori G. Identification and characterization of a prolactin-like hormone produced by the rat decidual tissue. *Proc Natl Acad Sci (USA)* 1984; 82:217-221.
6. Herz Z, Khan I, Jayatilak PG, Gibori G. Evidence for the synthesis and secretion of decidual luteotropin: a prolactin like hormone produced by rat decidual cells. *Endocrinology* 1985; 118:2203-2209.
7. Jayatilak PG, Gibori G. Ontogeny of prolactin receptors in rat decidual tissue: binding by locally produced prolactin-like hormone. *J Endocrinology* 1986; 110:115-121.

8. Gibori G, Rothchild I, Pepe GJ, Morishige WK, Lam P. Luteotrophic action of the decidual tissue in the rat. *Endocrinology* 1974; 95:1113-1118.
9. Gibori G, Basuray R, McReynolds B. Luteotropic role of the decidual tissue in the rat: dependency on intraluteal estradiol. *Endocrinology* 1981; 108:2060-2066.
10. Jayatilak PG, Glaser LA, Warshaw ML, Herz Z, Grueber JR, Gibori G. Relationship between luteinizing hormone and decidual luteotropin in the maintenance of luteal steroidogenesis. *Biol Reprod* 1984; 31:556-564.
11. Gibori G, Kalison B, Basuray R, Rao MC, Hunzicker-Dunn M. Endocrine role of the decidual tissue: decidual luteotropin regulation of luteal adenyl cyclase activity, luteinizing hormone receptors, and steroidogenesis. *Endocrinology* 1984; 115:1157-1163.
12. Gibori G, Kalison B, Warshaw ML, Basuray R, Glaser LA. Differential action of decidual luteotropin on luteal and follicular production of testosterone and estradiol. *Endocrinology* 1985; 116:1784-1791.
13. Gibori G, Jayatilak PG, Khan I, et al. Decidual luteotropin secretion and action: its role in pregnancy maintenance in the rat. In: Mahesh VB, Dhindsa DS, Anderson E, Kalra SP, eds. *Regulation of ovarian and testicular function*. Plenum Press NY, 1987:379-397.
14. Martel D, Monier MN, Psychoyos A, De Feo VJ. Estrogen and progesterone receptors in the endometrium, myometrium and metrial gland of the rat during the decidualization process. *Endocrinology* 1984; 114:1627-1634.
15. Cathala G, Savouret J-F, Mendez B, West BL, Karin M, Martial JA, Baxter JD. Laboratory methods. A method for isolation of intact translationally active ribonucleic acid. *DNA* 1983; 2:329-335.
16. Walter P, Blobel G. Preparation of microsomal membranes for cotranslational protein translocation. *Methods Enzymol* 1983; 96:84-93.
17. Laemmli UK. Cleavage of structural proteins during the assembly of the head of bacteriophage T_4. *Nature* 1970; 227:680-685.
18. Bell SC. Synthesis of decidualization associated proteins in tissues of the rat uterus and placenta during pregnancy. *J Reprod Fert* 1979; 49:177-181.
19. Bell SC. Immunochemical identity of decidualization-associated proteins and α_2 acute-phase macroglobulin in the pregnant rat. *J Reprod Immunol* 1979; 1:193-206.
20. Barrett AJ, Starkey PM. The interaction of α_2-macroglobulin with proteinases. Characteristics and specificity of the reaction, and a hypothesis concerning its molecular mechanism. *Biochem J* 1973; 133:709-724.
21. Linzer DIH, Lee S-J, Ogren L, Talamantes T, Nathans D. Identification of proliferin mRNA and protein in mouse placenta. *Proc Natl Acad Sci USA* 1985; 82:4356-4361.
22. Linzer DIH, Nathans D. A new member of the prolactin-growth hormone family expressed in mouse placenta. *EMBO J* 1985; 4:1419-1423.
23. Lee SJ, Talamentes F, Wilder E, Linzer DIH, Nathans D. Trophoblastic giant cells of the mouse placenta as the site of proliferin synthesis. *Endocrinology* 1988; 122:1761-1768.
24. Duckworth ML, Peden LM, Friesen HG. Isolation of a novel prolactin-like cDNA clone from developing rat placenta. *J Biol Chem* 1986; 261:10879-10884.
25. Freemark M, Comer M, Handwerger S. Placental lactogen and growth hormone receptors in sheep liver: Striking differences in ontogeny and function. *Am J Physiol* 1986; 251:E328-E333.
26. Freemark M, Handwerger S. The glycogenic effects of placental lactogen and growth hormone in ovine fetal liver are mediated through binding to specific fetal placental lactogen receptors. *Endocrinology* 1986; 118:613-618.
27. Freemark M, Comer M, Korner G, Handwerger S. A unique placental lactogen receptor: Implications for fetal growth. *Endocrinology* 1987; 120:1865-1872.
28. Jayatilak PG, Puryear TK, Herz Z, Fazleabas A, Gibori G, 1989. Protein secretion by mesometrial and antimesometrial rat decidual tissue: evidence for differential gene expression. *Endocrinology* 125: No. 2.

COMPARATIVE ASPECTS OF SECRETORY PROTEINS OF THE ENDOMETRIUM AND DECIDUA IN THE HUMAN AND NON-HUMAN PRIMATES

Stephen C. Bell,* Asgerally T. Fazleabas,† and Harold G. Verhage†

*Departments of Biochemistry and Obstetrics & Gynecology
The Medical School, University of Leicester
Leicester LE3 7LH, United Kingdom

†Department of Obstetrics & Gynecology
University of Illinois College of Medicine at Chicago
Chicago, Illinois 60680 USA

THE major function of the uterine endometrium in placental mammals is to support the conceptus from the pre-implantation morula/blastocyst stage until parturition. The nature of the interaction between this mucosal tissue—which in all species exhibits essentially similar cellular composition in its undifferentiated state—and the conceptus varies dramatically during implantation and pregnancy in different species. This is reflected by the structure of the placenta. For example, in species exhibiting epitheliochorial placentation, the luminal epithelium is not breached and the stromal compartment does not exhibit differentiation. Thus the conceptus is essentially dependent upon uterine secretions for nutrition. In contrast, in species with hemochorial placental structure, the endometrial stroma is penetrated during implantation by trophoblastic tissue and undergoes differentiation, termed decidualization. Additionally, within those species that exhibit decidualization, such as the human and a few closely related primates, some of these alterations are exhibited during the non-fertile cycle. Since in these species contact with maternal blood is established soon after implantation, and in the mature placenta the major maternal tissue in contact with trophoblastic tissue is maternal blood, it is thought that endometrial and decidual secretions do not play an important role. However, during the peri- and early implantation period, the glandular epithelial component exhibits secretory activity, and with the complex nature of cell populations associated with decidualization which are in intimate cellular contact with trophoblast populations throughout pregnancy, potential paracrine interactions mediated by secretory products may occur. A direct clinical value of these endometrial products would, of course, be apparent if they could be detected in an accessible compartment, since their measurement may provide an assessment of the functional activity of endometrial cell populations.[1] It is apparent, however, that elucidation of the nature and function of these secretory products and their role in endometrial-trophoblast interactions in the human at particular stages of pregnancy may be impractical. Therefore it will be of great value to assess the applicability of the study of closely related primate species to provide a more experimentally accessible model. As a first step towards this goal, it is necessary to establish the secretory profile of the endometrium and decidua in these species to identify analogous products. However, due to extreme species diversity in reproductive physiology, the fact that even available primates exhibit differences in endometrial-conceptus interactions must be considered.

COMPARATIVE ASPECTS OF ENDOMETRIAL-TROPHOBLAST INTERACTIONS IN HUMAN AND NON-HUMAN PRIMATES

Ultimately, to interpret the significance and function of secretory products of the endometrium, studies on these products must be related to the cellular populations in the endometrium during implantation and throughout pregnancy, and their anatomical relationship to trophoblast populations of the embryo and the developing and mature placenta. This is essential when these phenomena exhibit differences in the human and related primates since qualitative differences in the endometrial secretory phenotype may reflect these differences, and even be causally related, whereas production of common secretory proteins may be anticipated to relate to similar features exhibited in these species. Features that must be considered include the nature of endometrium present during the peri-implantation period, the nature of implantation of the blastocyst and extravillous trophoblast populations during pregnancy, and changes associated with the placental development through pregnancy. Studies on the rhesus macaque,[2] suggest that the endometrial changes are similar to the human. However, in contrast to the human, predecidualization of the stroma is less marked in the rhesus, and in the baboon it may be difficult to demonstrate.[3] Studies on implantation have not been as extensive in the baboon as in the macaque. In this latter species a dramatic difference is observed in the luminal epithelium compared to the human in that this population forms a transient epithelial plaque, a feature recently also described in the baboon.[4] In the rhesus macaque and baboon, implantation is superficial compared to the interstitial implantation in the human. In spite of this, however, maternal blood appears to be tapped more rapidly in the former species.[4] Analogous to the cycle, during pregnancy decidualization is less marked in terms of the extent of involvement of the stroma and the hypertrophy exhibited by the stromal cell compared to the human. Marked differences have been reported concerning the invasion of the endometrium and vasculature by cytotrophoblast cells with the phenomenon being more restricted to the rhesus macaque and baboon.[5]

PROTEIN SECRETION BY THE ENDOMETRIUM DURING THE MENSTRUAL CYCLE

Although secretory products of the endometrium have been identified by examination of the ability of this tissue to produce well-characterized proteins, this approach may fail to reveal the nature of the major secretory products produced by the tissue. Recently, however, techniques involving labeling of tissue explants with radiolabeled amino acid precursors, together with gel electrophoresis and fluorographic analysis of the medium, have successfully led to the identification of major secretory proteins of this tissue in the human and a non-human primate.

Human

A number of studies using these techniques have examined the nature of secretory proteins synthesized and secreted by the endometrium obtained during the menstrual cycle.[6-8] Direct comparison of the properties of these proteins is difficult because of the different techniques employed. When comparison of physiochemical properties together with features of the pattern and regulation of their synthesis and secretion during the cycle is possible, one can make initial comparisons of the previously described proteins (Table I). A feature of these studies is that no product appears uniquely associated with a particular phase of the cycle, but rather the quantitative rates of synthesis and secretion of certain proteins are modulated during the cycle and in some cases this can be related to regulation *in vitro* by steroids. Group I proteins are those secretory proteins that appear to be constitutively synthesized, although the rates of secretion, for example, of EP7 and EP8 appear to be slightly enhanced during the luteal phase. EP8 exhibits similar properties to a 70,000 molecular weight protein identified in peritoneal fluid of patients with severe endometriosis, whose levels appear elevated during the luteal phase,[9] and to a non-serum uterine fluid protein, whose levels are enhanced during the luteal phase.[10] Group II and III proteins were those that appeared to be hormonally regulated whether demonstrable by direct short-term *in vitro* exposure to steroid hormones, i.e., Group III, or implied by the association of enhanced synthesis and secretion with a particular phase of the cycle and thus, presumably, reflecting the effect of the hormonal milieu characteristic of that phase of the cycle, i.e., Group II. This distinction may be relevant since the production of Group II proteins may reflect the histologically defined phenotypic state of the endometrium, whereas Group III proteins may represent endometrial products whose synthesis is regulated irrespective of the stage of differentiation of the tissue.

A number of secretory proteins whose synthesis and secretion *in vitro* are regulated by progesterone have been identified. Progesterone-induced proteins include S1, S3 and S4.[7] S3 appears similar to EP11 and the secretory protein of molecular weight 51,000 identified in endometrial cell culture.[11] Progesterone-repressed proteins include S2, which appears analogous to EP9 and S5. It is of interest that EP9, a minor secretory product of proliferative endometrium and a major product of secretory endometrium cultured in the presence of progesterone, is detected as a major product of this latter tissue when cultured in the absence of progesterone.[6] It could be

Table I. *Proteins synthesized and secreted by the endometrium and decidua of human during menstrual cycle and pregnancy.*

Name of protein and equivalents (references)	M_r (native M_r)		Phase associated with maximal synthesis/secretion	Effect of progesterone in vitro
Group I				
1. EP6	120 000			
2. EP7	90 000			
3. EP8	66 000			
4. EP10	50 000			
50 kDa (29)	50 000			
5. EP12	40 000			
Group II				
1. EP13	33 000		follicular	
35kDa(8)	35 000			
2. EP15/α-PEG	28 000	(56000)	late-luteal, pregnancy	
25kDa(8)	25 000	(45000)		
<25kDa(29)	25 000	(55000)		
PEP,PP14,AUP				
3. EP14/α₁-PEG	32 000		pregnancy	
34kDa(29)	34 000			
IGF-BP,PP12				
Group III				
1. S1(7)	130 000		luteal	stimulation
2. EP11	45 000		luteal	stimulation
S3(7)	50 000			
43 kDa(29)	43 000			
3. S4(7)	35 000		luteal	stimulation
4. EP9	54 000		follicular	suppression
S2(7)	58 000			
59kDa(8)	59 000			
60kDa(29)	60 000			
5. S5(7)	28 000		follicular	suppression
28kDa(8)	28 000			

Based upon information in references 6, 23, and those cited above.

anticipated therefore that *in vivo* its secretion is inversely related to progesterone levels. It is not certain how these proteins relate to those described in another study[8] of molecular weights 28,000, 35,000, 50,000, and 59,000 in which both synthesis and secretion are elevated during the follicular phase. Protein EP15, which is isolated from first trimester pregnancy endometrium, has been characterized as a polymorphic dimeric glycoprotein termed pregnancy-associated endometrial α₂-globulin (α₂-PEG).[12] This protein has been isolated by a number of groups from a number of sources including amniotic fluid and term placenta (for reviews see refs. 1, and 13-15). However, we have noted that the protein secreted during the menstrual cycle exhibits a different degree of polymorphism compared to that secreted by pregnancy endometrium (unpublished observations). Amino acid analysis has revealed extensive sequence homology with the major milk whey proteins, the β-lactoglobulins, and it has been proposed that it is a member of the β-lactoglobulin-related secretory protein family, proteins possessing a calyx and involved in binding of hydrophobic labile ligands.[16] EP15/α₂-PEG is not immunocytochemically reactive with proteins of this family and the molecular weight is dissimilar; however, deglycosylation does produce a protein of similar size, i.e., 20,000 (unpublished observations). Although the nature of the putative ligand for EP15 has not been identified, and it does not appear to be retinol as suggested for β-lactoglobulin (unpublished observation), this ligand may be involved in the protein's postulated immunosuppressive properties.[17] During the menstrual cycle, a dramatic increase in synthesis and secretion is observed from 5 to 7 days post-ovulation and it is quantitatively the major product during the luteal phase.[6] The protein can be recovered from intrauterine luminal flushings or biopsies where levels reflect the pattern of *in vitro* synthesis. Therefore it appears to represent a secretory protein directed into the lumen.[18] Immunohistological localization studies employing monoclonal antibodies (Mabs) support this interpretation in that the protein is localized to the glandular epithelium and is present in secretions of the glandular lumen.[19] The protein is first detected during the mid-luteal phase in the functionalis zone and immunostaining increases in intensity toward the end of the late luteal phase. The staining is so intense during the luteal phase, that the staining observed during the early follicular phase, which is restricted to the basal zone, may merely reflect stored product synthesized during the luteal phase. Immunoreactive protein is detectable in peripheral serum where, when superimposed upon basal levels which are found in post-menopausal women in the absence of endometrial protein production, a cycle variation is observed which reflects the pattern of *in vitro* synthesis and localization.[6,19,20] These studies imply that EP15/α_2-PEG[25] is the major protein product of the glandular epithelium. It is not associated with the onset of histologically defined glandular secretion since this phenomenon is initiated earlier during the luteal phase in association with estradiol and progesterone hormone levels. Despite this disassociation with luteal estradiol and progesterone levels, its association with longer term progesterone-dependent action is supported by clinical studies where oral progesterone and exogenous progestogens increase serum levels[21] and uterine production.[22] In patients in whom inadequate luteal phase levels of hormones are produced, deficient serum levels of this protein are also observed. Thus this protein may be employed as a marker for endometrial function, particularly the glandular epithelium component, and also as an indication of the relative endometrial response to progesterone.[15,21] Its presence during the peri-implantation period, and its increase in synthesis after implantation suggests its intimate involvement with early pregnancy, although no evidence for its essential role has been obtained.

EP14 is initially a minor product during the menstrual cycle and becomes a major secretory product of pregnancy endometrium/decidua.[6,23,24] While synthesis and secretion of this protein, an insulin-like growth factor binding protein (IGF-BP),[25] is enhanced during the luteal phase, this synthesis is not sufficient to increase basal systemic levels which are presumably derived from other tissue sources. This protein has been localized to subpopulations of predecidualization, e.g., arteries (Fig. 1).[26] This localization implies a potentially important role for IGF-BP in early pregnancy even though it is quantitatively a minor secretory product of the whole tissue. This illustrates a potential limitation of the examination of total secretory products of whole tissue when synthesis of certain products may exhibit regional restriction or may be associated with a minor cell population. However, these studies have yet to be reconciled with the discrepant cellular localization reported for the identical or closely related protein, placental protein 12 (PP12).[21] Prolactin, another quantitatively minor product of the endometrium, has been detected as an immunoreactive protein in the incubation medium of endometrial explants from day 23 of the cycle, and its rate of secretion has been correlated with the extent of predecidualization. This may not imply a predecidual cell origin, since EP15 synthesis also exhibits a similar correlation. Incorporation studies have failed to detect labeled prolactin. However, one study reported the production of a glycosylated prolactin, and hence this form of prolactin must be considered in a discussion of the potential function of prolactin during the cycle.

Non-Human Primates

At present the most detailed information concerning the characterization of the synthesis and secretion of endometrial proteins during the menstrual cycle has been obtained from studies of the baboon.[27-28] On the basis of these studies, secretory proteins were also classified into two groups (Table II). Group I proteins were those that were constitutively synthesized throughout the cycle and only exhibited minor cyclic variations in synthesis and secretion. Group II proteins were those in which the synthesis appeared to be restricted to, or exhibited dramatic alterations associated with, a particular phase of the cycle and were therefore thought to be steroid hormone regulated. Group I proteins were comprised of several high molecular weight proteins ($M_r > 200,000$) and five proteins (protein 1-5) with M_r's of 37,000 to 80,000. The only major alteration in this group appeared to be enhanced synthesis and secretion of two of the high molecular weight proteins during the mid-cycle period. The synthesis and secretion of Group II proteins of molecular weight 33,000 were restricted to the follicular phase, whereas a number were associated specifically with the luteal phase endometrium. These included an acidic pro-

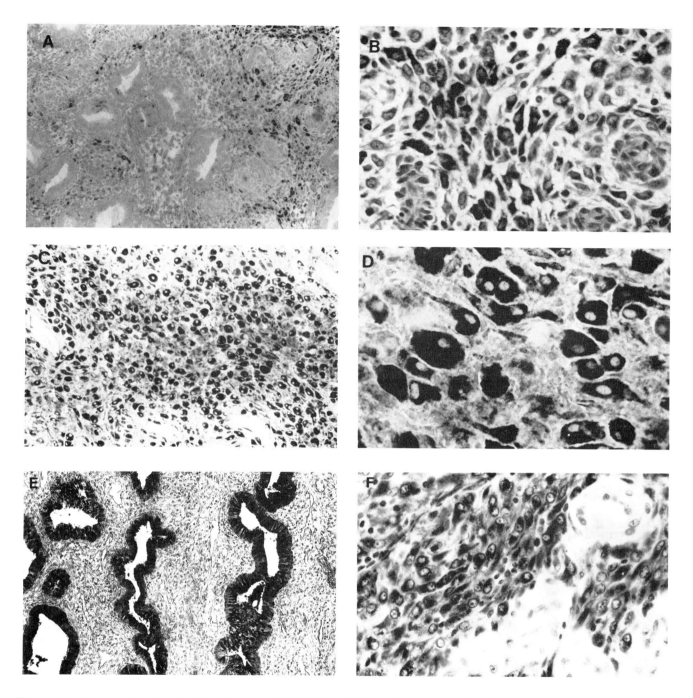

Figure 1. *Immunohistochemical localization of IGF-BP (α_1-PEG) employing monoclonal antibodies in the APAAP method in the human and baboon.* **A.** *Human late secretory endometrium, day 26 X82.* **B.** *X328 (Reproduced with permission from Waites et al., J Clin Endocrinol Metab 1988; 67:1100.* **C.** *Human first trimester pregnancy decidua compacta, X82.* **D.** *X328 (Reproduced with permission from Bell. J Reprod Fert Suppl. 1988; 36:109).* **E.** *Baboon late luteal pregnancy endometrium day 32, X92.* **F.** *Baboon third trimester decidual tissue, X275.*

tein of M_r 130,000, basic proteins 7 (M_r 88,000) and 9 (M_r 59-62,000) and another two proteins M_r 66,000 and M_r 40,000, which were more basic than proteins 2 and 4. Although not confirmed by the previous radiolabeled precursor incorporation experiments, presumably because they represent minor products, proteins immunochemically related to human placental protein 4, 7, 12 and 16 have been detected in culture medium with levels of 12 and 16 being detected only during the luteal phase. Similarly, immunoreactive prolactin was also detected, particularly during the mid-luteal phase.

Evidence that PP12 is synthesized by the luteal phase baboon endometrium has been provided by studies using Mabs to the human endometrial/decidual derived insulin-like growth factor binding protein, IGF-BP. IGF-BP was originally termed EP14 or pregnancy-associated endometrial α_1-globulin (α_1-PEG)[23,25] and was demonstrated to be immunocytochemically identical to PP12. Mabs in Western blots have detected immunoreactive protein in incubation medium of mid to late luteal phase endometrium. Its de novo synthesis is evidenced by the in vitro effect of cycloheximide on synthesis and the demonstration of specific mRNA in this tissue.[29] Immunocytochemical studies employing Mab's to the human protein have localized the protein to the deeper glandular epithelium during the mid to late luteal phase with no staining apparent in the stroma (Fig. 1).[29]

In ovariectomized steroid-treated animals, estradiol specifically induced synthesis of a protein (M_r 33,000) whose synthesis was also restricted to the follicular phase. Following estradiol priming, administration of progesterone maintained the synthesis and secretion of protein 7, M_r 88,000, protein 9, M_r 59-62,000, and the basic protein (M_r 40,000), as well as other proteins identified in ovariectomized animals. However, for synthesis and secretion of high molecular weight proteins (M_r > 200,000) and the acidic proteins of molecular weight 130,000, estradiol was required together with progesterone. The inclusion of estradiol with progesterone augmented the secretory potential of the endometrium for many of the proteins.[28] Similar hormone dependence has been demonstrated for IGF-BP/α_1-PEG synthesis and secretion by the endometrium.[29] The minimum requirement for induction of its synthesis was estradiol priming followed by progesterone administration. However, although this regimen induced production of the protein, the pattern of cellular localization and staining intensity which was observed during the late luteal phase was not achieved. This may reflect the failure in steroid-treated animals to achieve the appropriate changes in circulating steroid levels that are inherent to the normally cycling animal. Alternatively, the hormone induction studies in ovariectomized animals may also imply that an ovarian factor(s) may be essential for maximum synthesis of the IGF-BP.

PROTEIN SECRETION BY THE ENDOMETRIUM/DECIDUA DURING PREGNANCY

Human

The techniques that were used to identify secretory protein products of the endometrium during the menstrual cycle were also used to identify secretory products of the endometrium/decidua during the first and second trimester of pregnancy.[23,30] However, no products appeared to be unique to pregnancy. Rather, as during the cycle, major alterations in the rates of synthesis and secretion of specific proteins were observed. Of interest was the synthesis of EP15/α_2-PEG by the endometrial glands, which represented the quantitatively major product during early first trimester.[23] A gradual decline in in vitro synthesis and secretion during early pregnancy was observed which may be related to glandular involution within the decidua spongiosa region. This is supported by immunohistological localization studies employing monoclonal antibodies which demonstrated that the protein is localized primarily within the glandular epithelium of this region. Immunoreactive serum levels also reflect this pattern with peak levels being detected during weeks 8-10 of pregnancy. The high levels of authentic EP15/α_2-PEG detected in amniotic fluid during the first trimester, where concentrations exceed those in peripheral serum by over 100-fold, fall beyond week 15 of pregnancy.[31] α_2-PEG in amniotic fluid is thought to be derived from the endometrium. Similar data have been obtained from studies on PEP and PP14 proteins which are identical to α_2-PEG.[14,21] These studies suggest that this protein mediates some function of the glandular epithelium, that this function may be primarily restricted to early pregnancy, and that a non-decidualized stroma may be associated with this property of the glandular epithelium.

Another pregnancy protein of interest is α_1-PEG, a minor product during the menstrual cycle, which becomes the quantitatively major soluble protein product in second trimester endometrium/decidua specimens. The profile of in vitro synthesis and secretion by tissue suggests that this protein originates in the decidua compacta region. This observation is supported by immunohistological localization studies employing monoclonal antibodies, where the protein was principally localized to decidual cells, and implies that during this period it represents the major

Table II. *Proteins synthesized and secreted by the endometrium of the baboon (Papio anubis) during the menstrual cycle*[1]

Name of Protein	M_r	pI	Phase associated with maximal synthesis/secretion	Minimum steroid hormone regime required for optimal production
Group I				
High M_r proteins	>200 000		mid-luteal	(E_2-E_2+P)
Protein 1	80 000			
Protein 2	66 000	5.6-6.0	luteal	(E_2,P)
Protein 3	42-46 000	5.1		(E_2,E_2+P)
Protein 4	40 000			(E_2,E_2+P)
Protein 5(PP4)	37 000			(E_2,E_2+P)
Group II				
	130 000	acidic	mid-late luteal	E_2,E_2+P
Protein 7	88 000	basic	mid-late luteal	E_2,P
Protein 9	59-62 000	basic	mid-late luteal	E_2,P
	66 000	6.3	late luteal	E_2,P
	40 000	basic	mid luteal	E_2,P
	33 000	7.6	follicular	E_2
PP12*			mid-late luteal	
PP16*			mid-late luteal	
Prolactin*			mid luteal	
α_1-PEG/IGF-BP	32 000		mid-late luteal	E_2,P

[1]Based upon information in references 27, 28, 29.
*Evidence based upon immunoreactivity in Western blots.

product of a decidual population (Fig. 1).[32] EP15/α_1-PEG has been characterized as an insulin-like growth factor binding protein (IGF-BP) exhibiting identical IGF binding characteristics and N-terminal amino acid sequence to the 34,000 molecular weight IGF-BP isolated from amniotic fluid and the cDNA-derived sequence for this form.[33] The relationship of this protein to placental protein 12, and IGF-BP isolated from term placenta, with which α_1-PEG is immunochemically indistinguishable, is uncertain since minor discrepancies in amino acid sequence have been reported.[33]

α_1-PEG as synthesized by the endometrium of pregnancy exists in two forms which have identical molecular weights but different pI's, and although multiple molecular weight forms of PP12 have been reported, studies on α_1-PEG suggest that these could represent proteolytic fragments (unpublished observations). High levels of IGF-BP are also detected in amniotic fluid. The profile of IGF-BP in amniotic fluid appears to be reflective of the synthetic rate of the endometrium. Similarly, serum levels of immunoreactive protein are elevated above basal levels during pregnancy and the first peak at 15-20 weeks of the biphasic profile suggests that this could be accounted for by the endometrial/decidual origin. Whether elevated serum levels of this protein during the third trimester are related to this origin is uncertain since localization studies imply decreased endometrial production during this period. The production of this class of IGF-BP by many tissues and cell lines has been described[34] and this protein has been implicated in both inhibitory and stimulatory properties of IGF.[35,36] One can only speculate about the potential role this protein may play in pregnancy until the *in vitro* properties of the endometrial protein as well as the relative production of IGF by cell types within this tissue have been determined. However, a potential paracrine interaction with the trophoblast could be envisioned, since although no IGF-BP synthesis by placental tissue has been detected, IGF-1 mRNA has been localized to placental trophoblast and inferred to be present at highest levels during early pregnancy, the period of maximal endometrial IGF-BP synthesis and secretion.[36]

Other products have been identified by qualitative analysis of radiolabeled precursor incorporation; however, they have not been adequately characterized nor has their relationship to previously characterized products been determined.

Non-Human Primate

Studies characterizing the secretory endometrial/decidual proteins in the pregnant baboon have only been carried out with tissues obtained during the third trimester of gestation.[38] We have analyzed the secretory products of the decidua basalis, fetal membranes with associated tissues, and placental villi. The synthetic activity of the decidua is characterized by the presence of an acidic protein (M_r 33,000) that migrates as a fused doublet. Immunological, biochemical, and molecular studies have identified this protein as being identical to the IGF-BP synthesized by human decidual tissue.[38] None of the secretory proteins synthesized by the endometrium from the non-pregnant animal are readily identifiable in the fluorographs of decidual culture media. The IGF-BP is not synthesized by the placental villi. Third trimester baboon placental villi, however, do synthesize proteins that are immunoreactive with polyclonal antibodies to human placental lactogen, pregnancy-specific β_1-glycoprotein (SP_1), and placental protein 4 (PP_4). PP_4 has recently been cloned and shown to have homology with the lipocortin gene family.[39]

In human pregnancy, the first trimester is characterized by the continued synthesis of EP 15/α_2-PEG. By the 9th to 12th week of gestation EP 15/α_2-synthesis decreases and α_1-PEG/IGF-BP becomes the predominant secretory product. Significant levels of IGF-BP are also measurable in circulating plasma. Although the period during early pregnancy when α_1-PEG/IGF-BP becomes the major synthetic product of the baboon endometrium/decidua has not yet been established, radioimmunoassay (RIA) data from pregnant baboons show elevated peripheral plasma levels by the 6th week of gestation. Immunoreactive IGF-BP in peripheral plasma peaks at mid-gestation in the baboon (100-105 days; unpublished observations). The evidence that pregnant tissues contribute significantly to the circulating levels of IGF-BP is demonstrated by the fact that 3 hrs following removal of the fetus by caesarean section, peripheral plasma levels of IGF-BP drop dramatically and remain at baseline levels, at least out to 6 days post-partum. Thus, in the baboon as in the human, decidual IGF-BP is quantitatively the major product of pregnancy.

Table III. *Secretory proteins of baboon endometrium/decidua and their putative analogues in the human endometrium/decidua.*

	Baboon protein	Human protein*
1.	Protein 2 (66 000)	EP8 (66 000)
2.	Protein 3 (43-46 000)	EP10 (50 000)
3.	Protein 5 (37 000)	EP12 (40 000)
4.	Basic 40 000 protein mid-luteal P inducible (in vivo)	EP11 (45 000) luteal P inducible (in vitro)
5.	pI 7.6 33 000 protein follicular E_2 inducible (in vivo)	EP13 (33 000) follicular
6.	IGF-BP/α_1-PEG (33 000) late luteal pregnancy P inducible (in vivo)	EP14/α_1-PEG/IGF-BP (32 000) late luteal pregnancy

*See Table I and ref. for possible equivalents described in other studies.

COMPARISON BETWEEN HUMAN AND NON-HUMAN PRIMATES

Species Specific and Common Secretory Proteins

A comparison of proteins produced by identical tissues from different species is difficult at best. Putative identity when based upon crude biochemical properties such as molecular weight and pI is highly speculative, i.e., proteins 1-3 (Table III). However, one can be more confident when the hormonal regulation of their synthesis and secretion *in vitro* and their association with a specific phase of the cycle also appears similar, i.e., proteins 4 and 5.[28] Finally, purification of the proteins and the subsequent comparison of their immunochemical and molecular properties firmly establishes their relationships. We used this approach to successfully establish that the major secretory product of the baboon endometrium during pregnancy is an analogue of the human endometrial IGF-BP/α_1-PEG.[29,38]

Even though the histology of the endometrium is similar in both the baboon and human, and both establish a hemochorial placenta, dramatic differences are noted, especially during implantation and the development of that hemochorial placenta. If these interactions are mediated in part by secretory protein products it may be anticipated that both species-specific and common products may be identified which reflect these features and the relative roles of the endometrium's cellular constituents in these processes. Thus, it should not be surprising that incorporation studies reveal marked similarities and differences between the baboon and human, particularly during pregnancy. The most dramatic differences between the two species are observed during the luteal phase of the cycle, and this may be a reflection of the implantation process in these species. Although similarities exist in terms of several major secretory proteins in the human and baboon (Table III), the endometrium of the luteal phase in the human is characterized by the synthesis and secretion of a glandular epithelium-derived protein EP15/α_2-PEG, for which no apparent analogue exists in the baboon.[28,29] This is surprising since it would be anticipated that from the function proposed for this protein, i.e., immunosuppression, a similar functional analogue should be required in the baboon. A similar protein may indeed be absent in the baboon or it may simply illustrate the problems involved in selecting putative protein analogues on the basis of physiochemical and immunochemical criteria. EP15/α_2-PEG has been proposed to belong to a family of proteins which includes β-lactoglobulin and serum retinol binding protein. These proteins only exhibit limited sequence homology and no immunochemical cross-reactivity. However, they do possess a similar three-dimensional structure, a calyx, and a similar gene structure.[40] Therefore, a functional analogue for this protein may still exist in the baboon and it may be necessary to employ an *in vitro* functional assay for the human protein before it can be considered that this protein fulfills a function unique to implantation in the human.

Non-human Primate as a Model for Study of the Function of Human Endometrium/Decidual Insulin-like Growth Factor Binding Protein (IGF-BP)

The identification in the baboon and human of IGF-BP as both a product of the endometrium during the menstrual cycle and a major decidual protein during pregnancy illustrates the potential value of comparative studies of endometrial proteins in non-human primates and the human. However, interpretation of the observations made concerning this protein in these two species will be limited until the role of this IGF-BP in the action of IGF's has been fully elucidated. IGF's are potent mitogens and although they exhibit features of endocrine hormones, they are thought to act via autocrine and/or paracrine mechanisms. In serum, two major types of IGF binding or carrier binding proteins have been characterized, a growth hormone dependent 150,000 molecular weight form to which the majority of IGF is bound, and a low 30,000-40,000 molecular weight relatively less-saturated form.[34] It is the latter form that is detected in the endometrium and decidua. This is not surprising since synthesis and secretion of this form is a property of many cell types *in vitro*, and this form also is the major IGF-BP in many body fluids. This supports the contention that the low molecular weight form of IGF-BP is involved in the local action of IGF since most of these studies have also demonstrated a parallel synthesis and secretion of IGF. However, it must be noted that certain lines produce either IGF or IGF-BP. IGF-BP has been reported to exhibit either inhibitory or stimulatory activities upon IGF action. The stimulatory activity has been linked with the association of IGF-BP with the cell membrane, the IGF-BP being either endogenously produced by the cell or provided exogenously.[35,36] Recently, a molecular basis for this interaction has been suggested by the presence of—within the amino acid sequence of IGF-BP[41,42]—a tripeptide sequence which is involved in binding of proteins to the integrin class of membrane receptors.[43] The stimulatory activity of IGF-BP has been proposed as a mechanism which allows cells to differentially respond to stable endogenous levels of IGF.[35] This property of IGF-BP to differentially modulate IGF action may underly the features of IGF-BP production that are observed in the uterus and thus, elucidating their function in reproduction, may provide insight into the role of IGF in implantation and pregnancy.[44]

It is apparent that even the limited comparative studies performed to date on this protein suggest that differences in the nature of implantation in the baboon and human are reflected in differences in endometrial IGF-BP synthesis, and the similarities in the mature hemochorial placentation are reflected in essentially identical decidual production. In the non-pregnant baboon production of IGF-BP appears restricted to the glandular epithelium where immunohistological localization implies that it is a secretory product directed primarily into the uterine lumen prior to implantation. In contrast, in the non-pregnant human, staining was limited primarily to the peri-vascular stromal cells. It is tempting to hypothesize that this reflects differential roles of the epithelial and stromal cell populations in implantation in these species. In the human, predecidualization of the stromal cells is a feature of the luteal phase endometrium and is extensive in early pregnancy in contrast to the baboon.[45] In the baboon, implantation is of a superficial nature[46] and therefore the baboon embryo may potentially be more susceptible to exposure to the glandular secretions than the human embryo. During pregnancy the similarity between these two species is marked in that the major secretory product of the endometrium of pregnancy is IGF-BP in both species. IGF-BP originates from hypertrophied stromal cells in the baboon, and from decidual cells in the human. Although hypertrophied stromal cells are not histologically identical to human decidual cells, the hypertrophied stromal cells in the baboon are considered to represent analogues of the decidual cell by some investigators. Their biochemical properties suggest that they are identical and lead one to question whether this property of decidual cells extends to other species where, on histological grounds, decidualization of the stroma is not considered a prominent feature of the endometrium in pregnancy. Regardless, the production of IGF-BP in pregnancy reflects important and common functions of the endometrium associated with hemochorial placenta in these species, and thus, the baboon may provide a good model to examine the function of IGF-BP during pregnancy in primates.

CONCLUSIONS

Much progress has been made recently in the identification and characterization of the quantitatively major secretory proteins of the human endometrium and decidua during the menstrual cycle and pregnancy. The ability to detect a major product of the epithelial component of the endometrium in peripheral serum has facilitated clinical studies related to *in vitro* steroid hormone responsiveness of this tissue and assessment of endometrial function. Similarly, the identification of IGF-BP as a major product of the decidua has provided an opportunity to investigate the potential contribution of decidual dysfunction to abnormalities in pregnancy. It is apparent, however, that given the limitations of human studies, further progress toward understanding the function of these and other products produced by this tissue[47] will require animal models, particularly to investigate the inaccessible period of implantation and the establishment of the definite placenta. Although no non-human primate exhibits identical reproductive physiology during the establishment of pregnancy, early studies on the baboon suggest that the secretory phenotype of the decidua is very similar to the human, and thus the baboon may provide a suitable model for the study of decidual function. During the menstrual cycle, in spite of differences in the nature of the secretory protein species, candidates have been identified which may provide analogues for the study of steroid hormone action on the endometrium in the human. However, the differences identified may have equal relevance since they may reflect the different modes of implantation exhibited in these species and therefore provide an opportunity to analyze the potential contribution of the endometrium, its cellular constituents and secretions in the differential behavior of the blastocyst during implantation. In this respect, further studies on other non-human primate species may be particularly relevant.

Acknowledgment

The studies described in the authors' laboratories were financed by grants from the MRC (SCB), National Institutes of Health HD 21991 (ATF) and HD 20571 (HGV). The assistance of Ms. Margarita Guerrero in the preparation of this manuscript is gratefully acknowledged.

References

1. Bell SC. Secretory endometrial and decidual proteins: studies and clinical significance of a maternally derived group of pregnancy-associated serum proteins. *Hum Reprod* 1986; 1:129-143.
2. Brenner RM, Maslar IA. The primate oviduct and endometrium. In: Knobil E, Neill J et al. *The primate oviduct and endometrium.* New York: Raven Press Ltd., 1988:303-329.
3. Kraemer DC, Maqueo M, Hendrickx AG, Vera Cruz NC. Histology of the baboon endometrium during the menstrual cycle and pregnancy. *Fertil Steril* 1977; 28:482-487.
4. Enders AC, Schlafke S. Implantation in non-human primates and in the human. In: *Comparative primate biology. Vol 3: Reproduction and development.* New York: Alan R. Liss Inc., 1986:291-310.
5. Ramsey EM, Houston ML, Harris JWS. Interactions of the trophoblast and maternal tissues in three closely related primate species. *Amer J Obstet Gynecol* 1976; 124:647-652.
6. Bell SC, Patel SR, Kirwan PH, Drife JO. Protein synthesis and secretion by the human endometrium during the menstrual cycle and the effect of progesterone *in vitro*. *J Reprod Fert.* 1986; 77:221-231.
7. Strinden ST, Shapiro SS. Progesterone-altered secretory proteins from cultured endometrium. *Endocrinology* 1983; 112:862-870.
8. Heffner LJ, Iddenden DA, Lyttle CR. Electrophoretic analysis of secreted human endometrial proteins: identification and characterization of luteal phase prolactin. *J Clin Endocr Metab* 1986; 62:1288-1295.
9. Joshi SG, Zamah NM, Raiker RS, Buttram VC, Henriques ES, Gordon M. Serum and peritoneal fluid proteins in women with and without endometriosis. *Fertil Steril* 1986; 46:1077-1082.

10. MacLaughlin DT, Santaro NF, Bauer HH, Lawrence D, Richardson GS. Two dimensional gel electrophoresis of endometrial proteins in human uterine fluids: qualitative and quantitative analysis. *Biol Reprod* 1986; 34:579-586.
11. Maudelonde T, Rochefort H. A 51K progestin-regulated protein secreted by human endometrial cells in primary culture. *J Clin Endocr Metab* 1987; 64:1294-1301.
12. Bell SC. Purification of human secretory pregnancy-associated endometrial α_2-globulin from cytosol of first trimester pregnancy endometrium. *Hum Reprod* 1986; 1:313-318.
13. Bell SC. Synthesis and secretion of proteins by the endometrium and decidua. In: Chapman MG, Grudzinskas JG, Chard T, eds. *Implantation—biological and clinical aspects*. Berlin: Springer-Verlag 1988:95-118.
14. Joshi SG. A progestagen-associated protein of the human endometrium: basic studies and potential clinical applications. *J Steroid Biochem* 1983; 19:751-757.
15. Bell SC. Secretory endometrial/decidual proteins and their function in early pregnancy. *J Reprod Fert (Suppl)* 1988; 36:109-125.
16. Ali S, Clark AJ. Characterization of the gene encoding ovine beta-lactoglobulin. Similarity to the genes for retinol binding protein and other secretory proteins. *J Mol Biol* 1988; 199:415-426.
17. Bolton AE, Pockley AG, Clough KJ, Mowles EA, Stocker RJ, Westwood OMR, Chapman MG. Identification of placental protein 14 as an immunosuppressive factor in human reproduction. *Lancet* 1987;1:593-595.
18. Bell SC, Dore-Green F. Detection and characterization of human secretory "pregnancy-associated endometrial α_2-globulin" (α_2-PEG) in uterine luminal fluid. *J Reprod Immunol* 1987; 11:13-29.
19. Waites GT, Wood PL, Walker RA, Bell SC. Immunohistological localization of human endometrial secretory protein "pregnancy-associated endometrial α_2-globulin" (α_2-PEG) during the menstrual cycle. *J Reprod Fert* 1988; 82:665-672.
20. Wood PL, Walker RA, Bell SC. Serum levels of pregnancy-associated endometrial α_2-globulin (α_2-PEG) during normal menstrual and combined oral contraceptive cycles and relationship to immunohistological localization. *Human Reprod* 1989; in press.
21. Seppala M, Riittinen L, Julkunen M, Koistinen R, Wahlstrom T, Iino K, Alfthan H, Stenman UH, Huhtala ML. Structural studies, localization in tissue and clinical aspects of human endometrial proteins. *J Reprod Fert (Suppl)* 1988; 36:127-141.
22. Wood PL, Waites GT, MacVicar J, Davidson AC, Walker RA, Bell SC. Immunohistological localization of pregnancy-associated endometrial α_2-globulin (α_2-PEG) in endometrial adenocarcinoma and effect of medroxyprogesterone acetate. *Brit J Obstet Gynaecol* 1989; 95: in press.
23. Bell SC, Hales MW, Patel SR, Kirwan PH, Drife JO. Protein synthesis and secretion by the human endometrium and decidua during early pregnancy. *Br J Obstet Gynaecol* 1985; 92:793-803.
24. Bell SC, Patel SR, Hales MW, Kirwan PH, Drife JO. Immunochemical detection and characterization of pregnancy-associated endometrial α_1- and α_2-globulin secreted by the human endometrium. *J Reprod Fert* 1985; 74:261-270.
25. Bell SC, Patel SR, Jackson JA, Waites GT. Major secretory protein of human decidualization endometrium in pregnancy in an insulin-like growth factor binding protein. *J Endocr* 1988; 118:317-328.
26. Waites GT, James RFL, Bell SC. Immunohistological localization of the human secretory protein "pregnancy-associated endometrial α_2-globulin" (α_2-PEG), an insulin-like growth factor binding protein, during the menstrual cycle. *J Clin Endocrinol Metab* 1988; 67:1100-1104.
27. Fazleabas AT, Verhage HG. Synthesis and release of polypeptides by the baboon (Papio anubis) uterine endometrium in culture. *Biol Reprod* 1987; 37:979-988.
28. Fazleabas AT, Miller JB, Verhage HG. Synthesis and release of oestrogen and progesterone dependent proteins by the baboon (Papio anubis) uterine endometrium. *Biol Reprod* 1988; 39:729-736.
29. Fazleabas AT, Jaffe RC, Verhage HG, Waites GT, Bell SC. An insulin-like growth factor binding protein in the baboon (Papio anubis) endometrium: Synthesis, immunocytochemical localization and hormonal regulation. *Endocrinology* 1989; 124:2321-2329.
30. Kisalus LL, Nunley WC, Herr JC. Protein synthesis and secretion in human decidua of early pregnancy. *Biol Reprod* 1987; 36:785-798.
31. Bell SC, Hales MW, Patel SR, Kirwan PH, Drife JO, Mildford-Ward A. Amniotic fluid levels of secreted pregnancy-associated endometrial α_1- and α_2-globulins (α_1- and α_2-PEG). *Br J Obstet Gynaecol* 1986; 93:909-915.
32. Waites GT, James RFL, Bell SC. Human "pregnancy-associated endometrial α_1-globulin," an insulin-like growth factor binding protein: immunohistological localization in the decidua and placenta during pregnancy employing monoclonal antibodies. *J Endocr* 1989; 120:351-357.
33. Bell SC, Keyte JW. N-terminal amino acid sequence of human endometrial insulin-like growth factor binding protein—evidence for two forms of the small molecular

weight IGF binding protein. *Endocrinology* 1988; 123:1202-1204.
34. Ooi GT, Herington AC. The biological and structural characterization of specific binding proteins for the insulin-like growth factors. *J Endocr* 1988; 118:7-18.
35. Elgin RG, Busby WH, Clemmons DR. An insulin-like growth factor (IGF) binding protein enhances the biologic response to IGF-1. *Proc Natl Acad Sci USA* 1987; 84:3254-3258.
36. Busby WH Jr, Klapper DG, Clemmons DR. Purification of a 31,000-dalton insulin-like growth factor binding protein from human amniotic fluid. *J Biol Chem* 1988; 263:14203-14210.
37. Wang CY, Daimon M, Shen SJ, Engelmann GL, Ilan J. Insulin-like growth factor-1 messenger ribonucleic acid in the developing human placenta and term placenta of diabetics. *Mol Endocrinol* 1988; 2:217-229.
38. Fazleabas AT, Verhage HG, Waites GT, Bell SC. Characterization of an insulin-like growth factor binding protein (IGF-BP), analogous to human pregnancy-associated secreted endometrial α_1-PEG, in decidua of the baboon (Papio anubis) placenta. *Biol Reprod* 1989; in press.
39. Grundmann U, Abel KJ, Bohn H, Lobermann H, Lottspeich F, Kupper H. Characterization of cDNA encoding human placental anticoagulant protein (PP4): homology with the lipocortin family. *Proc Natl Acad Sci USA* 1988; 85: 3708-3712.
40. Julkunen M, Seppala M, Janne OA. Complete amino-acid sequence of human placental protein 14: A progesterone-regulated uterine protein homologous to β-lactoglobulins. *Proc Natl Acad Sci USA* 1988; 85:8845-8849.
41. Brewer MT, Stiler GL, Squires CH, Thompson RC, Busby WH, Clemmons DR. Cloning, characterization, and expression of a human insulin-like growth factor binding protein. *Biochem Biophys Res Commun* 1988; 152:1289-1297.
42. Lee YL, Hintz RL, James PM, Lee PDK, Snively JE, Powell DR. Insulin-like growth factor (IGF) binding protein complementary deoxyribonucleic acid from human HEP G2 hepatoma cells: predicted protein sequence suggests an IGF binding domain different from those of the IGF-I and IGF-II receptors. *Mol Endocrinol* 1988; 2:404-411.
43. Ruoslahti E, Pierschbacher MD. New prospectives in cell adhesion: RGD and integrins. *Science* 1987; 238:491-497.
44. Bell SC. Decidualization and insulin-like growth factor (IGF) binding protein: implications for its role in stromal cell differentiation and the decidual cell in haemochorial placentation. *Human Reprod* 1989; 4:125-130.
45. Bell SC. Comparative aspects of decidualization in rodents and humans: cell types, secreted products and associated function. In: Edwards RG, Purdy J, Steptoe PC, eds. *Implantation of the human embryo*. London: Academic Press 1985:71-122.
46. Hearn JP. The embryo-maternal dialogue during early pregnancy in primates. *J Reprod Fertil* 1986; 76:809-819.
47. Bell SC, Smith S. The endometrium as a paracrine organ. In: Chamberlain GVP, ed. *Contemporary obstetrics and gynaecology*. London: Butterworths Scientific Ltd., 1988:273-298.

THE BARRIER ROLE OF THE PRIMARY DECIDUAL ZONE

Margaret B. Parr and Earl L. Parr

Department of Anatomy
Southern Illinois University School of Medicine
Carbondale, Illinois 62901-6503 USA

IN many species, implantation of the blastocyst is marked by a striking transformation of the uterine endometrium into the decidua; it involves differentiation of fibroblasts into large, polyploid decidual cells with an epithelioid appearance and modification of components in the extracellular space. The decidua during early pregnancy in the rat demonstrates pronounced regional morphological differences. Based on light microscopic studies, Krehbiel[1] described two major areas of decidualized tissue: an antimesometrial decidual region consisting of primary and secondary zones and a mesometrial decidual region. More recent electron microscopic studies have confirmed and extended these early observations (see 2 for references). The fate of each region also varies. The primary decidual zone is short-lived, the secondary decidual zone develops into the decidua capsularis and the mesometrial zone becomes the decidua basalis. Thus, the uterine decidual tissue shows regional differentiation at different times during pregnancy.

While various aspects of decidualization have been extensively studied (see 3-6 for reviews), the function of decidual tissue is still speculative. A number of functions have been proposed, including: nourishing the developing embryo,[1] protecting maternal tissues from excessive trophoblast invasion,[7] isolating each embryo to ensure the development of separate vascular systems and protecting each from possible deleterious effects due to the failure of adjacent implantation sites,[3] protecting the embryo against immunological rejection by the mother,[8,9] acting as a barrier between embryonic and maternal circulation,[10-12] providing structural support for the embryo and remodeling the implantation chamber as embryogenesis ensues,[13] secreting a prolactin-like hormone[14-16] and playing a role in the immunology of pregnancy.[17-21] It is not unreasonable to assume that the decidual tissue, owing to its structural complexity, dynamic nature, regional variation, and diverse cell types, may play more than one functional role in the gravid uterus, and that each decidual zone may function in a different way.

The purpose of this report is to present the characteristic features of the primary decidual zone in the rat and to provide evidence suggesting that this zone acts as a partial permeability barrier during early pregnancy.

Morphology of the Primary Decidual Zone

In the rat, the fibroblasts immediately surrounding the implanting blastocyst and adjacent luminal epithelium at the antimesometrial side of the uterus became transformed into decidual cells, forming the primary decidual zone (PDZ).[1] This zone, which makes up part of the wall of the implantation chamber, consists of a narrow band of tightly-packed, elongated cells, 3 to 5 cells thick (Fig. 1). The cells are arranged more or less parallel to one another and to the long axis of the blastocyst in the mesometrial-antimesometrial direction. The zone first appears on day 6 of pregnancy and regresses by day 9. (Day 1 is the day

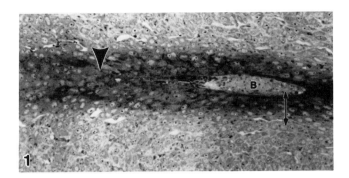

Figure 1. *A light micrograph of a transverse section through an implantation site in a rat uterine horn on day 6 of pregnancy. The primary decidual zone (arrowhead) surrounds both the blastocyst (B) in the uterine lumen and the remaining region of luminal epithelium at the antimesometrial side of the uterus (left side of photograph). An electron micrograph of a region similar to that indicated by the double arrow is presented in Fig. 2 X175.*

that sperm are found in the vagina after mating.) The PDZ appears to be devoid of blood vessels.[1,2,10-12,22] The combined vascular corrosion casting and scanning electron microscope technique clearly showed a region comparable to the PDZ free of capillaries at the implantation site in rats during normal pregnancy[10] or after estrogen activation following experimental delay of implantation.[23] However, Christofferson and Nilsson[23] have suggested that capillaries and vessels are present in the PDZ but are collapsed, do not conduct any blood flow, and can only be observed ultrastructurally. They have speculated further that the collapsed vessels eventually disintegrate and are phagocytosed by decidual cells.

Transmission electron microscope studies of the PDZ during normal pregnancy[2,12,22,24-27] showed that decidual cells of the PDZ are frequently binucleate and contain large ovoid euchromatic nuclei with one or more prominent nucleoli (Fig. 2). The cytoplasmic organelles include abundant rough endoplasmic reticulum with membrane profiles often oriented parallel to the long axis of the cell, lysosome-like bodies, scattered Golgi complexes, microfilaments, 10-nm filaments, numerous microtubules, lipid droplets, and glycogen granules. Annular gap junctions, coated vesicles, and small elongated dense organelles were also observed in the cytoplasm.

The PDZ consists of closely apposed cells. Adjoining cells exhibit long stretches of relatively straight surface membranes while in other places there are elaborate interdigitations with membranes from adjacent cells or even with portions of the same cells. Contacts between cells

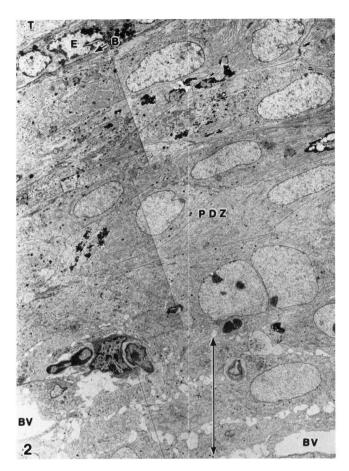

Figure 2. *A montage of electron micrographs showing the PDZ between the luminal epithelium (E) and secondary decidual zone (SDZ, double arrow). The PDZ is avascular and consists of elongated cells with little intercellular space, whereas the SDZ shows blood vessels (BV) and large spaces between the cells. T, trophoblast; B, basal lamina. X2,400.*

of the PDZ are frequent and include gap junctions, desmosome-like junctions and tight junctions[2,12](Figs. 3-5). The extracellular space at the sites of membrane interdigitations contains darkly stained amorphous material either alone or in combination with collagen fibrils. Bundles of collagen fibrils surrounded by plasma membrane are also present in deep invaginations of the decidual cell surface that appear to be continuous with the extracellular space. Such images suggest that the decidual cells may be involved in a reorganization of the collagen in the PDZ, perhaps including collagen degradation. This cellular activity may be required for the remodeling of the endometrium, including the formation of the PDZ, and

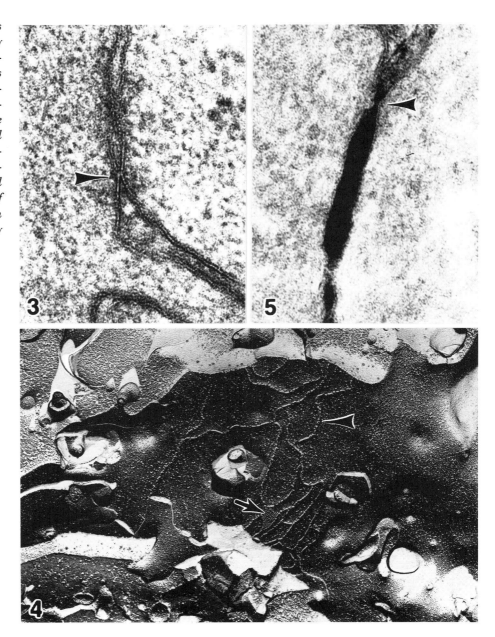

Figures 3-5. *Electron micrographs of cells in the PDZ from rats on day 7 of pregnancy.* **Fig. 3.** *A tight junction (arrow) between decidual cells showing fusion of the external membrane leaflets. X240,000.* **Fig. 4** *Lanthanum is present throughout the intercellular spaces between decidual cells except at the tight junction (arrowhead). X283,000.* **Fig. 5.** *A freeze fracture replica showing tight junctional strands (arrowhead) and a cluster of gap junctional particles (arrow) between cells of the PDZ. Approximately X40,000.*

for the normal growth and expansion of the developing embryo. Collagen remodeling has been proposed as an important part of decidualization in other parts of the decidua.[28,29]

Ultrastructural observations also suggest that decidual cells in the PDZ are invasive. Flange-like processes from decidual cells penetrate the basal lamina of the luminal epithelium adjacent to the mural trophoblast and also that of the endothelium lining the capillaries at the periphery of the PDZ.[2,12,13,26] Not only do portions of decidual cells abut the basal membrane of the endothelial cells without an intervening basal lamina,[2] but also the decidual cells themselves take up positions as part of the wall of the maternal blood vessels and form junctional attachments to adjacent endothelial cells.[13] Welsh and Enders[13] showed that decidual cells lining these vessels eventually degenerate and are replaced by trophoblast cells, allowing the latter to tap the maternal vessels. Thus, the invasive property of the cells of the PDZ in penetrating basal laminae may facilitate the invasion of the trophoblast into the uterine endometrium.

Fate of the PDZ

The PDZ is a transient region of cells; it develops on day 6 in the rat and shows signs of involution 2-3 days later.[1] Welsh and Enders[27] have demonstrated that on day 8 of pregnancy the decidual cells next to the trophoblast begin to show morphological features of apoptosis. This form of controlled physiological cell death is characterized by cell shrinkage, blebbing, or fragmentation of the cells, condensation of chromatin and fragmentation of nuclei and cytoplasmic organelles that appear intact.[30] The dying decidual cells detach from adjacent cells, become rounded, and are surrounded and phagocytosed by trophoblast cells (Fig. 6).[27,31] In this way, cells of the PDZ are removed and trophoblast cells occupy the space previously taken up by the decidual cells. This brings trophoblast cells into contact with the maternal vessels of the secondary decidual zone. Earlier in implantation the luminal epithelial cells next to the mural trophoblast also undergo apoptosis and are phagocytosed by trophoblast cells.[32] Thus, during this early period of implantation, the cells next to the mural trophoblast, initially the luminal epithelium and then the decidual cells of the PDZ, undergo apoptosis and are in turn phagocytosed by the proliferating trophoblast cells. The cause of cell death of these two cell types remains unknown but it is possible that trophoblast cells play a causal role.

Function of PDZ

The function of the PDZ is uncertain but evidence suggests that it acts as a partial permeability barrier between the blastocyst and maternal circulation during implantation.[11,12] This was demonstrated using fluorescein-conjugated (FITC) tracers of various molecular masses, including dextrans (17 kDa - 156 kDa) and proteins (40 kDa-450 kDa), administered i.v. to rats on days 6 to 9 of pregnancy. On days 6 or 7, tracers of 45 kDa or less penetrated the intercellular spaces of the PDZ within 10 min after i.v. administration, whereas FITC-BSA (66 kDa) and FITC-bovine hemoglobulin (64 kDa) had not penetrated up to 1 hr later. Only at 5 and 7 hrs was FITC-BSA detected in the PDZ and trophectoderm. FITC-bovine IgG (160 kDa) was absent or present only in small amounts in the PDZ and trophectoderm at 4 and 7 hrs (Fig. 7), while FITC-apoferritin did not penetrate into the zone 7 hrs after administration.

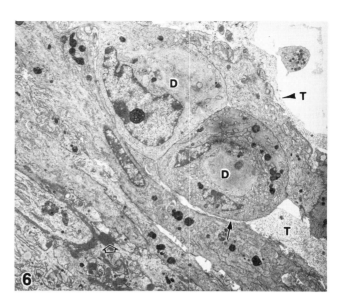

Figure 6. *Trophoblast (T) and decidual cells in the PDZ from a rat on day 8 of pregnancy. Some decidual cells (D) have lost their polarity and are rounded. Others are partially detached from one another. An arm of a trophoblast cell partially surrounds a decidual cell (arrow). X3,500.*

Further light and electron microscopic studies using horseradish peroxidase (HRP) and IgG-HRP as i.v. tracers on day 7 of pregnancy confirmed the previous results. HRP penetrated the PDZ within 30 min while IgG-HRP failed to penetrate this zone during 2 hrs (Fig. 8).[12] The peroxidase-tracing experiments indicated that the first barrier encountered by macromolecules passing between maternal blood and the implantation chamber was at the junctions between endothelial cells of the capillaries at the periphery of the PDZ. HRP readily penetrated the endothelial junction but the passage of IgG-HRP was impeded. The authors suggested that uterine capillaries near the PDZ exhibit differential permeability to macromolecules of various sizes. A second barrier occurs at the PDZ, inhibiting passage of IgG-HRP but not HRP alone. The morphological basis of the permeability barrier within the PDZ has not yet been established but several components of the PDZ may be involved, including discontinuous tight junctions between cells, extensive interdigitations of decidual cell membranes and the amorphous intercellular material. Collectively, these observations indicate that the PDZ is selectively permeable to blood-borne tracers on days 6 and 7 of pregnancy, with permeability decreasing with increasing molecular weight.

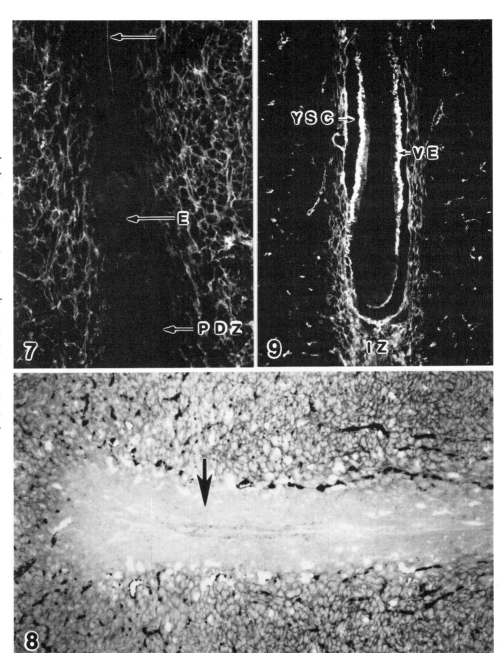

Figure 7. A uterus from a rat injected with FITC-IgG (i.v.) on day 7 of pregnancy and killed 4 hrs later shows bright fluorescence in the uterine lumen (arrow) and barely detectable fluorescence in the trophectoderm and PDZ. X150.

Figure 8. An unstained light micrograph shows the distribution of IgG-HRP in an implantation site of a rat uterus on day 7 of pregnancy 2 hrs after administration (i.v.). Reaction product is present in blood vessels and interstitial spaces of the endometrium but not in the PDZ (arrow). X105.

Figure 9. Photomicrograph of an embryo in the implantation site from a rat injected with FITC-IgG on day 9 of pregnancy and killed 1 hr later. There is bright fluorescence in the stromal blood vessels, PDZ, Reichert's membrane, parietal endoderm, and visceral endoderm (VE), but not in the underlying embryo. YSC, yolk sac cavity. X70.

The situation is quite different on day 9 of pregnancy when the PDZ is undergoing degeneration.[1,13] Vascular tracers, such as FITC-BSA and FITC-IgG administered at this time readily cross the PDZ, are endocytosed by the visceral yolk sac endoderm, but do not penetrate into the underlying embryonic cells (Fig. 9).[11] Similar results were obtained by Carpenter,[33] who administered HRP (i.v.) to hamsters on day 8 of pregnancy. The tracer readily penetrated the trophoblast, Reichert's membrane, and the parietal endoderm, but was endocytosed by the visceral yolk sac and did not enter the embryo proper. We agree with Carpenter[33] that at this time the visceral endoderm

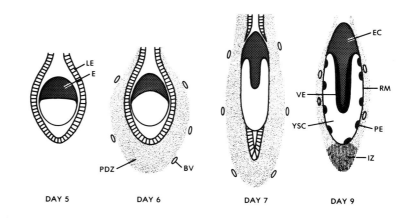

Figure 10. The tissue relationships in the rat implantation site between days 5 and 9 of pregnancy. The PDZ first appears on day 6 as an avascular zone of transformed fibroblasts separating the nearest blood vessels from the uterine luminal epithelium (LE). By day 7 the luminal epithelium adjacent to the embryo (E) is lost, and the trophectoderm comes into direct contact with the PDZ. The embryonic yolk sac at this time is not yet well developed, and the PDZ is the only significant barrier between maternal blood vessels (BV) and the embryo. On day 9 the PDZ is undergoing degeneration, and maternal blood spaces are closely adjacent to the parietal endoderm (PE) and Reichert's membrane (RM). At this stage the visceral endoderm (VE) appears to form an effective barrier between serum macromolecules and embryonic cells. The trophoblast has been omitted for clarity. YSC, yolk sac cavity; EC, ectoplacental cone; IZ, implantation zone.

is the critically selective element in the pathway for maternal-embryonic transfer of macromolecules.

The biological significance of the permeability barrier of the PDZ is speculative, but it may be related to the fact that the PDZ constitutes the only significant barrier between maternal blood and the embryo from the time when the luminal epithelium first begins to be lost from the implantation chamber until the visceral yolk sac is developed by days 8-9 of pregnancy (Fig. 10). The PDZ could protect the embryo during early implantation by limiting its exposure to maternal IgG, microorganisms, and immunocompetent cells. Tachi et al.[34] have reported that macrophages are absent from the PDZ but are aggregated around its periphery. They suggested that macrophages are unable to cross the PDZ and gain access to paternal antigens, thus resulting in blockage of the afferent arm of maternal immune recognition. While the PDZ may act as a partial barrier during implantation, it does allow the passage of smaller macromolecules between the embryo and the surrounding maternal tissues. Christofferson and Nilsson[23] have speculated that the vascular shut-down in the PDZ, in combination with the dilated subepithelial capillary plexus mesometrially, may set up a gradient of oxygen or other vascular factors which could facilitate the orientation of the inner cell mass mesometrially. Last, these studies underscore the view that morphologically distinguishable regions of the decidua are functionally distinct and play different roles during pregnancy.

Acknowledgment

The authors' original research reported in this review was supported by grant HD 17480 from the National Institute of Child Health & Human Development.

References

1. Krehbiel RH. Cytological studies of the decidual reaction in the rat during early pregnancy and the production of deciduomata. *Physiol Zool* 1937; 10:212-234.
2. Parr MB, Tung HN, Parr EL. The ultrastructure of the rat primary decidual zone. *Am J Anat* 1986; 176:423-436.
3. De Feo VJ. Decidualization. In: RM Wynn, ed. *Cellular biology of the uterus*. New York: Appleton-Century-Crofts, 1967:191-290.
4. Finn CA. The implantation reaction. In: RM Wynn, ed. *Biology of the uterus*. New York: Plenum Press, 1977: 245-308.
5. Glasser SR, McCormack SA. Separated cell types as analytical tools in the study of decidualization and implantation. In: Glasser SR and Bullock DW, eds. *Cellular and molecular aspects of implantation*. New York: Plenum Press, 1981:217-239.
6. Bell SC. Decidualization: Regional differentiation and associated function. *Oxford Rev Reprod Biol* 1983; 5:22-271.
7. Kirby DRS, Cowell TP. Trophoblast-host interactions, In: Fleischmajer R and Billingham RE, eds. *Epithelial-*

mesenchymal interactions. Baltimore: Williams & Wilkins, 1968:64-77.
8. Kirby DRS, Billington WD, James, DA. Transplantation of the eggs to the kidney and uterus of immunised mice. *Transplantation* 1966; 4:713-718.
9. Beer AE, Billingham RE. Host responses to intrauterine tissue, cellular and fetal allografts. *J Reprod Fertil (Suppl)* 1974; 21:59-88.
10. Rogers PAW, Murphy CR, Rogers AW, Gannon BG. Capillary patency and permeability in the endometrium surrounding the implanting rat blastocyst. *Int J Microcirc Clin Exp* 1983; 2:241-249.
11. Parr MB, Parr EL. Permeability of the primary decidual zone in the rat uterus: Studies using fluorescein-labeled proteins and dextrans. *Biol Reprod* 1986; 34:393-403.
12. Tung HN, Parr MB, Parr EL. The permeability of the primary decidual zone in the rat uterus: An ultrastructural tracer and freeze-fracture study. *Biol Reprod* 1986; 35:1045-1058.
13. Welsh AO, Enders AC. Trophoblast-decidual cell interactions and establishment of maternal blood circulation in the parietal yolk sac placenta of the rat. *Anat Rec* 1987; 217:203-219.
14. Kubota T, Kumasaka T, Yaoi Y, Suzuki A, Saito M. Study on immunoreactive prolactin of decidua in early pregnancy. *Acta Endocrinol* 1981; 96:258-264.
15. Basuray R, Gibori G. Luteotropic action of the decidual tissue of the pregnant rat. *Biol Reprod* 1980; 23:507-512.
16. Jayatilak RG, Glaser LA, Warshaw ML, Herz Z, Gruber JR, Gibori G. Relationship between luteinizing hormone and decidual luteotropin in the maintenance of luteal steroidogenesis. *Biol Reprod* 1984; 31:556-564.
17. Bernard O, Rachman F. Immunological aspects of the decidua cell reaction. In: Leroy F, Finn CA, Psychoyos A and Hubinont O, eds. *Progress in reproductive biology.* Volume 7. Basel: S Karger, 1980:135-142.
18. Rachman F, Bernard O, Scheid MP, Bennett D. Immunological studies of mouse decidual cells. II. Studies of cells in artificially induced decidua. *J Reprod Immunol* 1981; 3:41-48.
19. Lala PK, Parhar PS, Kearns M, Johnson S, Scodras JM. Immunologic aspects of the decidual response. In: Clark DA, Croy BA, eds. *Reproductive immunology.* New York: Elsevier, 1986:190-198.
20. Clark DA, Brierley J, Slapsys R, Daya S, Damji N, Chaput A, Rosenthal K. Trophoblast-dependent and trophoblast independent suppressor cells of maternal origin in murine and human decidua. In: Clark DA, Croy BA, eds. *Reproductive immunology.* New York: Elsevier, 1986:219-226.
21. Bulmer D, Peel S, Stewart I. The metrial gland *Cell Differ* 1987; 20:77-86.
22. Enders AC, Schlafke S. A morphological analysis of the early implantation stages in the rat. *Am J Anat* 1967; 120:185-226.
23. Christofferson RH, Nilsson BO. Morphology of the endometrial vasculature during early placentation in the rat. *Cell Tissue Res* 1988; 253:209-220.
24. Tachi C, Tachi S, Lindner HR. Ultrastructural features of blastocyst attachment and trophoblastic invasion in rat. *J Reprod Fertil* 1970; 21:37-56.
25. Sananes N, Le Goascogne C. Decidualization in prepubertal rat uterus. *Differentiation* 1976; 5:133-144.
26. Schlafke S, Welsh AO, Enders AC. Penetration of the basal lamina of the uterine luminal epithelium during implantation in the rat. *Anat Rec* 1985; 212:47-56.
27. Welsh AO, Enders AC. Trophoblast-decidual cell interactions and establishment of maternal blood circulation in the parietal yolk sac placenta of the rat. *Anat Rec* 1987; 172:203-219.
28. O'Shea JD, Kleinfeld RG, Morrow HA. Ultrastructure of decidualization in the pseudopregnant rat. *Am J Anat* 1983; 166:271-298.
29. Zorn TMT, Bevilacqua EMAF, Abrahamsohn PA. Collagen remodeling during decidualization in the mouse. *Cell Tissue Res* 1986; 244:443-448.
30. Wyllie AH. Cell death: A new classification separating apoptosis from necrosis. In: Bowen ID, Lockshin RA, eds. *Cell death in biology and pathology.* London: Chapman and Hall, 1981:9-34.
31. Katz S, Abrahamsohn PA. Involution of the antimesometrial decidua in the mouse. An ultrastructural study. *Anat Embryol* 1987; 176:251-258.
32. Parr EL, Tung HN, Parr MB. Apoptosis as the mode of uterine epithelial cell death embryo implantation in mice and rats. *Biol Reprod* 1987; 36:211-225.
33. Carpenter SJ. Placental permeability during early gestation in the hamster. Electron microscopic observations using horseradish peroxidase as a macro-molecular tracer. *Anat Rec* 1980; 197:221-238.
34. Tachi C, Tachi S, Knyszynski A, Lindner HR. Possible involvement of macrophages in embryo-maternal relationships during ovum implantation in the rat. *J Exp Zool* 1981; 217:81-92.

DETERMINANTS OF EMBRYO SURVIVAL IN THE PERI- AND POST- IMPLANTATION PERIOD

David A. Clark* and Gerard Chaouat†

*Departments of Medicine, Obstetrics & Gynecology
McMaster University
1200 Main Street West
Hamilton, Ontario, Canada L8N 3Z5

†INSERM U 262
Clinique Universitaire Baudelocque
Hôpital Cochin, 123 Boul. de Port Royal
75674 Paris Cédex 15, France

THE mammalian embryo to succeed must survive in utero and this requires a solution to two major problems (Table I). The need for growth is clear enough. The trophoblast that envelops the embryo and forms the feto-maternal interface after implantation must form a placenta capable of nourishing the fetus throughout gestation. Trophoblast cells bear receptors for growth factors such as colony stimulating factor, insulin-like growth factor, and epidermal growth factor.[1-3] In the case of epidermal growth factor, *in vivo* depletion by sialadenectomy of mice leads to subsequent abortion.[4] Colony stimulating factors (CSF-1 and GM-CSF) are made in decidual tissue (1 and unpublished data). Provided the maternal blood does not clot on contact with trophoblast, an effective dialysis of fetal blood in trophoblast-lined labyrinthine or villous placental tissue becomes possible and the fetus can grow.

The need for strategies to avoid active rejection by the mother is less self evident. There are, in fact, two modes of rejection that differ in important ways. When we use the term "rejection," it is traditional to think of the embryo as a type of graft that is antigenic to its host. Recognition of foreign (paternally-inherited or embryonic) antigens by the mother's immune system should trigger a cascade of events that leads to rejection just as when grafts of other types of paternal tissue (i.e., heart or kidney) fail when grafted to a genetically dissimilar recipient in the absence of potent immunosuppressive drug therapy. Indeed, the embryo, from the time it is initially fertilized until the time

Table I.

Problem to be solved	Solution(s)
1. Promote growth	Decidual growth factors for trophoblast cells.
	Angiogenesis
	Anti-clotting mechanism(s)
2. Avoid rejection (i.e., cytolysis and/or cytostasis)	Invulnerability
	Active suppression

of parturition, expresses on its cells antigens against which the mother can respond immunologically.[5] In most instances, the effectors stimulated by the embryo are not harmful, either because they are insufficiently potent, or because the embryo is inherently resistant to that type of effector. For example, pre-implantation embryos are resistant to lysis by cytotoxic lymphocytes (CTL) directed against paternal Class I major histocompatibility complex- (MHC-) type antigens due to zona pellucida or down-regulation of antigen expression after hatching.[6] Trophoblast cells are notoriously resistant to lysis by CTL even when Class I antigens are expressed on the cell surface.[7,8] Antibody usually requires participation of complement cells of the inflammatory response bearing receptors for the Fc end of the molecule or bearing receptors for complement[10]

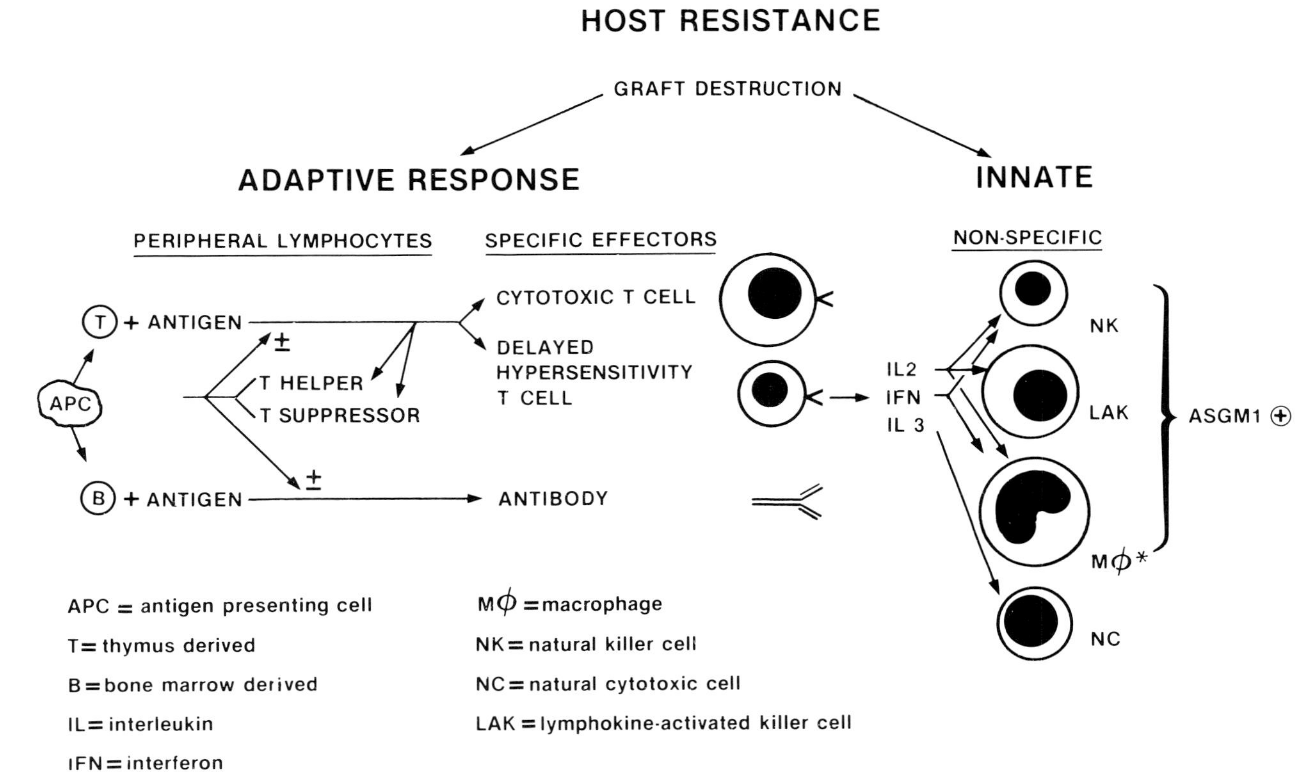

HOST RESISTANCE

Figure 1.

to produce damage, and in general, pre- and post-implantation embryos are not susceptible to this type of damage.[9,10] T cells producing delayed-type hypersensitivity by release of chemotactic and cell-activating cytokines have more potential to cause harm. The pre-implantation embryo appears sensitive to growth inhibition by cytokines, such as GM-CSF, and the products of activated macrophages, such as tumor necrosis factor alpha (TNF-α).[9,11] Indeed, it has been proposed that release of cytokines by peritoneal and fallopian tube macrophages in women with endometriosis explains the failure to implant and infertility.[12] We are now, however, dealing with a fundamentally different kind of rejection mechanism called the innate, natural, or para-immunological defence system. Figure 1 illustrates the relationship between the specific adaptive immune system and the innate or para-immune system.

The innate immune system is composed of cells that recognize and kill primitive cells such as tumor and embryonic cells. Included among the effector populations are macrophages, natural killer (NK) cells, and natural cytotoxic (NC) cells, some of which bear the asialo-GM1 surface marker. These cell populations employ primitive recognition mechanisms, do not require prior exposure to antigen to kill, but have no memory that enables a more vigorous response on second exposure. Killing may be mediated by H_2O_2 or enzymes in the case of macrophages, and by release of TNF-α.[13] The specific adaptive immune system has been added onto the innate mechanisms of host defence by the process of evolution, but while more specific, is not as rapid in its impact as the innate defences. Some of the cytotoxic capacities of the innate system are exploited by adaptive immunity (i.e., antibody-dependent targeting of NK and macrophage effector cell activity), and the activity of the innate effector cells can be boosted by lymphokines released by T-DTH cells. For example, GM-CSF, gamma-interferon, and IL-2 enhance the cytotoxic effects of monocytes-macrophages; interferon can boost NK activity; interleukin 2 (IL-2) can convert a subpopulation of NK cells into lymphokine-activated-killers (LAK cells); and IL-3 can activate NC-type cells.[14-16] While it is possible for cells such as trophoblast to possess an inherent resistance to many innate effector mechanisms,[9] a more active strategy is required if embryo survival is to be certain. The reasons are that certain innate effector cells can kill trophoblast[17,18] and both trophoblast and vascular endothelium (that lines the maternal blood supply to the embryo) may be sensitive to cytokines such as TNF-α.[19] Even if the "tumor" were "insusceptible," the blood supply could be thrombosed.[20] For this reason, we propose that active suppression of host rejection reactivity locally at the feto-maternal interface is crucial for the success of pregnancy. Both adaptive and innate systems must be inhibited, and the necessity is greatest when embryo-mother interaction is most intimate, that is, at and after implantation.

MECHANISMS OF SUPPRESSION

There are two possible ways the potentially harmful effects of rejection mechanisms of the embryo could be inhibited:

1. The embryo could directly suppress.
2. Suppressor cells could be activated in the mother.

Pre-implantation embryos may be associated with immunosuppressive factors but these appear likely to be sperm-derived,[21] and their spectrum of action has not been fully defined. We have not succeeded in obtaining inhibitory factors from blastocysts. In maternal pre-implantation endometrium, a large-sized non-specific suppressor cell develops both in mice and humans.[22,23] In the mouse, these suppressor cells appear to bear T cell surface markers such as Lyt 2 (CD 8). The possible importance of these cells is suggested by the observation that pre-implantation embryos are susceptible to inhibition by T cell and macrophage cytotoxins which can prevent implantation, that administration of monoclonal antibody to a T suppressor cell-inducer factor can produce subsequent pregnancy failure, and that anti-Lyt 2 antibody administered in a single dose 2 days after implantation or in several doses beginning 4 days after implantation can reduce placental cell function and increase the resorption rate.[24-26]

The period beginning with implantation may be divided into a 4 day peri-implantation phase in the mouse followed by development of the definitive fetus and placenta at 5 days after implantation. It is necessary to consider each phase separately.

Peri-implantation Phase

Blastocysts and peri-implantation ectoplacental cone trophoblast appear able to directly inhibit immune responses *in vitro*, but this inhibition is as effectively produced by fetal tissue.[27] Nevertheless, both fetal tissue and allogeneic blastocysts can be attacked by adaptive immune rejection mechanisms *in vivo*.[28,29] It has been suggested that trophoblast outgrowths can produce soluble inhibitory molecules,[30] but this is difficult to demonstrate using cultures of less than 96 hrs duration (Van Vlasselaer & Vandeputte, personal communication) and such factors as may be produced with formation of trophoblast giant cells are best discussed with respect to the post-implant phase that begins 5 days after implantation. In the peri-implant period, in contrast, two aspects of maternal decidualization appear important in the protection of the conceptus. First, macrophages and lymphatics appear to be excluded from the primary decidua (decidua capsularis) and delayed type hypersensitivity (cellular immunity) against such organisms as listeria cannot be expressed, even in immunized mice.[31,32] Any expression of immunity against minor histocompatibility antigens or embryonal antigens expressed on the conceptus[29,33] would be limited and restricted to the junction of decidua with uterus where there would be macrophages capable of presenting these antigens to maternal T cells. (Maternal T cells require MHC expression for such recognition and there is no surface MHC on the conceptus at this time.) Antibody that could interact with the embryo would not have macrophages available to complete the killing. The second feature of peri-implant decidua is that the hormonally activated non-specific suppressor cells bearing Lyt 2 persist (manuscript in preparation). The peri-implant embryo is susceptible to induced failure under 3 conditions:

1. Indomethacin is administered. Indomethacin blocks production of prostaglandins that are important in decidualization and also activates macrophages to cytotoxicity.[34,35] Indomethacin treatment leads to abortion by day 8.5 (3 days post-implantation) in association with an infiltrate of non-specific killer cells.[36]
2. Administration of poly I:C on day 6.5 of pregnancy terminates the embryos (G. unpublished data). Poly I:C is a potent activator of the innate effector system and provides a cleaner experimental system than indomethacin which may have several mechanisms of action.
3. Administration of antibody to Lyt 2 (CD 8) as previously mentioned.[26]

Post-implantation Phase

The post-implantation phase is particularly interesting as it is during this period that most spontaneous abortions occur in mice. While the peri-implantation phase of mouse pregnancy can be related to the stages of human embryo development at which occult miscarriages occur (abortion of chemical pregnancies),[37] the post-implantation phase involves development of a distinct fetus and placenta together with a circulation to connect the two. The majority of clinically evident first trimester miscarriages in humans occur in connection with this phase of development.[26,37] At this time, there is expression of a variety of antigens on trophoblast cells including expression of Class 1 MHC-like molecules on extravillous trophoblast.[38,39] The latter is in contact with maternal decidua and by invading the walls of the maternal arterial feed to the placenta come in contact with maternal blood. The cells of the fetus also begin to express paternal MHC antigens and become susceptible to lysis by CTL. What protects the developing embryo at this stage?

There is good evidence that placental trophoblast plays a key role in determining the success of pregnancy at this stage of development. An intact and functional healthy trophoblast appears able to block access of potentially aggressive maternal lymphocytes to the fetus, and except in unusual cases, small numbers of maternal cells entering the fetus are eliminated.[40-42] However, it has been suggested that maternal alloreactive lymphocytes entering placental villi may trigger thrombosis of the villous blood supply and harm the fetus indirectly (43 and personal communication). Trophoblast as well as vascular endothelium possess receptors for TNF-α and trophoblast cells may be sensitive to killing by IL-2 activated killers (LAKs)[17,18,26] and TNF-α (19 and manuscript in preparation). Further, abortion can be increased by injecting lipopolysaccharides (LPS), an activator of TNF-α production, and by injecting recombinant TNF-α (manuscript in preparation). Further, macrophages as well as polymorphonuclear leukocytes attracted to areas where TNF-α is being produced,[44] can produce lytic enzymes and toxic oxygen metabolites to which all cells are susceptible. Evidence that natural (innate) effector cells play an important role in some forms of spontaneous abortion is provided by the CBA/J X DBA/2 system. Female CBA/J mice mated to DBA/2 suffer a high rate of spontaneous abortion and this can be prevented by injecting antibody against the asialo-GM1 marker[26,45] that is found on a variety of natural effector cells (Fig. 1). Although an infiltrate of ASGM1-positive cells develops at the outer margin of the primary decidua by day 6.5 of pregnancy,[45] injection of antibody as late as day 9.5-10.5 prevents abortion (manuscript in preparation) so that lethal damage is not apparently inflicted until the post-implantation phase of pregnancy. Several mechanisms may be able to protect the embryo against the diverse variety of cells that may mediate "rejection" during the post-implantation phase:

1. Placental trophoblast cells may produce soluble factors that inhibit the cytolytic action of effector cells such as CTL, antibody-dependent K cells, NK cells, and LAKs.[7,46] Whilst such factors might confer resistance to some types of effectors, they clearly do not produce a state of invulnerability to all types of effectors and could not be expected to protect the placental vascular supply from TNF-α. Placental trophoblast also appear to produce molecules that suppress the generation and activation of effector cells by cytokines[46] and the case is particularly strong in this respect for trophoblastic tumors (i.e., hydatidiform moles and choriocarcinoma cell lines) which may produce molecules inhibiting IL-2.[47] However, suppressive activity of this type recovered from the normal mouse placenta is not very potent and 4-8 times greater immunosuppressive activity is obtainable from the underlying decidua and metrial gland tissue (manuscript in preparation).

2. On day 9.5, a potent non-T suppressor cell bearing Fc receptors accumulates at the implantation site at the mesometrial side of the murine uterus.[48] The dominant suppressor population appears to be a small lymphocytic cell with cytoplasmic granules, but a population of large-sized suppressor cells may also be present.[48] A feature distinguishing these cells from the large sized pre- and peri-implantation suppressor T-like cells is that the post-implantation suppressor cells do not bear T cell markers and both the large and small cells in post-implantation decidua release a soluble suppressor factor.[48] The soluble suppressor activity has been characterized and is related to TGF-β-2.[49,50] However, the factor isolated from decidua appears to differ in molecular weight from TGF-β-2 and may therefore represent a new member of the TGF-β family.[50]

Evidence That a Unique TGF-β Molecule is Relevant to Preventing Abortion

First, development of this unique type of suppression in decidua depends upon soluble signals from trophoblast cells.[48,51] The signal is not related to TGF-β but appears rather to activate target cells in decidua (or pre-decidual human luteal phase endometrium) to produce the suppressor factor.[50] Activation of suppression confers upon the tissue the ability to inhibit to some extent the expression of pre-existing transplantation immunity. For example, allografts placed on decidua in pseudopregnant mice or on decidua in pregnant mice at a site distant from trophoblast are protected temporarily by impairment of the ability of the graft to sensitize the host. If the animals are immunized against the graft, however, prompt rejection occurs.[52] Nevertheless, allografts placed at the choriodecidual junction appear protected to some extent, even in immune recipients (average survival 28.4% on days 4, 6, 8 compared to 7.4% expected based on studies of skin grafts on pseudopregnancy decidua, P = 0.016 by Fisher's Exact Test).[52,53] More satisfactory data than that provided by meta-analysis was provided by histologic comparison of skin grafts placed on pregnancy decidua in one horn of a rat uterus devoid of fetuses (due to ligation before mating) to similar grafts at the choriodecidual junction of successful implants in the opposite horn. 75% of 4 grafts on remote decidua showed a lymphocytic infiltrate on day 4-8, but in spite of this low grade expression of an active immune response, there was no infiltration in grafts at 17 separate choriodecidual sites (P = 0.017).[53] Further, the suppressor factor isolated from trophoblast-conditioned decidua has been shown to inhibit the destruction of labeled allogeneic tumor cells injected into immune mice with protection evident as early as 24 hrs after injection (manuscript in preparation).

Second, the TGF-β-like suppressor factor is capable of inhibiting a wide variety of effector cells potentially relevant to embryo rejection. Thus, CTL generation, NK activity, IL-3-dependent NC cell activation, and macrophage activation are all blocked (49, 54 and in preparation). These are all effects known to be within the spectrum of action of the TGF-β family of molecules. Indeed, TGF-β is reported to be an immunosuppressive 10,000 times more potent than cyclosporine A and to have a Yin-Yang relationship with TNF-α in regulating the immune response and in the killing of certain target cells.[49,55] TGF-β can inhibit the growth of a variety of cells including vascular endothelial cells.[56] While this might imply a threat to the developing embryo, recent data indicate that TGF-β-2, to which the decidual factor is related, has minimal inhibitory activity on endothelial cell growth compared to TGF-β-1.[57]

Third, the activity of suppression at individual implantation sites follows a distribution curve, and it is those implants with the least suppressive activity that appear most likely to resorb.[26] Indeed, in animal systems such as the CBA/J X DBA/2J system, a relative deficiency of suppressor cell activity predicts subsequent resorption.[26,48] Certain forms of alloimmunization can diminish the rate of resorption and this "rescue" is associated with boosting of local suppressor cell activity.[26,48] Further, injection of an antibody against pregnancy-associated null-type suppressor cells (i.e., cells typical of the trophoblast-dependent suppressor cell in the decidua) produces spontaneous abortion.[58]

Taken together, the foregoing observations strongly support the idea that suppressor cells and their factors play a key role in protecting the embryo from rejection. Indeed, during normal pregnancy there is evidence for activation of NK, NC, and macrophage-type cells that could be interpreted as Mother Nature attempting to ensure that the least fit of the implants (i.e., subnormal ability to activate suppressor cells) are eliminated (59 and in preparation). The balance point that determines success vs. abortion is then decided by the level of suppressor activity vs. the level or intensity of maternal natural effector activity during the post-implantation period. What has yet to be determined is the extent to which events in the peri-implantation period determine the functional ability of the trophoblast to activate suppressor cells on day 9.5 of murine pregnancy. The increase in the post-implant phase abortion rate by injecting anti-Lyt 2 in the peri-implant phase implies that suppressor cells and maternal effector mechanisms on day 6.5 of murine pregnancy are important but not the final arbiter.

GROWTH FACTORS AND EMBRYO SURVIVAL

At the outset we stated that to survive, the embryo had to grow. Most of the subsequent discussion has focused on the identification and regulation of "stop" signals. Could not pregnancy failure also be explained by suboptimal growth factor production?

A major growth factor for trophoblast is believed to be CSF-1.[1] This factor is produced primarily by gland epithelium and levels of CSF-1 increase 1000-fold during pregnancy.[1] This is thought to be a result of the decidual response. Since the decidual response is determined by gestational hormones and the intensity of trauma (produced by the trophoblast), it would follow that subnormal embryo-trophoblast growth due to excessive "stop" signals would lead to subnormal decidualization and hence, less growth factor production. Thus, it would be extremely difficult to decide if lower levels of growth factor production represented a primary defect rather than an epiphenomenon. Other types of CSF such as GM-CSF are also produced in decidua, presumably by a variety of cell types.[26] Injection of low doses of GM-CSF into CBA/J mice pregnant by DBA/2 dramatically reduces the rate of abortion (26, submitted for publication). While it has been suggested that the benefit might be mediated by a direct growth stimulating effect on trophoblast cells, for a variety of reasons[26] an indirect mechanism seems more likely. CBA/J X DBA/2J do not have a genetically determined high abortion rate; rather, the susceptibility to abortion is only manifest when the mice are maintained in nongonobiotic (i.e., dirty) cages.[60] The flora is a major stimulus to natural effector cell activity in these mice, and GM-CSF has the ability to down-regulate TNF-α production from macrophages activated by bacterial LPS.[26] We have recently discovered that recombinant human GM-CSF that has no stimulatory effects on murine trophoblast proliferation *in vitro* can also prevent abortion in the CBA/J X DBA/2 system.[26] Of interest, both the murine and human recombinant GM-CSFs can inhibit the *in vitro* activation of cells capable of killing a mouse trophoblast cell line (manuscript in preparation). Suppression of cells capable of giving "stop" signals to trophoblast could explain the *in vivo* prevention of growth retardation and abortion by GM-CSF. Since a single dose of GM-CSF given in the peri-implantation phase of pregnancy is protective, and since CSF-type molecules[1] but not TGF-β type suppressor factors would be present at this time, it is tempting to suggest that GM-CSF may represent both a growth stimulating and a major suppressive molecule for this phase of mouse pregnancy. It now becomes necessary to ask if other putative growth factors might also act to suppress certain cell functions, and whether suppressive factors such as the TGF-β-related factor might have other growth stimulatory effects important for pregnancy? The embryo appears to dwell in a sea of diverse cytokines. Identification of all of the participants, their interactions and effects on cells of the embryo and decidua will lead to a full appreciation of how survival in the peri- and post-implantation phases of pregnancy is determined.

Acknowledgment

Supported by grants from MRC Canada and INSERM France.

References

1. Pollard JA, Bartocci R, Orlofsky A, Ladner MB, Stanley ER. Apparent role of the macrophage growth factor, CSF-1, in placental development. *Nature* 1987; 330:484-489.
2. Jonas HA, Harrison LC. The human placenta contains two distinct binding and immunoreactive species of insulin-like growth factor-1 receptors. *J Biol Chem* 1985; 260:2288-2294.
3. Morrish DW, Bhardway D, Dabbagh LK, Marusyk H, Siy O. Epidermal growth factor induces differentiation and secretion of human chorionic gonadotropin and placental lactogen in normal human placentae. *J Clin Endocr Metab* 1987; 65:1282-1290.
4. Tsutsumi O, Oka T. Epidermal growth factor deficiency causes abortion in mice. *Amer J Obstet Gynec* 1987; 156:241-244.
5. Clark DA. Current concepts of immunoregulation of implantation. In: Chapman M, Grudzinskas G, Chard T, eds. *Implantation, biological and clinical aspects*. London: Springer-Verlag, 1988:163-175.
6. Warner CM, Brownell MS, Ewoldsen MA. Why aren't embryos immunologically rejected by their mothers? *Biol Reprod* 1988; 38:17-29.
7. Kolb JP, Chaouat G, Chassoux D. Immunoactive products of placenta. III. Suppression of natural killer activity. *J Immunol* 1984; 12:2305-2310.
8. Zuckerman FA, Head JR. Murine trophoblast resists cell-mediated lysis I. Resistance to allospecific cytotoxic T lymphocytes. *J Immunol* 1987; 139:2856-2864.
9. Zuckerman FA, Head JR. Murine trophoblast resists cell-mediated lysis. II. Resistance to natural cell-mediated lysis. *Cell Immunol* 1988; 116:274-286.
10. Croy BA, Gambel P, Rossant J, Wegmann TG. Characterization of murine decidual natural killer (NK) cells and their relevance to the success of pregnancy. *Cell Immunol* 1985; 93:315-326.
11. Hill JA, Haimovici F, Anderson DJ. Products of activated lymphocytes and macrophages inhibit murine embryo development in vitro. *J Immunol* 1987; 139:2250-2254.
12. Fakih H, Baggett B, Holz G, Tsang KY, Lee JC, Williamson HO. Interleukin 1: a possible role in the infertility associated with endometriosis. *Fertil Steril* 1987; 47:213-217.
13. Clark DA, Daya S. Macrophages and other migratory cells in endometrium: relevance to uterine bleeding. In: White J, Fraser IS, eds. *Contraception and mechanisms of uterine bleeding*. WHO Symposium 28 November-2 December, 1988, in press.
14. Grabstein KH, Urdal DL, Tushinski RJ, Mochizuki DY, Price VL, Cantrell MA, Gillis S, Conlon PJ. Induction of macrophage tumoricidal activity by granulocyte-macrophage colony-stimulating factor. *Science* 1986; 232:506-508.
15. Malkovsky M, Loveland B, North M, Asherson GL, Gaw L, Ward P, Fiers W. Recombinant interleukin-2 directly augments the cytotoxicity of human monocytes. *Nature* 1987; 325:262-265.
16. Djeu JY, Lanza E, Pastore S, Hapel AJ. Selective growth of natural cytotoxic but not natural killer effector cells in interleukin-3. *Nature* 1983; 306:788-791.

17. Drake BL, Head JR. Murine trophoblast cells are susceptible to lymphocyte-activated killer (LAK) cell lysis. *Amer J Reprod Immunol Microbiol* 1988; 16:414.
18. Clark DA, Croy BA, Rossant J, Chaouat G. Immune presensitization and intrauterine defences as determinants of success or failure of murine interspecies pregnancies. *J Reprod Fertil* 1986; 77:633-643.
19. Eades DK, Cornelius P, Pekala PH. Characterization of the tumor necrosis factor receptor in human placenta. *Placenta* 1988; 9:247-251.
20. Shiomura K, Manda T, Mukumoto S, Robayashi K, Nakano K, Mori J. Recombinant human tumor necrosis factor-a: thrombus formation is a cause of anti-tumor activity. *Int J Cancer* 1988; 41:243-247.
21. Clark DA, Lee S, Fishell S, Mahadevan M, Goodhall L, Ah-Moye M, Schechter O, Stedronska-Clark J, Daya S, Underwood J, Craft I, Mowbray J. Immuno-suppressive activity in human IVF culture supernatants and prediction of outcome of embryo transfer—a multicenter trial. *J In Vitro Fert Embryo Transfer* 1988; 6:51-58.
22. Brierley J, Clark DA. Characterization of hormone-dependent suppressor cells in the uterus of pregnant and pseudopregnant mice. *J Reprod Immunol* 1987; 10:201-218.
23. Daya S, Clark DA, Devlin MC, Jarrell J, Chaput A. Preliminary characterization of two types of suppressor cells in the human uterus. *Fertil Steril* 1985; 44:778-785.
24. Ribbing SL, Hoversland RC, Beaman KD. T-cell suppressor factor plays an integral role in preventing fetal rejection. *J Reprod Immunol* 1988; 14:83-95.
25. Athanassakis I, Wegmann TG. The immunotrophic interaction between maternal T cells and fetal trophoblast/macrophages during gestation. In: Clark DA, Croy BA, eds. *Reproductive immunology.* 1986. Amsterdam: Elsevier, 1986:99-105.
26. Clark DA, Chaouat G. What do we know about spontaneous abortion mechanisms? *Amer J Reprod Immunol Microbiol* 1988, in press.
27. Croy BA, Rossant J, Clark DA, Wegmann TG. Nonspecific suppression of in vitro generation of cytotoxic lymphocytes by allogeneic and xenogeneic embryonic tissue. *Transplantation* 198 ; 35:627-629.
28. Simmons RL, Russell PS. The histocompatibility antigens of fertilized mouse eggs and trophoblast. *Ann New York Acad Sci* 1966; 129:35-45.
29. Searle RF, Johnson MH, Billington WD, Elson J, Clutterbuck-Jackson S. Investigation of H-2 and non-H-2 antigens on the mouse blastocyst. *Transplantation* 1974; 18:136-141.
30. Van Vlasselaer P, Vandeputte M. Immunosuppressive properties of mouse trophoblast. *Cell Immunol* 1984; 83:422-432.
31. Head JR. Lymphoid components in the rodent uterus. In: Gill TJ, Wegmann TG, eds. *Immunoregulation and fetal survival.* New York: Oxford Univ Press, 1987:46-59.
32. Redline RW, Shea CM, Papaioannou VE, Lu CY. Defective anti-listerial responses in deciduoma of pseudopregnant mice. *Amer J Pathol* 1988; 133:485-497.
33. Hamilton MS, Vernon RB, Eddy EM. A monoclonal antibody derived from syngeneically multiparous mouse alters in vitro fertilization and development. *J Reprod Immunol* 1985; 8:45-49.
34. Kennedy TG. Intrauterine infusion of prostaglandins and decidualization in rats with uteri differentially sensitized for the decidual cell reaction. *Biol Reprod* 1986; 4:327-335.
35. Voth R, Storch E, Huller K, Kirchner H. Activation of cytotoxic activity in culture of bone marrow-derived macrophages by indomethacin. *Eur J Immunol* 1987; 17:145-148.
36. Scodras JM, Lala PK. Reactivation of natural killer lymphocytes in the decidua with indomethacin, IL 2, or combination therapy is associated with embryonic demise. *Amer J Reprod Immunol Microbiol* 1987; 14:12.
37. Clark DA. Immunology of Recurrent Abortion. In: Bonnar J, ed. *Advances in obstetrics & gynecology,* Volume 16. London: Churchill Livingstone, 1989; in press.
38. Hsi BL, Yeh JG, Faulk WP. Class 1 antigens of the major histocompatibility couples on cytotrophoblast and human chorion laeve. *Immunol* 1984; 52:621-629.
39. Ellis SA, Sargent IL, Redman CWG, McMichael AJ. Evidence for a novel HLA antigen found on extravillous trophoblast and a choriocarcinoma cell line. *Immunol* 1986; 59:595-601.
40. Hunziker RD, Gambel P, Wegmann TG. Placenta as a selective barrier to cellular traffic. *J Immunol* 1984; 133:667-671.
41. Jadus MR, Peck AB. Naturally occurring spleen-associated suppressor activity of the newborn mouse. *Scand J Immunol* 1986; 23:35-44.
42. Ammann AJ. Fetal and neonatal graft-vs.-host and immunodeficiency disease. In: Clark DA, Croy BA, eds. *Reproductive immunology 1986.* Amsterdam: Elsevier, 1986:19-26.
43. Faulk WP. Haemostasis and fibrinolysis in human normal placenta. In: Beard RW, Sharp F, eds. *Early pregnancy failure, mechanisms and treatment.* Ashton-under-Lyne (UK): Peacock Press, 1988:193-198.
44. Sayers TJ, Wiltrout TA, Bull CA, Pilaro AM, Lohesa B. Effects of cytokines on polymorphonuclear infiltration in the mouse. *J Immunol* 1988; 141:1670-1677.

45. Gendron RL, Baines MG. Immunohistochemical analysis of decidual natural killer cells during spontaneous abortion in mice. *Cell Immunol* 1988; 113:261-267.
46. Chaouat G. Placental immunoregulatory factors. *J Reprod Immunol* 1987; 10:179-188.
47. Bennett WA, Ellsaesser CF, Cowan BD. Hydatidiform mole macromolecules inhibit interleukin-2 mediated murine lymphocyte proliferation in vitro. *Amer J Reprod Immunol Microbiol* 1988, 18:76-80.
48. Clark DA, Damji N, Chaput A, Daya S, Rosenthal KL, Brierley J. Decidua-associated suppressor cells and suppressor factors regulating interleukin 2: their role in the survival of the "fetal allograft." In: Cinader B, Miller RG, eds. *Progress in Immunology VI*. New York: Academic Press, 1986:1089-1099.
49. Clark DA, Falbo M, Rowley RB, Banwatt D, Stedronska-Clark J. Active suppression of host-versus-graft reaction in pregnant mice. IX. Soluble suppressor activity obtained from allopregnant mouse decidua that blocks the response to interleukin 2 is related to TGF-beta. *J Immunol* 1988; 141:3833-3840.
50. Clark DA, Harley C, Book W, Flanders K. Suppressor factor in murine decidua is related to transforming growth factor beta-2. *Fed Proc* 1989; 3:A503.
51. Slapsys RM, Younglai E, Clark DA. A novel suppressor cell is recruited to decidua by fetal trophoblast-type cells. *Regional Immunol* 1988; 1:182-189.
52. Beer AE, Billingham RE. Host responses to intrauterine tissue, cellular and fetal allografts. *J Reprod Fertil* 1974; Suppl 21:59-88.
53. Sio J. Allograft reactivity and progesterone involvement at the choriodecidual junction. *Ph.D. Thesis*. Dallas (USA): Univ Texas, 1985.
54. Tsunawaki S, Sporn M, Ding A, Nathan C. Deactivation of macrophages by transforming growth factor-beta. *Nature* 1988; 334:260-262.
55. Sugarman BJ, Lewis GD, Eessalu TE, Aggarwal BB, Shepard HM. Effects of growth factors on the antiproliferative activity of tumor necrosis factors. *Cancer Res* 1987; 47:780-786.
56. Bensaid M, Tauber MT, Melecaze F, Prots H, Bayard F, Tauber JP. Effect of basic and acidic FGF and TGF-beta in controlling the proliferation of retinal capillary endothelial cells. *Acta Paed Scand* 1988;Suppl 343:230-231.
57. Jennings JC, Mohan S. Linkhart TA, Widstrom R, Baylink DJ. Comparison of the biologic actions of TGF beta-1 and TGF beta-2: differential activity in endothelial cells. *J Cell Physiol* 1988; 137:167-172.
58. Gronvik KO, Hoskin DW, Murgita RA. Monoclonal antibodies against murine neonatal and pregnancy-associated natural suppressor cells induce resorption of the fetus. *Scand J Immunol* 1987; 25:533-542.
59. Gambel P, Croy BA, Moore WD, Hunziker RD, Wegmann TG, Rossant J. Characterization of effector cells present in early murine decidua. *Cell Immunol* 1985; 93:303-314.
60. Hamilton MS, Hamilton BL. Environmental influences on immunologically associated spontaneous abortion in CBA/J mice. *J Reprod Immunol* 1987; 11:237-241.

HORMONAL DEPENDENCE OF THE METRIAL GLAND

D. Martel, M.N. Monier, V.J. De Feo* and A. Psychoyos

Laboratoire de Physiologie de la Reproduction
CNRS UA 549, Hôpital de Bicêtre, Bat. INSERM
78 rue du Général Leclerc
94270 Le Kremlin Bicêtre, France

*Department of Anatomy and Reproductive Biology
University of Hawaii, School of Medicine
Honolulu, Hawaii 96822 USA

The metrial gland develops in the mesometrial part of the uterus during pregnancy in the rat, or during pseudopregnancy after a traumatic decidualizing stimulus. In that case, the metrial gland becomes noticeable by day 5 after stimulation and grows considerably thereafter.[1-3] In the past, several functions have been postulated for the metrial gland, but there is now strong evidence that the granulated metrial gland cells differentiate from lymphocytes of bone marrow origin,[4,3] thus implicating this gland in the immunology of pregnancy. The development of this gland has been shown to be highly dependent on progesterone;[5,6] further, the concentration of the progesterone receptor has been shown to be elevated in this tissue during pseudopregnancy.[7]

The aim of the present study is to analyze the dependence of the metrial gland on ovarian steroidal hormones. The main aim is to attempt to understand how the progesterone response of this tissue can be maintained for a long period in a hormonal environment which is dominated by progesterone, since progesterone is known to down regulate its own receptor. For this purpose, rats were ovariectomized on day 13 of pseudopregnancy, when the gland had reached its maximal development, and were then submitted to hormonal therapy. The influences of estradiol and/or progesterone on the evolution of the metrial gland and on the tissue concentrations of estradiol and progesterone receptors were studied.

METHODS

Animals

On day 4 of pseudopregnancy (last day of estrus = day 0 of pseudopregnancy), rats were lightly anesthetized with ether and each uterine horn was injected with 50 µl of sesame oil via the cervical canals between 09:00 and 09:30 hrs. A *second* identical injection was given between 13:15 and 13:30 hrs. By giving animals two stimuli/cornu, the quality of tissue development which followed was found less variable and the tissue growth was two to three times greater than that obtained when using a knife-scratch traumatization. On day 13 of pseudopregnancy, animals were ovariectomized and received or did not receive implants of progesterone and/or estradiol.

Subcutaneous Implants

On the day of ovariectomy, six silastic implants each containing a 30 mm column of crystalline progesterone were introduced s.c.[8] These implants produced circulating plasma progesterone levels in the same range as those measured during pregnancy in the rat.

We found that it was difficult to induce a plasma estradiol concentration in the range of physiological values when ovariectomized animals received one s.c. implant filled with crystalline estradiol. We obtained better results when the implant was filled with a 30 mm column of estradiol dissolved in sesame oil. The amount of estradiol released can be simply and finely controlled by diluting the solu-

Table I. *Plasma estradiol and progesterone concentrations in pseudopregnant rats that underwent massive decidualization.*

	Plasma Progesterone nmol/l	Plasma Estradiol pmol/l
Pseudopregnant day 13		
Controls	202.38 ± 53.55	31.78 ± 9.47
Pseudopregnant day 17		
Controls	160.59 ± 63.31	25.36 ± 6.60
OVX	19.08 ± 6.07	32.70 ± 21.98
OVX plus P	238.40 ± 90.09	————
OVX plus E2 (1 mg/ml)	————	312.10 ± 43.30
OVX plus E2 (0.1 mg/ml)	————	77.65 ± 26.90
Pseudopregnant day 19		
Controls	163.77 ± 40.73	23.12 ± 4.22
OVX	23.59 ± 11.73	17.06 ± 5.69
OVX plus P	222.35 ± 49.35	————
OVX plus E2 (1 mg/ml)	————	298.55 ± 55.42
OVX plus E2 (0.1 mg/ml)	————	55.86 ± 2.57
Pseudopregnant day 21		
Controls	93.55 ± 41.34	37.98 ± 18.35
OVX	17.81 ± 8.36	16.11 ± 4.77
OVX plus P	212.87 ± 54.82	————
OVX plus E2 (1 mg/ml)	————	261.78 ± 33.40
OVX plus E2 (0.1 mg/ml)	————	59.23 ± 12.11

Values are means ± S.D. for 5 to 15 animals. OVX is ovariectomy on day 13 of pseudopregnancy; P is six progesterone implants on day 13 of pseudopregnancy; E2 is one estradiol implant on day 13 of pseudopregnancy.

tion in the implants. Thus, two types of estradiol implants have been tested: the implant contained either a 1 mg/ml or a 0.1 mg/ml estradiol solution.

Plasma Estradiol and Progesterone Measurements

Plasma samples were extracted twice with ether, and the steroid concentrations determined using commercial radioimmunoassays (Centre de l'Energie Atomique, Saclay, France).

Measurements of Estradiol and Progesterone Receptor Levels

The concentrations of the cytosoluble estradiol receptor were estimated from Scatchard plots[8] using estradiol as ligand, as previously described.[9] The concentrations of the nuclear estradiol receptor were estimated using an exchange assay.[7]

Concerning the progesterone receptor, the present work measures the concentration of the total KCl (0.5 mol/l)-soluble progesterone receptor (cytosol and nuclei). We did not measure the subcellular distribution of the receptor because of the rapid dissociation time of the natural ligand from its receptor in the rat ($t\frac{1}{2}$ = 8 min.). Thus, any variations in the times of preparation of the subcellular extracts would result in the dissociation of an unknown fraction of the nuclear complexes, and consequently, in a modification of the receptor repartition between the cytosolic and nuclear fractions. The concentrations of the progesterone receptor were measured in 0.5 mol/l KCl-extract of the tissue as described previously.[10] Briefly: after removal of endogenous progesterone (free and/or bound) with charcoal dextran suspension, the concentrations of the progesterone receptor were estimated from Scatchard plots,[8] using ORG 2058 as ligand.

The DNA content of the tissues were measured according to the procedure described by Burton,[11] and used for the expression of the receptor levels.

Statistical Analysis

All assessments of statistical significance were calculated using the Student's t-test.

EVOLUTION OF THE METRIAL GLAND DURING THE LAST WEEK OF PSEUDOPREGNANCY IN INTACT ANIMALS AND FOLLOWING OVARIECTOMY ON DAY 13

During the last week of pseudopregnancy, two phases can be distinguished in the evolution of the metrial gland in intact animals. During the first phase which lasts from day 13 to day 19 of pseudopregnancy the tissue was maintained and little variations were noted in the weight (Fig. 1). This phase was characterized by the absence of variation of the other parameters studied; the plasma progesterone levels were high ($\cong 175$ nmol/l) and the estradiol levels were low ($\cong 19$ pmol/l) at the limit of the assay. The concentration of the progesterone receptor in the tissue was high ($\cong 3$-4 fmol/μg DNA) and that of the estradiol receptor was low ($\cong 1.5$ fmol/μg DNA). The second phase, between day 19 and 21 of pseudopregnancy, coincided with the regression of the gland. The dramatic fall in the metrial gland weight (passing from 2000 to 200 mg) was accompanied by a significant decrease of the plasma progesterone level ($P < 0.001$) and by a slight but not significant increase of the estradiol plasma concentration. During this period, the concentration of the progesterone receptor decreased significantly ($P < 0.01$) in the gland to reach the value of $\cong 1.6$ fmol/μg DNA. No variation was observed in the concentration of the estradiol receptor which remains low in the tissue.

Ovariectomy on day 13 of pseudopregnancy was followed by rapid regression of the gland, similar to that occurring at the end of pseudopregnancy. This observation confirms in the rat, the hormonal dependency of the gland. The fall in the plasma concentration was more marked for progesterone (passing from 202 to 19 nmol/l before and after ovariectomy) than for estradiol (passing from 32 to 16 pmol/l). Ovariectomy resulted in the total disappearance of the progesterone receptor from the tissue and surprisingly, in a persistent increase in tissue estradiol receptor

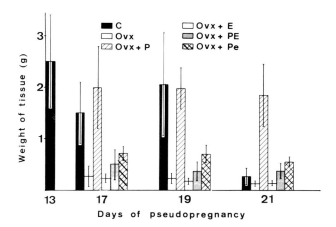

Figure 1. Metrial gland weight (means ± S.D.; both cornua) in pseudopregnant rats that underwent massive decidualization. C, control group; OVX, after ovariectomy on day 13 of pseudopregnancy; OVX, followed by hormonal treatment; P, six progesterone implants; e, one 0.1 mg/ml estradiol implant; E, one 1 mg/ml estradiol implant. In each group separate samples from 5 to 15 animals were measured.

concentration, most of this receptor being present in a cytosoluble form (Fig. 2). It thus appears that receptors for both hormones are not regulated in the same way. The results suggested that the production of the estrogen receptor was repressed before the ovariectomy. It can be suggested that it was under the influence of the high levels of progesterone.

EVOLUTION OF THE METRIAL GLAND FOLLOWING OVARIECTOMY ON DAY 13 OF PSEUDOPREGNANCY AND HORMONAL REPLACEMENT

Supplementation With Progesterone or Estradiol

Animals ovariectomized on day 13 of pseudopregnancy and given six s.c. implants of progesterone exhibited a stable and high plasma concentration of progesterone of $\cong 225$ nmol/l. This mean value was slightly higher than that measured in the control groups between day 13 and 19 of pseudopregnancy (Table I). The supplementation with progesterone totally abolished the effects of ovariectomy on the metrial gland weight (Fig. 1) and on progesterone and estradiol receptor contents in the tissue (Fig. 2). Thus, for these three parameters there were no significant differences between the control groups on days 17 and 19 of pseudopregnancy and the progesterone treated groups on days 17, 19, and 21. In contrast to deciduo-

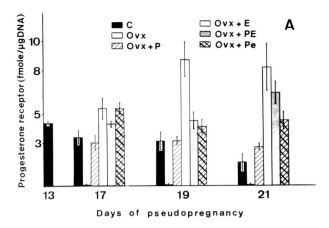

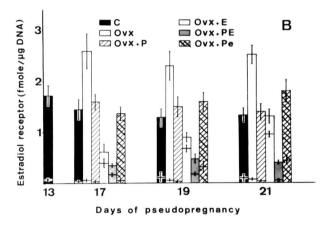

Figure 2. A. *Changes (means ± S.D.) in the total (nuclear and cytosolic) KCl (0.5 mol/l)-soluble progesterone receptor concentrations in the metrial gland.* B. *Changes of estradiol receptor concentrations in the metrial gland; the total heights of the columns are the values of total receptor concentrations (cytosoluble and nuclear) and the internal columns are values of the nuclear receptor concentrations. The groups were C, control group, normal pseudopregnant rats that underwent massive decidualization; OVX, after ovariectomy on day 13 of pseudopregnancy, and after OVX on day 13 of pseudopregnancy followed by hormonal treatment; P, six progesterone implants; e, one 0.1 mg/ml estradiol implant; E, one 1 mg/ml estradiol implant. In each group separate samples from 5 to 15 animals were measured.*

mata, which regress spontaneously even if progesterone is given,[1,2] the metrial gland is perfectly maintained as long as progesterone is given well after the period of normal regression in intact animals.

Animals ovariectomized on day 13 of pseuodpregnancy and given one s.c. implant containing an estradiol solution of 1 mg/ml showed a constant and high plasma concentration of estradiol ($\cong$ 262-312 pmol/l) (Table I). The estradiol treatment failed to prevent the metrial gland regression which followed the ovariectomy (Fig. 1). The weights of the gland in treated animals were not significantly different from those of ovariectomized animals. In contrast, the estradiol prevented the progesterone receptor disappearance observed after overiectomy, and in spite of the tissue regression, it induced a gradual increase of the progesterone receptor concentrations which became significantly higher than those measured in the corresponding intact animals. The estradiol receptor concentration in the metrial gland decreased soon (on day 17) after estradiol replacement and a gradual increase occurred thereafter, most ($\cong$ 80%) of the total estradiol receptor was found in the cell nuclei. In all cases the total levels reached remained low, indicating that estrogen receptor is poorly expressed in this tissue.

Supplementation With Progesterone and Estradiol

Because estradiol treatment after ovariectomy on day 13 of pseudopregnancy had induced a significant increase in the progesterone receptor concentration, it was expected that the effect of progesterone on the metrial gland would be enhanced by a simultaneous estradiol treatment.

In this set of experiments two types of s.c. estradiol implants were tested. Animals received, together with the six progesterone implants, either a high-dose estradiol implant (1 mg/ml) which resulted in estradiol circulating levels of $\cong$ 290 pmol/l, or a low-dose estradiol implant resulting in estradiol circulating levels of 64 pmol/l. Even with the low-dose estradiol implant, the plasma estradiol concentrations were higher than those found in the corresponding pseudopregnant groups. Both treatments resulted in a reduction in the size of the gland which was dose dependent; the highest estradiol dose resulting in the highest size reduction. However, the metrial gland weight loss after treatment with the low dose was already considerable, indicating that the tissue was highly sensitive to estradiol. Treatment associating progesterone with the low dose of estradiol maintained or slightly increased (after a week of treatment) both the estradiol and the progesterone receptor concentrations in the tissue. Treatment associating progesterone with the high dose of estradiol resulted in opposite effects on both receptors: estradiol receptor content which was already low was dramatically decreased and progesterone receptor content was significantly increased. It is obvious from our results that in spite of the fact that estradiol increases the progesterone receptor content in the gland, both hormones exert antagonistic effects on the size of the gland.

CONCLUSIONS

Our results demonstrate that maintenance of the metrial gland appears to be strictly dependent on progesterone. What is intriguing, however, is the presence of a stable and high level of progesterone receptor ($\cong 3$ fmol/μg DNA) in the metrial gland of animals that were maintained on progesterone alone. Thus it appears that in this tissue progesterone does not down regulate its own receptor as has been described for other uterine tissues.[12,13] Further, in this system, progesterone receptor production which is, of course, over increased by estradiol treatment as described for other uterine tissue, does not require the presence of estradiol in order to be maintained. An attractive hypothesis is that the progesterone receptor is constitutively produced, as has already been described[14] in the hamster uterus under sustained progesterone treatment.

Not only is estradiol not required to maintain the progesterone response, but also its action results in a reduction of the size of the gland. Based on the observation that circulating estrogen levels are not negligible during pregnancy, it can be suggested that estradiol during normal pregnancy may serve to modulate the system by controlling the proliferation of the gland. The balance between progesterone and estradiol may be crucial in the immunology of pregnancy in light of the unfolding role of granulated metrial gland cells in the process.[3,15]

References

1. De Feo VJ. Decidualization. In: Wynn RM ed. *Cellular biology of the uterus.* 1967:191-290.
2. Finn C, Porter DG. *The uterus.* London: *Elek Sciences* 1975:74-85.
3. Bulmer D, Peel S, Stewart I. The metrial gland—a review. *Cell differentiation* 1987; 20:77-86.
4. Peel S, Stewart I. The differentiation of granulated metrial gland cells in chimeric mice and the effect of uterine shielding during irradiation. *J Anat* 1984; 139:593-598.
5. Sely H, Borduas A, Masson G. Studies concerning the hormonal control of deciduomata and metrial glands. *Anatomical Record* 1942; 82:199-210.
6. Sharma R, Bulmer D, Peel S. Effects of exogenous progesterone following ovariectomy on the metrial glands of pregnant mice. *J Anat* 1986; 144:189-199.
7. Martel D, Monier MN, Psychoyos A, De Feo VJ. Estrogen and progesterone receptors in the endometrium, myometrium and metrial gland of the rat following decidualization process. *Endocrinology* 1984; 1627-1633.
8. Bridges RG. A quantitative analysis of the role of dosage, sequence and duration of estradiol and progesterone exposure in the regulation of maternal behavior in the rat. *Endocrinology* 1984; 114:930-940.
9. Martel D, Psychoyos A. Progesterone induced estrogen receptor in the rat uterus. *J Endocrinol* 1978; 76:145-154.
10. Martel D, Monier MN, Roche D, De Feo VJ, Psychoyos A. Hormonal dependence of the metrial gland: further studies on estradiol and progesterone receptor levels in the rat. *J Endocr* 1988; 120:465-472.
11. Burton K. A study of the conditions and mechanism of the diphenylamine reaction for the colorimetric examination of deoxyribonucleic acid. *Biochem J* 1956: 117:433-450.
12. Milgrom E, Luu Thi MT, Atger M, Baulieu EE. Mechanism regulating the concentration of progesterone receptor(s) in the uterus. *J Biol Chem* 1973; 248:6366-6374.
13. Walters MR, Clark KJH. Cytosol and nuclear compartmentalization of progesterone receptor of the rat uterus. *Endocrinology* 1978; 103:601-603.
14. Okulicz WC. Progesterone receptor replenishment during sustained progesterone treatment in the hamster uterus. *Endocrinology* 1986; 188:2488-2494.
15. Parr EL, Parr MB, Din-E Young J. Localization of a pore forming protein (perforin) in granulated metrial gland cells. *Biol Reprod* 1987; 37:1327-1335.

A POSSIBLE IMMUNOLOGICAL ACTION MECHANISM OF OVINE TROPHOBLAST PROTEIN-1 (oTP-1)

Koji Yoshinaga

Reproductive Sciences Branch
Center for Population Research
NICHD, National Institutes of Health
Bethesda, Maryland 20892 USA

IT has been documented in the sheep and cow that the embryonic signal for maternal recognition of pregnancy is mainly a protein produced by the trophoblast cells of the blastocyst (see Dr. Roberts' article in this volume). The protein is named oTP-1 in the sheep and bTP-1 in the cow. The mechanism of action of oTP-1 has been shown to rescue the corpus luteum of the fertile cycle from luteolysis by preventing the release of a potent luteolytic factor, prostaglandin F_2-α from the endometrial epithelial cells. Besides this endocrine action mechanism, oTP-1 has been suggested to exert immunological action to secure the establishment of pregnancy. In this article, I will suggest a possible immunological action mechanism of oTP-1.

SIMILARITY OF BLASTOCYST IMPLANTATION TO TUMOR METASTASIS

Blastocyst implantation and tumor metastasis are similar in terms of one biological phenomenon, namely, translocation of specialized cells through, or invasion of, established tissues. In metastasis, tumor cells translocate through and invade a variety of tissues. While, in blastocyst implantation, trophoblast cells attach the luminal surface of the endometrial epithelial cells and exert a variety of invasive activities, the degree of which varies depending on the species of animals (see Dr. Finn's article in this volume).

Immunologically, the implanting blastocyst behaves as if it is "self" and not "foreign" because the maternal system does not immunologically reject it. When mouse, rat, or rabbit blastocysts are collected from the uterus of one animal and transferred into the uterus appropriately conditioned with ovarian steroid hormones of another animal of the same species, these blastocysts implant into the host uterus, continue to develop until term, and the babies will be delivered. Thus, antigenicity of the transferred blastocysts is masked by some mechanism.

When malignant tumor cells are innoculated to a host animal, the tumor cells are not rejected by the host and metastasis takes place. On the basis of this similarity, one may equate the question "what makes a tumor cell metastatic?" to "what makes a blastocyst implant?"

IMMUNOLOGICAL MECHANISM OF TUMOR METASTASIS

Each living cell is said to have an immunological marker on its surface (the major histocompatibility complex). When a living cell is transplanted into a living individual, its immunological surveillance system checks the marker of the cell and decides whether the cell is "self" or "foreign." When it is determined to be "foreign," cytotoxic or "killer" T lymphocytes attack the cell and it is destroyed. Therefore, the immunological marker plays an important role in tumor metastasis and blastocyst implantation.

In their comprehensive article, Feldman and Eisenbach[1] explain the relationship between the composition of the marker, namely, major histocompatibility complex component molecules, and the metastatic ability of the tumor cells when they are transplanted into a mouse. There are two types of cell surface molecules (H-2D and H-2K) that decide whether or not a tumor cell is to be metastatic, that is, to make the cell look like a "self" or leave it as a "foreign" cell. In normal cells there is a certain ratio of the amounts of H-2D and H-2K on the cell surface, and the immune surveillance system recognizes this ratio as "foreign." On a highly malignant tumor cell (D122), on the other hand, most of the surface molecules are H-2D; a few H-2K molecules are found on the cell. These cells with H-2D molecules on the surface are metastatic and, therefore, the host immune system does not recognize them as "foreign." Since these cell surface molecules are produced by transcription of the respective genes, one can manipulate the amount of surface molecules by introducing these genes. When the H-2K gene is inserted into the DNA of highly metastatic D122 cells, the inserted H-2K gene promotes the production of H-2K molecules, resulting in a significant change in the H-2D/H-2K ratio. Thus, the transgenic D122 cells lose their metastatic ability.

The most interesting finding pertinent to this topic, described in the same article by Feldman and Eisenbach is that, when ordinarily non-metastasizing A9 cells are treated with a combination of interferons alpha and beta, the H-2D gene is switched on more than the H-2K gene, more H-2D molecules are produced, and the cells become metastatic. On the other hand, interferon gamma switches on the H-2K gene and the treated D122 cells become less metastatic.

DOES oTP-1 PROMOTE H-2D?

If the immunological role of oTP-1 in sheep implantation is similar to that of interferon alpha and beta in mouse tumor cells, it is conceivable that the oTP-1 produced by trophoblast cells act on themselves as an autocrine, stimulating the production of cell surface molecules equivalent to the mouse H-2D through activation of the corresponding gene. Like metastatic tumor cells, sheep trophoblast cells may be masked with molecules equivalent to the mouse H-2D. If so, the blastocyst, which is about to invade or interact with the uterine endometrium, may be sending the signal that it is not "foreign," but is a part of the mother.

Whether this possible mechanism actually operates during sheep implantation remains to be investigated. Many experiments can be designed. But, if one can prevent implantation of sheep blastocyst by treating locally with interferon gamma, close examination of the sheep trophoblast major histocompatibility molecules would appear to be warranted.

References

1. Feldman M, Eisenbach L. What makes a tumor cell metastatic? *Scientific American* November, 1988, 60-85.

SECTION V: MAINTENANCE OF PREGNANCY

ROLE OF THE MAMMALIAN CORPUS LUTEUM IN THE MAINTENANCE OF EARLY PREGNANCY

Rodney A. Mead

Department of Biological Sciences
University of Idaho
Moscow, Idaho 83843 USA

IT has long been recognized that bilateral ovariectomy of mammals within a few days after conception results in termination of pregnancy (see 1 for review). Fraenkel[2] was the first of several investigators to extirpate the corpora lutea (CL) from mammals, thereby providing experimental evidence that this ovarian compartment was essential for the maintenance of pregnancy. The pioneering studies of Allen and Corner[3] demonstrated that luteal extracts could maintain pregnancy in ovariectomized rabbits and virtually all studies have implicated progesterone as being the primary luteal product responsible for the maintenance of pregnancy. However, progesterone is not the only luteal secretory product. Estrogens, prostaglandins, relaxin, oxytocin, basic fibroblast growth factor, angiogenic factor(s), and a luteal implantation factor have been reported to be secretory products of the corpus luteum of various eutherian mammals. The primary objective of this review will be to explore the role of progesterone, relaxin, and a luteal implantation factor in the maintenance of early pregnancy.

PROGESTERONE

Effects on Oviductal Functions

Prior to and immediately after ovulation, the female reproductive tract is predominantly under the influence of estrogen, which stimulates synthesis of receptor sites for itself and for progesterone.[4,5] Formation of the CL results in increased progesterone secretion and reduction in estrogen levels. One of the first effects of progesterone is to modulate the action of estrogen by inhibiting replenishment of both cytoplasmic and nuclear estrogen receptors in the uterus of rodents.[6,7,8] In the oviduct, nuclear estrogen receptor levels are higher during the follicular phase than during the luteal phase of the cycle,[9] thus suggesting that progesterone may also modulate estrogen receptor concentration in the oviduct. Consequently, one would predict that neutralization of progesterone in early pregnancy would modify oviductal secretion and motility and thus might alter the rate of embryonic development and/or tubal transport. Several lines of evidence suggest that this is the case. Oviductal fluid secretion is maximal during estrus in rabbits, sheep, and pigs and during peak vaginal cornification in the rhesus monkey, but it is greatly reduced during the luteal phase.[10] Estrogen induces increased formation of oviductal fluid and stimulates synthesis of sulphated glycoproteins in ovariectomized rabbits, whereas progesterone causes the release of these proteins and an overall reduction in oviductal fluid formation.[10,11] Therefore the volume and composition of the medium in which early mammalian embryonic development occurs is in part controlled by progesterone. Post-coital administration of antiprogesterone monoclonal antibodies to mice or ferrets resulted in developmental arrest of most embryos prior to cavitation.[12,13] These results have been interpreted as indicating that neutralization of progesterone resulted in the formation of an unfavorable oviductal environment as *in vitro* culture of mouse embryos in the presence of the monoclonal antibody did not inhibit cleavage.[12] Stone and Hamner[14] reported that few zygotes developed to morulae when retained in oviducts of ovariectomized-estrogen-treated rabbits whereas normal cleavage was obtained when zygotes were retained in ovariectomized or ovariectomized-progesterone-treated does. Other experiments suggested the presence of an estrogen induced low molecular weight inhibitor of embryo development in oviductal fluid.[15] Thus it would appear that one of the early actions of progesterone in the maintenance of pregnancy is to modulate the inhibitory effects of estrogen and thereby provide an oviductal environment which is conducive to cleavage.

Alteration of tubal transport and the subsequent interruption of pregnancy by administration of pharmacological doses of steroids has been reported by several investigators.[1,7,6] Conversely, neutralization of progesterone by monoclonal antibodies had little or no effect on rate of tubal transport in mice or ferrets.[12,13] However, the antibodies were not administered until 22 hrs (in mice) to 46 hrs (in ferrets) after ovulation. Consequently, the complete role played by progesterone in modulating tubal transport and the delivery of the embryo to the uterus at the most favorable time still remains to be determined.

Effect on Blocking Further Ovulations

It is now well recognized that another important early action of progesterone in most mammals is to inhibit further ovulations (see 17 for review). Progesterone is believed to exert its inhibitory effect on ovulation by altering gonadotropin releasing hormone (GnRH) secretion from the hypothalamus,[18] and perhaps more importantly, by reducing pituitary responsiveness to GnRH, thereby suppressing the preovulatory luteinizing hormone surge.[19-21] Moderately high physiological levels of progesterone are required to prevent ovulation. This fact is nicely demonstrated in pregnant mink, which return to estrus within 6 to 10 days after ovulation and will ovulate for a second time if permitted to copulate.[22] This occurs because CL from the first ovulation are not yet fully functional and secrete insufficient progesterone to inhibit ovulation.[23]

Effects of Progesterone on Uterine Physiology

Progesterone enhances long-term embryo viability as indicated by its ability to maintain blastocyst survival for 45 days in ovariectomized-progesterone-treated rats. These embryos subsequently implanted when exposed to a low dose of estrogen.[24] Nutting and Meyer[25] reported a dose dependent increase in embryo viability when progesterone was administered to ovariectomized rats. Similar results have been reported for mice[26] and a variety of species exhibiting obligate delay of implantation.[27] This effect is postulated to be indirectly mediated through the action of progesterone on the uterus rather than through a direct effect on the blastocyst.[28,29] Although the precise mechanism by which progesterone achieves increased embryo viability is currently unknown, several non-mutually exclusive possibilities exist. Progesterone might modulate or inhibit synthesis of estrogen induced uterine or oviductal specific proteins, some of which may be detrimental to the embryos, by preventing replenishment of estrogen receptors.[7] Alternatively, progesterone can stimulate the synthesis and secretion of uterine specific proteins which might enhance embryo viability (see 30 for review). Some progesterone-induced uterine specific proteins, such as uteroferrin, uteroglobin, and retinol-binding protein, are believed to transfer products from the maternal system to the fetus. Others appear to act as potent inhibitors of protease activity.[31-34] It is also presumed that proteins from the uterine lumen can contribute to the overall nutritional requirements of the embryo. Lysozyme presumably exerts a bactericidal effect[30,35] whereas others may exert an immunosuppressive effect.[36,37] Uteroglobin may play an immunosuppressive role by masking antigens on the surface of the embryo, suppressing chemotaxis and phagocytic activity of leukocytes, and by inhibiting phospholipase-A_2 and thrombin-induced platelet aggregation (see 38 for review). Alternatively, uteroglobin's immunosuppressive action could be due to its ability to bind and maintain high intrauterine levels of progesterone as Siiteri et al.[39] have proposed that progesterone might exert a local immunosuppressive effect and thus prevent rejection of the embryo. It has also been reported that progesterone induces a 10-fold increase in the selective movement of IgG into the uterine lumen of rats possessing decidual tissue.[40] It has been suggested that IgG might coat the blastocyst and mask its foreign antigens or prevent complement fixation. However, virtually all reports of immunosuppression by numerous endogenous substances that are present during pregnancy rest on inadequately tested assumptions and/or results from *in vitro* experiments.[41]

Effect of Progesterone on Uterine Contractility

Excessive uterine motility can lead to expulsion of unimplanted embryos, hasten transport of embryos to the uterus such that embryonic and uterine development are out of synchrony, or dislodge the placenta and thus terminate pregnancy. Progesterone may act in a variety of ways to decrease the response of the myometrium to numerous compounds which enhance uterine contractility. Progesterone can inhibit replenishment of nuclear estrogen receptors which are presumably required for estrogen to enhance uterine motility via up regulation of oxytocin,[42] angiotensin II,[43] and adrenergic receptors.[44] Moreover, progesterone reportedly decreases uterine receptor sites for each of the above compounds, although it is not clear whether it does so directly or through its action on estrogen receptors. Other mechanisms by which progesterone has been proposed to induce refractoriness to myometrial excitation include reduction of intracellular Ca^{++}[45] and inhibition of myometrial cyclooxygenase and/or synthetase systems of rats.[46] Thus the net effect of increased levels of progesterone during pregnancy is to decrease the overall sensitivity of the uterus to a variety of known stimulants to uterine contractility and thus aid in retention of the developing embryos within the uterus.

Effect of Progesterone on Decidual Formation

During pregnancy, progesterone acts on the estrogen-primed endometrium of rodents to shift mitotic division from the uterine epithelium to the stroma. The ability of progesterone to stimulate proliferation of the endometrial stroma is obviously of paramount importance in the attainment of uterine sensitivity to decidualization.[47,48] The essentiality of progesterone in the development of the decidual response has recently been reconfirmed by administration of anti-progesterone monoclonal antibodies to pregnant mice. This blocked the expected increase in endometrial stromal cell mitotic activity, prevented increased endometrial vascular permeability at the normal time, inhibited decidualization, and ultimately prevented implantation.[49,50] Prostaglandins, presumably PGE_2, are essential for increased endometrial vascular permeability and induction of decidualization in rodents and rabbits (see 51 for review). Pretreatment with progesterone is essential for estrogens to maximally stimulate uterine prostaglandin synthesis in ovariectomized rats.[52] Consequently, insufficient prostaglandin synthesis in the absence of progesterone might account for the observed decrease in vascular permeability prior to implantation and failure of stromal cells to decidualize.

RELAXIN

Relaxin is known to be secreted by the CL of pigs, rats, cows, and humans during pregnancy and by the fetoplacental unit of other species.[53] In most species, immunoreactive levels of relaxin are not detectable in plasma until the latter half of pregnancy, whereas plasma levels are elevated throughout most of pregnancy in primates.[53] It has long been known that relaxin suppresses uterine motility and this may be its primary function during early pregnancy in primates. Relaxin has been reported to induce a rapid efflux of radiolabeled Ca^{++}, decrease activity of myosin light chain kinase, and increase intracellular levels of cAMP in rat myometrial cells, all of which are correlated with reduced uterine contractility.[54-56] Administration of relaxin prior to implantation results in irregular spacing of blastocysts, interference with the normal antimesometrial positioning of the embryos, and reduction of the decidual cell response in rats.[57,58] Such observations may explain why relaxin has not been detected in the peripheral circulation of any species prior to implantation. Relaxin has also been demonstrated to promote uterine growth and distensibility by increasing uterine water and glycogen content and altering the fluid matrix of the connective tissue framework of both the endometrium and myometrium of rats.[59-61] Thus relaxin may play an important role in the ability of the uterus to accommodate the developing fetus during the latter half of pregnancy.

LUTEAL IMPLANTATION FACTOR

Corpora lutea of mustelid carnivores play an additional role in the maintenance of pregnancy in that they appear to secrete a nonsteroidal hormone that is essential for successful induction of blastocyst implantation.[62,63] Administration of progesterone alone or in combination with estrogens to intact or ovariectomized mink, European badgers, long-tailed and short-tailed weasels, and western spotted skunks during the period of delayed implantation has consistently failed to induce nidation (see 62 for review). Yet the CL are the only ovarian compartment in these species that undergo a dramatic change in both structure and function prior to implantation, thus suggesting that they secrete some factor which is required for nidation.[62] Blastocyst implantation will occur at the normal time in ferrets, which do not exhibit delayed implantation, that have been ovariectomized on day 8 of pregnancy and treated with progesterone. However, if ovariectomy is performed on day 6 implantation, as evidenced by the attachment of the trophoblast to the uterine epithelium, it cannot be induced with progesterone alone or in combination with estrogens.[64,65] Wu and Chang interpreted these results to indicate that there was a critical period of ovarian function that occurred between days 6 and 8 of pregnancy, during which the ovaries secreted some factor in addition to progesterone that was essential to induce nidation.[64] We have subsequently demonstrated that implantation will occur in both ferrets and mink bearing ectopic CL that have been ovariectomized on day 6.[65,66] Such experiments unequivocally establish the essential role played by the CL. Detailed studies of steroid metabolism in CL of spotted skunks and ferrets suggest that the CL of these species have exceedingly limited capability to synthesize steroids other than progesterone, but can convert androgens obtained from other sources to estrogens.[62] This suggests that something other than steroids may be involved as estrogen and/or progesterone will not induce implantation. We have recently demonstrated that aqueous extracts of CL obtained from ferrets on day 9 of pseudopregnancy will induce implantation in ferrets that have been ovariectomized on day 6 of pregnancy and treated with progesterone. However, identically prepared extracts of nonluteal ovarian tissue had no effect on implantation. The active factor is retained on ultrafiltration membranes with a MW cutoff of 50,000 and its biological activity is destroyed when treated with a broad spectrum protease.[63] Biological activity is retained after DEAE anion exchange or gel filtration chromatography and after preparative isoelectric focusing. Results from the latter procedure suggest that the factor is a basic protein. Nothing is currently known about the site or mode of action of this factor. It might act directly upon the blastocyst. Alternatively, it may act on the uterus to create an environment that is more conducive to continued embryonic development and implantation.

SUMMARY

This brief review of the recent literature clearly indicates that several hormones secreted by the CL participate in the establishment and maintenance of early pregnancy in mammals. Our understanding of the various events in pregnancy that are affected by these hormones has been enhanced by new techniques which selectively remove a single hormone. Many of the sites of action of these hormones are now known. Although many hypotheses have been advanced to explain the way in which these hormones act to maintain pregnancy, much more work will be required to determine which hypotheses are correct, which mechanisms are species specific, and which are applicable to most mammals.

Acknowledgment

A portion of this work has been supported by a grant from the National Institute of Child Health and Human Development (HD 06556).

References

1. Amoroso EC, Finn CA. Ovarian activity during gestation, ovum transport and implantation. In: Zuckerman S, Mandl AM, Eckstein P, eds. *The ovary.* New York: Academic Press, 1962:451-537.
2. Fraenkel L. Die Function des Corpus luteum. *Arch Gynaek* 1903; 68:438-535.
3. Allen WM, Corner GW. Physiology of the corpus luteum. III. Normal growth and implantation of the embryos after very early ablation of the ovaries, under the influence of extracts of the corpus luteum. *Am J Physiol* 1929; 88:340-346.
4. Sarff M, Gorski J. Control of estrogen binding protein under basal conditions and after estrogen administration. *Biochemistry* 1971; 10:2257-2263.
5. Leavitt WW, Toft DO, Strott CA, O'Malley BW. A specific progesterone receptor in the hamster uterus: physiological properties and regulation during the estrous cycle. *Endocrinology* 1974; 94:1041-1053.
6. Clark JH, Hsueh AJW, Peck EJ Jr. Regulation of estrogen receptor replenishment by progesterone. *Annals NY Acad Sci* 1977; 286:161-179.
7. Evans RW, Leavitt WW. Progesterone action in hamster uterus: rapid inhibition of ³H-estradiol retention by nuclear fraction. *Endocrinology* 1980; 107:1261-1263.
8. Leavitt WW, MacDonald RG, Okulicz WC. Hormonal regulation of estrogen and progesterone receptor systems. In: Litwack G, ed. *Biochemical actions of hormones.* Vol. 10 New York: Academic Press, 1983:323-356.
9. West NB, Brenner RM. Estrogen receptor levels in the oviducts and endometria of cynomolgus macaques during the menstrual cycle. *Biol Reprod* 1983; 29:1303-1312.
10. Hamner CE, Fox SB. Biochemistry of oviductal secretions. In: Hafez ESE, Blandau RJ, eds. *The mammalian oviduct comparative biology and methodology.* Chicago: University of Chicago Press, 1969:333-355.
11. Greenwald GC. Endocrine regulation of the secretion of mucin in the tubal epithelium of the rabbit. *Anat Rec* 1958; 130:447-495.
12. Rider V, Heap RB, Wang MY, Feinstein A. Antiprogesterone monoclonal antibody affects early cleavage and implantation in the mouse by mechanisms that are influenced by genotype. *J Reprod Fertil* 1987; 79:33-43.
13. Rider V, Heap RB. Heterologous antiprogesterone monoclonal antibody arrests early embryonic development and implantation in the ferret (*Mustela putorius*). *J Reprod Fertil* 1986; 76:459-470.
14. Stone SL, Hamner CE. Hormonal and regional influences of the oviduct on the development of rabbit embryos. *Biol*

Reprod 1977; 16:638-646.
15. Stone SL, Richardson LL, Hamner CE, Oliphant G. Partial characterization of hormone-mediated inhibition of embryo development in rabbit oviduct fluid. *Biol Reprod* 1977; 16:647-653.
16. Pauerstein CJ, Hodgson BJ, Kramen MA. The anatomy and physiology of the oviduct. In Wynn RM, ed. *Obstetrics and gynecology annual.* New York: Appleton-Century-Crofts, 1974:137-201.
17. Rothchild I. Interrelations between progesterone and the ovary, pituitary, and central nervous system in the control of ovulation and the regulation of progesterone secretion. *Vitamins and Hormones* 1965; 23:209-325.
18. Ramirez VD, Kim K, Dluzen D. Progesterone action on the LHRH and nigrostriatal dopamine neuronal systems: *in vitro* and *in vivo* studies. *Recent Prog Horm Res* 1985; 41:421-472.
19. Hilliard J, Schally AV, Sawyer CH. Progesterone blockade of the ovulatory response to intrapituitary infusion of LH-RH in rabbits. *Endocrinology* 1971; 88:730-736.
20. Labrie F, Drouin J, Lean AD, Lagace L, Ferland L, Beaulieu M. Mechanism of action of luteinizing hormone releasing hormone and thyrotropin releasing hormone in the anterior pituitary gland and modulation of their activity by peripheral hormones. In: Porter JC, ed. *Hypothalamic peptide hormones and pituitary regulation. Advances in experimental medicine and biology.* New York: Plenum Press, 1977:157-179.
21. Batra SK, Miller WL. Progesterone decreases the responsiveness of ovine pituitary cultures to luteinizing hormone-releasing hormone. *Endocrinology* 1985; 117:1436-1440.
22. Hansson A. The physiology of reproduction in mink (*Mustela vison*, Schreb.) with special reference to delayed implantation. *Acta Zool* 1947; 28:1-136.
23. Moller OM. The progesterone concentrations in the peripheral plasma of the mink (*Mustela vison*) during pregnancy. *J Endocrinol* 1973; 56:121-132.
24. Cochrane RL, Meyer RK. Delayed nidation in the rat induced by progesterone. *Proc Soc Exp Biol Med* 1957; 96:155-159.
25. Nutting EF, Meyer RK. Implantation delay, nidation, and embryonal survival in rats treated with ovarian hormones. In: Enders AC, ed. *Delayed implantation.* Chicago: University of Chicago Press, 1963:233-252.
26. Weitlauf HM. Effect of progesterone on survival of blastocysts in the uteri of ovariectomized mice. *J Endocrinol* 1971; 51:375-380.
27. Mead RA, Concannon PW, McRae M. Effect of progestins on implantation in the western spotted skunk. *Biol Reprod* 1981; 25:128-133.
28. Dickmann Z. Hormonal requirements for the survival of blastocysts in the uterus of the rat. *J Endocrinol* 1967; 37:455-461.
29. Weitlauf HM. Protein synthesis by blastocysts in the uteri and oviducts of intact and hypophysectomized mice. *J Exp Zool* 1971; 176:35-40.
30. Roberts RM, Bazer FW. The functions of uterine secretions. *J Reprod Fertil* 1988; 82:875-892.
31. Mullins DE, Bazer FW, Roberts RM. Secretion of a progesterone-induced inhibitor of plasminogen activator by the porcine uterus. *Cell* 1980; 20:865-872.
32. Fazleabas AT, Bazer FW, Roberts RM. Purification and properties of a progesterone-induced plasmin/trypsin inhibitor from uterine secretions of pigs and its immunochemical localization in the pregnant uterus. *J Biol Chem* 1982; 257:6886-6897.
33. Fazleabas AT, Geisert RD, Bazer FW, Roberts RM. The relationship between the release of plasminogen activator and estrogen by blastocysts and secretion of plasmin inhibitor by uterine endometrium in the pregnant pig. *Biol Reprod* 1983; 29:225-238.
34. Fazleabas AT, Mead RA, Rourke AW, Roberts RM. Presence of an inhibitor of plasminogen activator in uterine fluid of the western spotted skunk during delayed implantation. *Biol Reprod* 1984; 30:311-322.
35. Roberts RM, Bazer FW, Baldwin N, Pollard WE. Induction of lysozyme and leucine amino-peptidase activities in the uterine flushings of pigs by progesterone. *Archs Biochem Biophys* 1976; 177:499-507.
36. Murray FA, Segerson EC, Brown FT. Suppression of lymphocytes *in vitro* by porcine uterine secretory protein. *Biol Reprod* 1978; 19:15-25.
37. Hansen PJ, Segerson EC, Bazer FW. Characterization of immunosuppressive substances in the basic protein fraction of uterine secretions from pregnant ewes. *Biol Reprod* 1987; 36:393-404.
38. Miele L, Cordella-Miele E, Mukherjee AB. Uteroglobin: structure, molecular biology, and new perspectives on its function as a phospholipase A2 inhibitor. *Endocr Rev* 1987; 8:474-490.
39. Siiteri PK, Febres F, Clemens LE, Chang RJ, Gondos B, Stites D. Progesterone and maintenance of pregnancy: is progesterone nature's immunosuppressant? *Ann NY Acad Sci* 1977; 286:384-397.
40. Stern JE, Wira CR. Immunoglobulin and secretory component regulation in the rat uterus at the time of decidualization. *Endocrinology* 1986; 119:2427-2432.
41. Gill TJ III. Immunological and genetic factors influencing pregnancy. In: Knobil E, Neill, JD, eds. *The physiology of reproduction.* New York: Raven Press, 1988; 2:2033-2042.

42. Nissenson R, Flouret G, Hechter O. Opposing effects of estradiol and progesterone on oxytocin receptors in rabbit uterus. *Proc Natl Acad Sci USA* 1978; 75:2044-2048.
43. Schirar A, Capponi A, Catt KJ. Regulation of uterine angiotensin II receptors by estrogen and progesterone. *Endocrinology* 1980; 106:5-12.
44. Williams LT, Lefkowitz RJ. Regulation of rabbit myometrial alpha adrenergic receptors by estrogen and progesterone. *J Clin Invest* 1977; 60:815-818.
45. Csapo AI. The "see-saw" theory of parturition. In: Knight J, O'Connor M, eds. *The fetus and birth*. A Ciba Foundation Symposium. Amsterdam: Elsevier, 1977:159-195.
46. Jeremy JY, Dandona P. RU 486 antagonizes the inhibitory action of progesterone on prostacyclin and thromboxane A_2 synthesis in cultured rat myometrial explants. *Endocrinology* 1986; 119:655-660.
47. Finn CA, Martin L. The control of implantation. *J Reprod Fertil* 1974; 39:195-205.
48. Glasser SR, Clark JH. A determinant role for progesterone in the development of uterine sensitivity to decidualization and ovo-implantation. In: Markert CL, Papaconstantinou J, eds. *The developmental biology of reproduction*. New York: Academic Press, 1975; 311-345.
49. Rider V, McRae A, Heap RB, Feinstein A. Passive immunization against progesterone inhibits endometrial sensitization in pseudopregnant mice and has antifertility effects in pregnant mice which are reversible by steroid treatment. *J. Endocrinol* 1985; 104:153-158.
50. Rider V, Wang MY, Finn C, Heap RB, Feinstein A. Antifertility effect of passive immunization against progesterone is influenced by genotype. *J Endocrinol* 1986; 108:117-121.
51. Kennedy TG. Prostaglandins and the endometrial vascular permeability changes preceding blastocyst implantantation and decidualization. *Prog Reprod Biol* 1980; 7:234-243.
52. Castracane VD, Jordan VC. The effect of estrogen and progesterone on uterine prostaglandin biosynthesis in the ovariectomized rat. *Biol Reprod* 1975; 13:587-596.
53. Sherwood OD, Downing SJ. The chemistry and physiology of relaxin. In: Greenwald GS, Terranova PF, eds. *Factors regulating ovarian function*. New York: Raven Press, 1983:381-410.
54. Hsu CJ, Sanborn BM. Relaxin treatment alters the kinetic properties of myosin light chain kinase activity in rat myometrial cells in culture. *Endocrinology* 1986; 118:499-505.
55. Rao MR, Sanborn BM. Relaxin increases calcium efflux from rat myometrial cells in culture. *Endocrinology* 1986; 119:435-437.
56. Hsu CJ, McCormack SM, Sanborn BM. The effect of relaxin on cyclic adenosine 3′,5′-monophosphate concentrations in rat myometrial cells in culture. *Endocrinology* 1985; 116:2029-2035.
57. Pusey J, Kelly WA, Bradshaw JMC, Porter DG. Myometrial activity and the distribution of blastocysts in the uterus of the rat: interference by relaxin. *Biol Reprod* 1980; 23:394-397.
58. Rogers PAW, Murphy CR, Squires KR, MacLennan AH. Effects of relaxin on the intrauterine distribution and antimesometrial positioning and orientation of rat blastocysts before implantation. *J Reprod Fertil* 1983; 68:431-435.
59. Vasilenko P, Mead JP, Weidmann JE. Uterine growth-promoting effects of relaxin; a morphometric and histological analysis. *Biol Reprod* 1986; 35:987-995.
60. Vasilenko P, Mead JP. Growth-promoting effects of relaxin and related compositional changes in the uterus, cervix, and vagina of the rat. *Endocrinology* 1987; 120:1370-1376.
61. Vasilenko P, Adams WC, Frieden EH. Uterine size and glycogen content in cycling and pregnant rats: influence of relaxin. *Biol Reprod* 1981; 25:162-169.
62. Mead RA. Role of the corpus luteum in controlling implantation in mustelid carnivores. *Ann NY Acad Sci* 1986; 476:25-35.
63. Mead RA, Joseph MM, Neirinckx S, Berria M. Partial characterization of a luteal factor that induces implantation in the ferret. *Biol Reprod* 1988; 38:798-803.
64. Wu JT, Chang MC. Effects of progesterone and estrogen on the fate of blastocysts in ovariectomized pregnant ferrets: a preliminary study. *Biol Reprod* 1972; 7:231-237.
65. Foresman KR, Mead RA. Luteal control of nidation in the ferret (*Mustela putorius*). *Biol Reprod* 1978; 18:490-496.
66. Murphy BD, Mead RA, McKibbin PE. Luteal contribution to the termination of preimplantation delay in mink. *Biol Reprod* 1983; 28:497-503.

HORMONAL REQUIREMENT FOR THE ESTABLISHMENT OF PREGNANCY IN PRIMATES

N. Ravindranath and N.R. Moudgal

Centre for Advanced Research in Reproductive Biology
Primate Research Laboratory
Indian Institute of Science
Bangalore 560 012, India

In most primates, implantation occurs between days 7 and 9 post-fertilization, and this coincides with days 21 to 24 of cycle. Fertilization itself occurs in the ampullary region of the fallopian tube within 24 to 36 hrs of the luteinizing hormone (LH) peak. Subsequent development into the eight-cell stage in the ampulla takes about 48 to 72 hrs. The developmental stages of fertilized ovum to blastocyst in the rhesus macaque have been described by Lewis and Hartman[1] and by Heuser and Streeter.[2] Implantation and pregnancy establishment requires synchronous development of the embryo and the uterus. This precisely tuned event is dependent on an intricate interplay of hormones at the uterine end. The hormonal requirements for ovum implantation in the primate appear not well defined, and consequently, an attempt has been made in this paper to review the current status of our knowledge in this area.

PREPARATION OF THE ENDOMETRIUM FOR IMPLANTATION

The uterine receptivity to the blastocyst is attained as a result of a complex interaction between estrogen and progesterone which affects the pattern of cell proliferation, macromolecular synthesis, and secretory activity of the endometrium. Decidualization is normally provoked by the blastocyst. In the monkey, mechanical traumatization, as well as injection of oil into the uterine lumen, has been shown to induce a superficial decidual reaction under appropriate hormonal conditions.[3-5] The nature of the signal for initiating decidualization during the normal implantation process is thought to be a humoral factor(s),[6] the possible candidates being estrogen,[7] histamine,[8,9] and/or prostaglandin.[10] The changes in the uterine metabolic and secretory activity during cycle and early pregnancy have been attributed to the combined action of estrogen and progesterone. The type of biochemical changes occurring at the site of implantation in the primate, however, are yet to be documented.

HORMONAL CHANGES DURING THE PERI-IMPLANTATION PERIOD

Ovarian Steroids in Circulation

Available information suggests that with implantation and initiation of chorionic gonadotropin secretion, the corpus luteum of the cycle is converted to that of pregnancy and is rescued from luteolysis. The corpus luteum is presumably needed for early pregnancy maintenance, i.e., until the placenta takes over the function of producing progesterone. The period of placental takeover seems to differ for different species of primates. Neill et al.[11] observed that the circulating patterns of progesterone in both fertile and nonfertile cycling rhesus monkeys are indistinguishable until day 22 to 24 of cycle. This appears to be true also for the cynomolgus monkey[12] and the human.[13] Around this time, in contrast to the corpus luteum of the nonfertile cycle, the corpus luteum of the fertile cycle shows an increase in progesterone secretion. Plasma progesterone patterns during the post-implantation period have been described for the rhesus[14-16] and the bonnet monkey.[17,18] Similarly, Hearn et al.[19] have observed an increase in serum progesterone concentration in pregnant marmosets. In addition, the serum levels of progesterone of fertile cycles in chimpanzees,[20] baboons,[21] bonnets,[18] and marmosets[19] show increment even before implantation and this is attributed to the unimplanted blastocyst sending 'rescue' signals to the corpus luteum.[22] Evidence is now forthcoming to show that blastocysts in culture in the case of the human[23] as well as the rabbit[24] secrete chorionic gonadotropin-like material which is luteotropic.

The general pattern of circulating estradiol-17β or total estrogen concentration during the fertile cycle in rhesus monkeys, chimpanzees, and marmosets is markedly different when compared to that of the nonfertile cycles. While no change has been observed in circulating estrogen levels before implantation in the rhesus monkey,[25] this has been shown to increase in the early post-implantation period.[15,16] Similarly, chimpanzee exhibits increased estrogen levels during the immediate post-implantation period.[20] In the human[13] and baboon,[21] however, there is a delay in increase of estradiol levels beyond the implantation period. Even though the bonnet monkey[26] and the marmoset[19] show an early increase in estradiol levels as in the rhesus monkey, lack of information on the actual timing of implantation in these species limits further discussion.

Chorionic Gonadotropin in Circulation

The elevation in the level of ovarian steroids, estrogen and progesterone, in circulation during a fertile cycle has been attributed to a luteotropic stimulus provided by the implanting embryo.[27] This luteotropic stimulus has been identified as chorionic gonadotropin (CG) released by the preimplantation blastocyst, initially,[28] and later by the syncytial trophoblastic cells of the placenta. The resurgence of luteal functionality under its stimulus is termed "rescue" of the corpus luteum. The relationship between the appearance of CG and the increase in serum sex steroid levels appears well correlated in the case of the rhesus monkey[16,28] and the human.[13] In the bonnet monkey, however, chorionic gonadotropin has been detected in the serum only by day 28, much after the increase in serum progesterone and estrogen levels during the fertile cycle.[26] This is probably due either to the blastocyst secreting too small amounts of CG before and during the immediate post-implantation period, making it difficult to detect, or perhaps the CG assay system in use was not sensitive enough to detect CG before day 28 of the cycle. Chorionic gonadotropin in a fertile bonnet monkey is secreted in maximum concentrations from day 28 to 40 of the cycle. It slowly declines to undetectable levels beyond day 50 of the cycle. However, Mukku and Moudgal[29] have shown that LH antibody capable of cross-reacting with CG does not terminate pregnancy or reduce progesterone if given after day 35 of the fertile cycle, indicating that already by this time the functional importance of CG is waning.

Generally, primates which have undergone a fertile mating show an increase over the nonfertile cycle in the levels of both serum estrogen and progesterone, and this, in some species of primates, can be seen even a couple of days before implantation.[18-21] In the bonnet monkey, we have observed a distinct change in the ratio of serum estrogen:progesterone (E:P) levels (ng/ml) in cycling monkeys undergoing fertile vs. nonfertile mating. Although the E:P ratios increase in both nonfertile and fertile cycles beyond day 24 of cycle, the ratios for days 24 to 28 range between 0.04 and 0.1 in fertile cycles and between 0.1 and 1.0 in nonfertile cycles. Besides, there is ample evidence to suggest that 'luteal rescue' by exogenous human chorionic gonadotropin (hCG) results in an increase not only in serum progesterone but also in serum estrogen, and the latter is also a product of the corpus luteum.[30] What then is the role of estrogen? It remains to be determined if it is required for sustaining estrogen and progesterone receptors in the endometrium and/or myometrium of the uterus during the peri-implantation period.

STEROID RECEPTOR CONCENTRATIONS IN UTERUS DURING PERI-IMPLANTATION PERIOD

Uterine progesterone and estradiol receptor concentrations change during the menstrual cycle. These changes have been correlated to serum or plasma concentrations of progesterone in primates.[31,32] Total estrogen and progesterone receptors were high during proliferation of the endometrium in the follicular phase of the human menstrual cycle. Estradiol receptors were concentrated in the nuclear fraction, whereas progesterone receptors were primarily in the cytoplasm. In the early luteal phase, both estrogen and progesterone receptors were high in the nuclear fraction. The receptors to both these steroids dropped to low levels in the nuclei as well as cytoplasm in the late luteal phase.[31] Similar results have been reported in cynomolgus monkeys.[32] However, at the end of the cycle (i.e., beyond day 25 of cycle), when serum concentrations of both estrogen and progesterone are low, the elevation in estrogen receptor levels is attributed to a decline in progesterone levels.[33] During gestation, endometrial estrogen and progesterone receptor concentrations have been studied in human females at around 8 to 10 weeks of gestation. At this time, estrogen receptor levels are low and progesterone receptor levels are comparable to that seen during the mid-luteal phase of cycle.[34] But Levy et al.[35] have observed an increase in progesterone receptor concentration during the same period of gestation.

Information available on the progesterone:estrogen receptor concentration during the peri-implantation period in the primate is limited. The studies in the rhesus monkey[36] have shown that during a fertile cycle, the ratio of endometrial estrone/estradiol receptors around the peri-implantation period (day 18 to 24 of fertile cycle) is high. Recently, Ghosh and Sengupta[37] have observed that levels of endometrial nuclear progesterone receptors are significantly high on days 4, 5, and 6 of gestation in rhesus monkeys. While total cytoplasmic estrogen receptor concentrations register an increase from day 4 of gestation, the nuclear estrogen receptors show a change by day 3 of gestation itself. These authors have suggested that, during the pre-nidatory stage, increased endometrial concentrations of nuclear estrogen and progesterone receptors indicate a higher degree of occupancy required for endometrial differentiation permitting blastocyst implantation.

The role of circulating estrogen and progesterone in regulating the receptor concentrations of either of the hormones in the endometrium has been studied to a limited extent in both the human and macaque. The endometrial progesterone receptor concentrations have been shown to be under the control of both estrogen and progesterone.[38] It has also been suggested that not only circulating estrogen but also its own tissue receptor levels regulate progesterone receptor concentration.[39] Progesterone has been shown to suppress both estrogen and its own receptor levels in the reproductive tract of the cynomolgus macaque.[40] However, the mechanism of induction of estrogen receptors by estrogen itself is not well understood.

Most model systems used to induce progesterone receptors require initial treatment with estrogen. What is not known is whether continuous estrogen support is required for maintenance of progesterone receptors. This particularly needs to be demonstrated during the luteal phase of the primate.

MODEL SYSTEMS AVAILABLE FOR DETERMINING THE HORMONAL REQUIREMENTS FOR IMPLANTATION

Several model systems have been used to determine the actual requirement of hormones for pregnancy established in primates. The results of these studies are discussed briefly below.

Ovariectomy and Steroid Hormone Replacement

The requirement of progesterone for implantation has been demonstrated in the rhesus monkey by Meyer et al.[41] They initially observed that ovariectomy during early postcoitum in rhesus monkeys led to blockade of pregnancy. Similarly, luteectomy performed on day 6 of gestation in rhesus monkeys failed to induce implantation.[42] However, Meyer et al.[41] reported the ability of supplementation with progesterone alone to maintain pregnancy in 7 out of 10 ovariectomized rhesus monkeys, suggesting the absolute need for progesterone for maintaining pregnancy. In contrast, Bosu and Johannson,[42] using the same protocol, could maintain pregnancy in only 1 out of 6 monkeys on progesterone supplementation alone. They noted that in those monkeys in which progesterone supplementation was successful, the sera was observed to contain low levels of estrogen, raising the possibility that this steroid is also required for implantation and maintenance of pregnancy. If this is correct, the threshold of the estrogen requirement should be very low.

Blocking Steroid Hormone Production Followed by Hormone Replacement

In the luteal phase, the corpus luteum is the primary source of ovarian progesterone and estrogen. While luteectomy results in a drastic reduction of both these hormones, exogenous hCG/LH injection brings about an increase in secretion of both steroid hormones.[30] Characterized gonadotropin antibodies (to LH/CG) have been successfully used during the luteal phase of monkeys to block ovarian steroid hormone production.[18,43,44] However, in most cases supplementation with progesterone alone has been shown to override the 'abortifacient' effect of the LH antibody thus casting doubts as to the requirement for estrogen.[30] All the same, analyzing the effect of LH antibody more carefully, we observed recently that while LH neutralization results in an 80% reduction of progesterone levels, during the same period it reduces estrogen levels by only 30%, again suggesting that the threshold requirement for estrogen, if any, could be quite low.

Besides, in most experiments where LH antibody has been administered, it is used during the immediate post-implantation phase (i.e., beyond day 25 of cycle).

Use of Steroid Hormone Antagonists

Steroid hormone antagonists have also been used to determine the hormonal requirements during the peri-implantation period. It is assumed that the major site of action of these antagonists is the uterus whose receptor concentrations for estrogen and progesterone during day 18-24 of the cycle have been shown to vary depending upon whether the monkey has experienced an infertile or fertile cycle.[36,45] Progesterone receptor blockers (RU-486 and ZK-734) have been successfully used for early termination of pregnancy.[46,47] Studies using synthetic antiestrogens for prevention of pregnancy establishment, however, have been very few. Morris et al.[48] have shown that a variety of antiestrogenic compounds effective in blocking implantation in the rat can also inhibit pregnancy establishment in rhesus monkeys. These compounds have been observed to elicit, in addition to antiestrogenic activity, pronounced estrogenic activity. Sankaran et al.[49] administered Zuclomiphene to cycling female rhesus monkeys exposed to males from days 5 to 10 of 3 consecutive cycles. The dosage used did not block ovulation but prevented 4 out of 5 monkeys from becoming pregnant. They suggested that preovulatory estrogen, itself, could have a role in adequately preparing the uterus for implantation to occur.

During the last few years, we have successfully used Tamoxifen, a potent antiestrogen, in proven fertile bonnet monkeys to obtain proof of the requirement of estrogen for the establishment of pregnancy. In brief, the results show that administration of Tamoxifen in a post-ovulatory mode for either 1, 5, or 13 days starting from day 14, 16, or 18 of the cycle protects against conception in over 80% of the mated monkeys. In addition to Tamoxifen not having any effect on luteal function *per se*, exogenous progesterone supplementation also was unable to override the antiestrogen effect.[50-52]

Use of Steroid Antibodies

It was our feeling that conclusive evidence for the requirement of estrogen for implantation perhaps could be obtained by selectively neutralizing that hormone alone. We achieved this by using specific antibodies against estradiol-17β-BSA conjugate (raised in a donor male monkey) in a proven fertile female bonnet monkey model system.

Proven fertile monkeys (n = 5), which had cohabitated with proven fertile males from days 9 to 14 of the cycle, received, from day 14 through 18 of the cycle, 5 ml of estrogen antiserum/day/monkey i.p. A control group of 5 mated monkeys received daily 5 ml of normal monkey serum from day 14 through 18. The pregnancy establishment was assessed based on serum progesterone levels beyond day 25 of the cycle and chorionic gonadotropin levels from day 28 to 36 of the cycle. Whereas in the control group, 3 out of 5 monkeys conceived following 1 ovulatory cycle exposure to the male (normal for the colony), none became pregnant in the estrogen antiserum treated group. This study, while providing unequivocal evidence for estrogen requirement for implantation in the primate, particularly emphasizes the need of post-ovulatory estrogen in the implantation process. The estrogen antiserum used, in addition to providing near total neutralization of endogenous estrogen, was specific in its effect in that it did not interfere with luteal function.

CONCLUSION

While reviewing the current state of our knowledge on the relative requirements for progesterone and estrogen in pregnancy establishment in primates, we have described recent experimental evidence supporting the need for estrogen for implantation. The dependence of pregnancy on progesterone has not been discussed in depth here, as it is a well-established phenomenon. Since total neutralization of estrogen leads to blockade of conception, progesterone alone in the total absence of estrogen appears unable to establish pregnancy. However, the results thus far suggest that the threshold of estrogen requirement is low and may be satisfied very early in the post-ovulatory period. The actual role of estrogen remains to be established.

Acknowledgment

Aided by grants from the HRP WHO, Geneva (No. 85012) and the DBT, Government of India.

References

1. Lewis WH, Hartman CG. Tubal ova of the rhesus monkey. *Carnegie Inst Wash Contrib Embryol* 1941; 29:9-15.
2. Heuser CH, Streeter GL. Development of the macaque embryo. *Carnegie Inst Wash Contrib Embryol* 1941; 29:17-228.
3. Hisaw FL. The physiology of menstruation in macacus rhesus monkey. 1. Influence of the follicular and corpus luteum hormones. 2. Effects of anterior pituitary extracts. *Am J Obstet Gynecol* 1935; 93:1301-1307.

4. Wislocki GB, Streeter GL. On the placentation of macaque (*Macaca radiata*) from the time of implantation until the formation of the definitive placenta. *Contrib Embryol Carnegie Inst* 1938; 27:1-66.
5. Marston JH, Kelly WA, Eckstein P. Decidual reaction induced in rhesus monkeys by tubal injection of arachis oil and by the presence of an intrauterine device. *J Reprod Fertil* 1971; 25:451-454.
6. Siddiqui UA, Heald PJ. Mechanisms of action of the antifertility agents U11, 100 A and U11, 555A in the rat. *J Reprod Fertil* 1976; 47:251-254.
7. Sengupta J, Roy SK, Manchanda SK. Effect of an antiestrogen on implantation of mouse blastocyst. *J Reprod Fertil* 1981; 62(2):433-436.
8. Shelesnyak MC. Nidation of the fertilized ovum. *Endeavour* 1960; 19:81-87.
9. Dey SK, Johnson DC, Santos JC. Is histamine production by the blastocyst required for implantation in the rabbit? *Biol Reprod* 1979; 21:1169-1173.
10. Kennedy TG. Timing of uterine sensitivity for the decidual cell reaction: Role of prostaglandins. *Biol Reprod* 1980; 22:519-525.
11. Neill JD, Johansson EDB, Knobil E. Patterns of circulating progesterone concentrations during the fertile menstrual cycle and remainder of gestation in the rhesus monkey. *Endocrinology* 1969; 84:45-48.
12. Stabenfeldt GH, Hendrickx, AG. Progesterone studies in the *Macaca fascicularis*. *Endocrinology* 1973; 92:1296-1300.
13. Thomas K, De Hertogh R, Pizzarro M, Van Exter C, Ferin J. Plasma LH-hCG, 17-β oestradiol, oestrone and progesterone monitoring around ovulation and subsequent nidation. *Int J Fertil* 1973; 18:65-73.
14. Hodgen GD, Dufau ML, Catt KJ, Tullner WW. Estrogen, progesterone and chorionic gonadotropin in pregnant rhesus monkeys. *Endocrinology* 1972; 91:896-900.
15. Bosu WTK, Johannson EDB, Gemzell C. Patterns of circulating oesterone, oestradiol 17-β and progesterone during pregnancy in the rhesus monkey. *Acta Endocrinol (kbh)* 1973; 74:348-352.
16. Atkinson LE, Hotchkiss J, Fritz GR, Surve AH, Neill JD, Knobil E. Circulating levels of steroids and chorionic gonadotropins during pregnancy in the rhesus monkey, with special attention to the rescue of the corpus luteum in early pregnancy. *Biol Reprod* 1975; 12:335-345.
17. Stabenfeldt GH, Hendrickx AG. Progesterone levels in the bonnet monkeys (*Macaca radiata*) during the menstrual cycle and pregnancy. *Endocrinology* 1972; 91:614-619.
18. Prahalada S, Mukku Venkatramaiah, Jagannadha Rao A, Moudgal NR. Termination of pregnancy in macaques (*Macaca radiata*) using monkey antiserum to ovine luteinizing hormone. *Contraception* 1975; 12:137-147.
19. Hearn JP, Abbot DH, Chambers PC, Hodges JK, Lunn SF. Use of the common marmosets, callithrix facchus, in reproductive research. *Primate Med* 1978; 10:40-49.
20. Reyes FI, Winter JS, Faiman C, Hobson WC. Serial serum levels of gonadotropins, prolactin and sex steroids in the nonpregnant and pregnant chimpanzee. *Endocrinology* 1975; 96:1447-1455.
21. Shaikh AA, Allen-Rowland C, Dozier T, Kraemer DC, Goldzeiher, JW. Diagnosis of early pregnancy in the baboon. *Contraception* 1976; 14:391-402.
22. Moudgal NR. Corpus luteum of the nonhuman primate. *Adv Vet Sci Comp Med* 1984; 28:343-366.
23. Fischel SB, Edwards RG, Evans CJ. Human chorionic gonadotropin secreted by preimplantation embryos cultured *in vitro*. *Science* 1984; 223:816-818.
24. Saxena BB, Hasan SH, Haour F, Schmidt Gollwitzer M. Radioreceptor assay of human chorionic gonadotropin: Detection of early pregnancy. *Science* 1974; 184:793-795.
25. Reinius S, Fritz GR, Knobil E. Ultrastructure and endocrinological correlates of an early implantation site in the rhesus monkey. *J Reprod Fertil* 1973; 32:171-173.
26. Jagannadha Rao A, Kotagi SG, Moudgal NR. Serum concentrations of chorionic gonadotropin, estradiol 17 β and progesterone during early pregnancy in the south Indian bonnet monkey (*Macaca radiata*). *J Reprod Fert* 1984; 70:449-455.
27. Neill JD, Knobil E. On the nature of the initial luteotropic stimulus of pregnancy in rhesus monkey. *Endocrinology* 1972; 90:34-38.
28. Hodgen GD, Tullner WM, Vaitukaitis JL, Ward DN, Ross GT. Specific radioimmunoassay of chorionic gonadotropin during implantation in rhesus monkey. *J Clin Endocrinol Metab* 1975; 39:457-464.
29. Venkatramaiah Mukku, Moudgal NR. Studies on luteolysis: Effect of antiserum to luteinizing hormone on sterols and steroid levels in pregnant hamsters. *Endocrinology* 1975; 97:1455-1459.
30. Ravindranath N. Studies on reproductive endocrinology of the female bonnet monkey (*Macaca radiata*): Hormonal regulation of follicular maturation, luteal function and implantation. Ph.D. Thesis, Indian Institute of Science, Bangalore, India, 1988.
31. Bayard F, Damilano S, Robel P, Baulieu EE. Cytoplasmic and nuclear estradiol and progesterone receptors in endometrium. *J Clin Endocrinol Metab* 1978; 46:635-648.
32. West NB, Brenner RM. Estrogen receptor levels in the oviducts and endometria of cynomolgus macaques during the menstrual cycle. *Biol Reprod* 1983; 29:1303-1312.

33. McClennan MC, West NB, Brenner RM. Immunocytochemical localization of estrogen receptors in the macaque endometrium during the luteal follicular transition. *Endocrinology* 1986; 119:2467-2475.
34. Kreitmann B, Bayard F. Oestrogen and progesterone receptor concentrations in human endometrium during gestation. *Acta Endocrinol* 1979; 92:547-552.
35. Levy C, Robel P, Gautray JP, et al. Estradiol and progesterone receptors in human endometrium: Normal and abnormal menstrual cycles and early pregnancy. *Am J Obstet Gynecol* 1980; 136:646-651.
36. Kreitman-Gimbal B, Bayard F, Hodgen GD. Changing ratios of nuclear estrone to estradiol binding in endometrium at implantation: Regulation by chorionic gonadotropin and progesterone during rescue of primate corpus luteum. *J Clin Endocrinol Metab* 1981; 52:133-137.
37. Ghosh D, Sengupta J. Patterns of estrogen and progesterone receptors in rhesus monkey endometrium during secretory phase of normal menstrual cycle and preimplantation stages of gestation. *J Steroid Biochem* 1988; 31(2):223-229.
38. Kreitmann B, Bugat R, Bayard F. Estrogen and progestin regulation of the progesterone receptor concentration in human endometrium. *J Clin Endocrinol Metab* 1979; 49:926-929.
39. Barile G, Sica G, Montemurro A, Lacobelli S, Corradini M. Levels of estrogen and progesterone receptors in human endometrium during the menstrual cycle. *Europ J Obstet Gynec Reprod* 1979; 94:243-246.
40. West NB, Hess DL, Brenner RM. Differential suppression of progesterone receptors by progesterone in the reproductive tract of female macaques. *J Steroid Biochem* 1986; 25:497-503.
41. Meyer RK, Wolf RC, Arslan M. Implantation and maintenance of pregnancy in progesterone treated ovariectomized monkeys (*Macaca mulatta*). In: Hoffer S, ed. *Recent advances in primatology.* Basel: Karger, 1969; 2:30-35.
42. Bosu WTK, Johansson EDB. Implantation and maintenance of pregnancy in mated rhesus monkeys following bilateral oophorectomy or luteectomy with and without progesterone replacement. *Acta Endocrinol Copenh* 1975; 79:598-609.
43. Moudgal NR, Macdonald GJ, Greep RO. Effect of human chorionic gonadotropin antiserum on ovulation and corpus luteum formation in the monkey (Macaca fascicularis). *J Clin Endocrinol Metab* 1971; 32:579-581.
44. Mukku VR, Moudgal NR. Regulation of corpus luteum function in the subhuman primate—a study in bonnet monkeys. In: Talwar GP, ed. *Recent advances in reproduction and regulation of fertility.* Amsterdam: Elsevier/North Holland, 1979: 135-142.
45. Martel D, Malet C, Olmedo C, Monier MN, Dubouch P. Oestrogen receptor in the baboon endometrium: Cytosolic receptor detection, characterization and variation of its concentration during the menstrual cycle. *J Endocrinol* 1980; 84:261-272.
46. Philibert D, Moguilewsky M, Mary I. In: Baulieu EE, Segal SJ, eds. *The antiprogestin steroid RU 486 and human fertility control.* New York: Plenum Press, 1986:49-68.
47. Puri CP, Pongubala JMR, Jayaraman S, Hinduja IN, Elger WG. Antifertility action of progestins [Abstract]. In: *XI Congress of the International Primatological Society.* Gottingen FRG: 1986:191.
48. Morris JM, Van Wagenen G, McCann T, Jacob D. Compounds interfering with ovum implantation and development (ii) synthetic estrogens and antiestrogens. *Fertil Steril* 1967; 18:18-34.
49. Sankaran MS, Prahalada S, Hendrickx AG. Effects of zuclomiphene citrate on the nonfertile and fertile menstrual cycles in the rhesus monkey (*Macaca mulatta*). An experimental approach to the understanding of the role of periovulatory estrogens in implantation in primates [Abstract]. *Am J Primatol* 1984; 7:309.
50. Ravindranath N, Moudgal NR. Antifertility effect of Tamoxifen as tested in the female bonnet monkey (*Macaca radiata*) *J Biosci* 1986; 10:167-170.
51. Ravindranath N, Moudgal NR. Use of Tamoxifen, an antiestrogen, in establishing a need for oestrogen in early pregnancy in the bonnet monkey (*Macaca radiata*). *J Reprod Fertil* 1987; 81:327-336.
52. Moudgal NR, Ravindranath N. Requirement for estrogen in implantation and post-implantation survival of blastocyst in the bonnet monkey. In: Yoshinaga K, Mori T, eds. *Development of Preimplantation Embryos and Their Environment.* New York: Alan R. Liss, Inc., 1989:277-288.

PREGNANCY DEFERRED: AN UNUSUAL ROLE FOR PROLACTIN IN A MARSUPIAL

L.A. Hinds

CSIRO Division of Wildlife and Ecology
P.O. Box 84, Lyneham, A.C.T., 2602
Australia

THE regulation of the mammalian corpus luteum (CL) has been the subject of study for many years. After ovulation, the persistence of the CL depends upon interactions between the ovary, pituitary, uterus, and/or conceptus. Progesterone, the major steroid secreted by the CL, is essential for the establishment and maintenance of early pregnancy in all mammalian species. However, the significance of the CL, and its ability to secrete progesterone in the later stages of pregnancy, differs between species. Some species (sheep, guinea pig) can dispense with the CL when the placenta begins to produce progesterone, while other species such as the goat and rabbit depend on the CL throughout gestation. The maintenance of progesterone synthesis by the CL is largely regulated by pituitary hormones, and thus, hypophysectomy can disrupt pregnancy. For example, hypophysectomy before mid-pregnancy often leads to fetal death and resorption due to the loss of anterior lobe secretions (rabbit, rat, mouse, guinea pig, rhesus monkey). After implantation, however, hypophysectomy has different effects in different species depending on whether the placenta assumes a luteotrophic role. In some species the placenta produces progesterone and/or luteotrophic hormones, and consequently, in the later stages of pregnancy the presence of the pituitary is not essential. In many other species, however, prolactin, either alone or in conjunction with luteinizing hormone (LH) and/or follicle stimulating hormone (FSH), forms a luteotrophic complex which is essential for the support and maintenance of the early stages of pregnancy and/or the estrous cycle.[1]

Studies of luteal function in marsupials have been extensive (see 2 for review) and have shown, with minor exceptions, that the CL is short-lived and its life-span is neither extended by pregnancy, nor apparently influenced by luteotrophins or luteolysins. For these reasons, the marsupial CL most nearly conforms to the ancestral pattern as proposed by Rothchild[3] (see below). Thus, marsupials provide a unique opportunity for the study of basic principles of endocrine control from which concepts concerning the regulation of luteal function in Eutheria can be derived. The most detailed information of luteal function in marsupials has been gained from the study of the tammar wallaby, *Macropus eugenii*. Before outlining the endocrine regulation of the CL of this species, its breeding pattern is described.

BREEDING BIOLOGY OF THE TAMMAR

The tammar exhibits embryonic diapause and is a strictly seasonal breeder.[4] The gestation period is almost the same length as the estrous cycle and pregnancy does not inhibit follicular growth. Thus, parturition is followed by a postpartum estrus. In the southern hemisphere these events occur in most females in late January to early February, shortly after the summer solstice. Ovulation occurs between 30 to 40 hrs post-coitum[5] and the CL forms within 3 to

4 days.[6] By day 8 after fertilization, the embryo has developed to a unilaminar blastocyst comprising 80-160 cells.[7] Further development of the CL and blastocyst is arrested during lactation due to the sucking stimulus of the pouch young. This period of facultative diapause, when sucking is the proximate stimulus arresting ovarian activity, is typical of all macropodid species exhibiting diapause and is known as lactational quiescence. Thus, from February to June loss or removal of the sucking pouch young results in reaction of the CL and development of the embryo to term. Birth and post-partum estrus occur 26 to 27 days later.[8]

After reactivation, the CL increases in weight from about 10 mg to 60 mg. The progesterone concentration of luteal tissue remains relatively constant at 10-11 ng/mg until about day 13 to 15, rising thereafter to about 32 ng/mg by day 22.[9,10] Circulating progesterone levels remain at about 200 pg/ml until day 5 or 6 when there is a transient increase to about 500 pg/ml (Fig. 1).[11] Levels revert to basal until day 10 then steadily increase to a plateau after day 16 with maximum concentrations of 500-600 pg/ml. Coincident with parturition, which invariably occurs 21-22 days after the progesterone peak, there is a marked decrease in plasma progesterone (Fig. 1), as well as progesterone content of the CL.[9,11,12] The early transient peak of progesterone, which occurs in both the pregnant and non-pregnant cycle, provides the first evidence that a female is undergoing an active reproductive cycle and so is a useful criterion of reactivation and a precise indicator of CL function.

In the tammar, lactational quiescence is followed by a period of obligate diapause known as seasonal quiescence. During this time, from July to December in the Southern hemisphere, seasonal factors predominate and loss, removal, or weaning of the pouch young does not induce reactivation of the CL. It is termed seasonal quiescence rather than seasonal anestrus because the CL remains viable throughout the period[6] and spontaneously reactivates after the summer solstice. Hence a CL formed at post-partum estrus in one breeding season may remain in quiescence for up to 11 months.[4]

In the tammar, therefore, the activity of the CL is inhibited during both periods of quiescence. How is this suppression of the growth and secretory activity of the CL maintained? Is the suppression at the pituitary level or at the luteal cell? If the latter, is it tonic inhibition or lack of a particular stimulus?

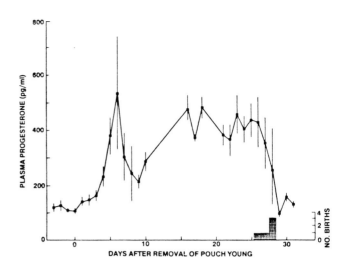

Figure 1. *Progesterone concentrations (mean ± SEM) in peripheral plasma of 5 tammars through delayed pregnancy, initiated by removal of pouch young. Note the pulse of progesterone on days 5-6.*[11]

ENDOCRINE CONTROL OF THE CORPUS LUTEUM

Lactational and Seasonal Quiescence

The first report of the role of the pituitary in maintaining quiescence appeared in 1973;[13] during lactational quiescence removal of the pituitary caused lactation to fail within 2 days and, unexpectedly, induced reactivation of the quiescent CL and dormant blastocyst. This result did not discriminate between the effects of the loss of the sucking stimulus and the loss of the pituitary. However, when hypophysectomy was performed on non-lactating females in seasonal quiescence, reactivation of the CL also occurred. Thus, hypophysectomy during either period of quiescence resulted in resumption of the growth and activity of the CL, and the embryo developed to term. However, parturition failed, and follicular growth, estrus and ovulation were abolished.[13] Furthermore, the pattern and concentration of plasma progesterone was equivalent to that observed in females undergoing active pregnancy; the magnitude of the early peak of progesterone, which occurred on day 7 or 8, was not significantly different from the peak occurring after removal of pouch young and concentrations were elevated in the later stages of pregnancy.[14] This extraordinary effect of hypophysectomy indicated that the CL is under a tonic inhibition directed by the pituitary but, once released, it requires no luteotrophic support to maintain progesterone production during pregnancy. Is the tammar CL autonomous?

Autonomy of the Corpus Luteum

Luteal tissue taken from quiescent and reactivated CL and cultured *in vitro* actively secreted progesterone into the medium.[10,15] The addition of luteotrophic hormones (prolactin and LH) did not affect the rate of progesterone production *in vitro*, or the tissue progesterone content of quiescent CL or CL incubated 5 days after removal of pouch young.[10,15] Luteal tissue from the latter CL (day 5) showed an increased secretion rate compared to CL incubated on day 0, 9, or 16 after resumption of development. Thus the increased peripheral concentrations of progesterone at day 5 (Fig. 1) are probably due to this change in progesterone secretion rate since there is no change in the mass of the CL at this time.[10] The subsequent increase in peripheral progesterone later in pregnancy, however, is a reflection of an increased mass of luteal tissue.

These results, which are in marked contrast with most other mammals, suggest that the CL is autonomous and capable of independently expressing its full development once reactivated. Three other observations support this view. First, the CL is virtually devoid of LH receptors, although there are abundant prolactin receptors.[16] Second, in females immunized against gonadotrophin releasing hormone (GnRH) in early pregnancy, follicular development, estrus, and ovulation are prevented but the CL grows, pregnancy is sustained, and parturition occurs.[17] Third, the changes in progesterone secretion rate occur *in vivo* several days after hypophysectomy, as indicated by the presence of the early progesterone peak.[14]

As shown above, there is substantial evidence indicating that the tammar CL is independent once reactivated. Indeed the *in vitro* changes in secretion rate of progesterone which result in the transient peripheral progesterone peak may occur because the CL has an intrinsic ability to regulate its progesterone production rather than any ability to respond to extrinsic factors of hypophysial origin. In many other mammals, hypophysectomy before midpregnancy results in abortion due to lack of luteotrophic support for the CL. However, during the estrous cycle the effects of hypophysectomy vary and in some species can be interpreted as an ability of the CL to function independently; regression of the CL is delayed after hypophysectomy in the dog, guinea pig, and pig but in none of these do peripheral progesterone levels or luteal tissue progesterone concentrations remain at normal, elevated levels.[18-20] *In vitro* studies of porcine CL indicate that it is independent in the early stages of its life-span following a single luteotrophic stimulus at the time of ovulation, but after day 12 of the estrous cycle it becomes responsive to LH.[21] Similarly, in the marsupials, the pre-ovulatory surge of LH may provide the single stimulus essential for development of the CL of pregnancy/estrous cycle. Alternatively, tammar LH may have a very high affinity for the few LH receptors on the CL and this LH may be irreversibly bound, in the absence of sufficient circulating levels, such that it can exert a luteotrophic effect even several days after reactivation is delayed by hypophysectomy and 7 days of prolactin treatment (see below, 22). Despite this long delay and lack of endogenous circulating LH, the CL subsequently grows and supports a pregnancy to term. Irreversible binding of LH to its receptor has not been excluded, although it appears unlikely, especially because passive immunization against GnRH does not influence the activity of the CL but does inhibit follicular growth.[17]

One of the models[3] proposed for the evolution of control of the CL requires that the ancestral CL was autonomous. Secretion of both progesterone and prostaglandin was controlled by positive feedback mechanisms, such that when a critical ratio of these hormones was reached in the luteal tissue, luteolysis occurred—thus a typical progesterone profile consisted of a rising, plateau, and regressing phase. Since the evolution of viviparity, the CL has become sensitive to extrinsic factors so that its life-span is prolonged during the plateau phase.[3] In marsupials, as in carnivores, the plateau phase of progesterone secretion is not extended during pregnancy and the progesterone profile largely resembles that proposed as ancestral by Rothchild.[3] However, in the macropodid marsupials (kangaroos and wallabies), in which the progesterone profile is bimodal (Fig. 1),[2,11] it is not possible to explain the increase and decrease in progesterone secretion rate around day 5 using a self-regulating positive feedback system which also incorporates the luteolytic effects of prostaglandin.

Role of prolactin in the inhibition of the CL

Clearly, in the tammar, the main role of the pituitary is not to stimulate the activity of the CL, as in most other mammals. Instead, the pituitary tonically inhibits the CL, not by affecting the rate of steroidogenesis but apparently by preventing hyperplasia and hypertrophy of the CL. What is the pituitary factor that maintains this tonic inhibition?

Several studies have suggested that the pituitary factor involved in the inhibition is prolactin. Injections of ovine prolactin or oxytocin three times daily for 7 days after removal of pouch young delayed reactivation for this interval.[22] However, because these were intact animals, the results did not discriminate between a direct effect of the hormones or an indirect effect, perhaps mediated via the pituitary. Therefore, non-lactating females were treated with prolactin, oxytocin, or saline after hypophysectomy or anterior hypophysectomy during seasonal quiescence. Reactivation was delayed in animals given prolactin but not in those treated with oxytocin or saline alone.[22] Thus, prolactin was the most likely pituitary agent inhibiting the CL, a most unusual role for this hormone in mammals.

The dopamine agonist, bromocriptine, inhibits the release of prolactin by the pituitary and has been used in many species to demonstrate the role of prolactin in luteal function. The results of treatment of the tammar with bromocriptine (Sandoz Australia) supported the hypothesis that prolactin is the inhibitor of luteal function,[23] but also raised some paradoxes. A single intramuscular injection of bromocriptine (5 mg/kg) between February and early September induced reactivation; the early progesterone pulse occurred on day 5 or 6 and birth and/or estrus 26 to 27 days later, the same intervals as after removal of pouch young.[23,24] Between September and December, when bromocriptine treatment is ineffective, basal prolactin levels in non-lactating females are 2-3 fold higher than in lactational quiescence.[23] However, no effect of bromocriptine on plasma prolactin concentrations could be demonstrated in either lactating animals during lactational quiescence (although lactation failed in some females), or non-lactating females in seasonal quiescence.[23] In addition, plasma prolactin levels have not been observed to change after removal of pouch young during lactational quiescence.[25,26] Another macropodid marsupial, the Bennett's wallaby, *Macropus rufogriseus rufogriseus*, has a similar pattern of seasonal breeding as the tammar.[27] It responds similarly to bromocriptine treatment and there are no effects of bromocriptine on plasma prolactin levels in lactational quiescence, although in lactating females in seasonal quiescence prolactin levels decrease after treatment with bromocriptine.[28] However, in seasonal quiescence, prolactin concentrations in lactating females are significantly elevated compared to non-lactating females.[28,29] Thus, in both species, it is not clear whether the effect of bromocriptine is via the hypothalamus or pituitary or is directed at the CL itself.[23] Nevertheless, since the rate of recovery of the CL, as determined by the presence of the early progesterone peak, is the same as after removal of pouch young, both hypophysectomy and bromocriptine treatment must affect the same pathway of inhibition. These results also suggest that the basal level of prolactin may not be the most important factor maintaining the inhibition.

What is this pathway of inhibition during seasonal quiescence, when neither removal of pouch young nor bromocriptine treatment will induce reactivation[23] while hypophysectomy does?[22] A photoperiodic component was first recognized when tammars transferred to the northern hemisphere continued to breed after the summer solstice (i.e., June 22).[30]

Experimental manipulations of photoregimens have confirmed that tammars and Bennett's wallabies are responsive to specific changes in photoperiod.[31,32] When tammars are held on a summer solstitial daylength of 15L:9D, they remain in quiescence but reactivation can be induced if the daylength is reduced to 12L:12D.[31] Births and/or estrus occur about 32 to 34 days later, an interval which is approximately 6 days longer than after removal of pouch young. This longer interval to birth is due to a delay in the appearance of the early progesterone peak and not to a delay in the later stages of the cycle; the progesterone peak occurs on day 10 but the interval from the peak to birth remains at 22 days.[33] Subsequent studies[24] have shown that the tammar responds to a change in the duration of elevated melatonin concentrations and not to elevated melatonin at a specific time of day. Furthermore, a change in duration of elevated melatonin experienced for only 3 days is sufficient to induce reactivation. Thus, during the first 3 days after a stimulatory photoperiod change, the melatonin message is being transduced by the brain and transmitted to the pituitary before affecting the ovaries.[24] What then is this signal from the pituitary which leads to an ovarian response?

Recently, we have observed a daily pulse of plasma prolactin lasting less than 2 hrs and with a magnitude ranging from 30 to 100 ng/ml in tammars held on an inhibitory photoperiod of 15L:9D. This morning prolactin peak was absent 5 days after tammars began experiencing a stimulatory photoperiod of 12L:12D (Fig. 2).[34] When this prolactin peak was artificially maintained in tammars that were experiencing a stimulatory photoperiod, reactivation was delayed for the duration of the 10-day treatment.[35] The control females showed early peaks of progesterone between days 6 and 9 and gave birth 27 to 30 days after the change in daylength. The prolactin-treated females had peaks of progesterone on day 14 or 15 after the start of treatment, or 4 to 5 days after the last prolactin injection, and gave birth on day 36 or 37. These results indicate

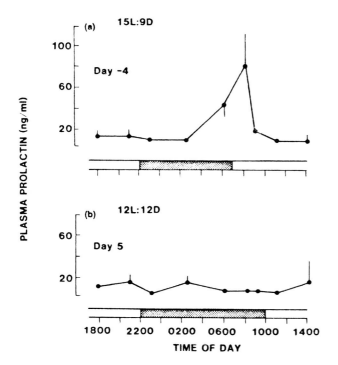

Figure 2. *Concentrations (mean ± SEM) of plasma prolactin in 6 tammars held on (a) an inhibitory photoperiod (15L:9D) and (b) 5 days after a change to a stimulatory photoperiod (12L:12D).*[34]

that the early morning prolactin peak is directly implicated in the inhibition of the CL during inhibitory photoperiods. Thus, it is not a change in basal levels that is important for the maintenance of the tonic inhibition, but the occurrence of a peak of prolactin once a day. The finding of this morning peak helps to explain the main paradox raised by the earlier studies with bromocriptine; the injections of bromocriptine in seasonal quiescence were probably ineffective because they were administered after the morning peak of prolactin would have occurred.

CONCLUSION

Prolactin plays a significant role in the regulation of the function of the CL of the tammar. In contrast with other mammals, in which prolactin often plays a luteotrophic role, its major role in this marsupial is to tonically inhibit luteal activity. Moreover, the presence of a single, daily pulse of prolactin appears to be critical for the maintenance of this quiescence. In the absence of this peak, reactivation of the CL occurs, and the subsequent activity of the CL is then independent of hypophysial support; once released from inhibition, it is apparently autonomous as its growth and secretion of progesterone are equivalent in intact and hypophysectomized females, and luteal tissue *in vitro* shows changes in secretion rate of progesterone independent of added luteotrophic hormones. Thus, the role of prolactin appears to be to prevent growth and development of the CL and so defer pregnancy.

SUMMARY

The corpora lutea of marsupials, like those of other mammals, are essential for the maintenance of pregnancy. In macropodid marsupials, such as the tammar wallaby, *Macropus eugenii*, the CL remains undeveloped and plasma progesterone concentrations low during lactation and associated embryonic diapause. Removal of the sucking stimulus induces reactivation and, once reactivated, the CL undergoes hyperplasia and hypertrophy, and increases its secretion of progesterone. The factors that inhibit the CL during diapause are central to our understanding of its endocrine control.

The pituitary tonically inhibits the CL; removal of this inhibition induces reactivation of the CL which then proceeds irreversibly to completion of its development. In contrast to other mammals, the tammar CL, once reactivated, is autonomous, requiring no luteotrophic support (luteinizing hormone or prolactin) to grow or to secrete progesterone at concentrations equivalent to those in intact females undergoing active pregnancy. The pituitary factor involved in the inhibition has been shown to be prolactin—daily treatment with prolactin delays reactivation after hypophysectomy or removal of the sucking stimulus. Recent studies have shown that it is not the basal concentration of prolactin but the daily presence of a brief peak of prolactin that maintains the inhibition of the CL and prevents it from expressing its full development. Thus, prolactin has a novel role in this species in that it prevents hyperplasia and hypertrophy of luteal cells during diapause but does not provide any luteotrophic support after the inhibition has been removed.

References

1. Amoroso EC, Perry JS. Ovarian activity during gestation. In: Zuckerman S, Weir BJ, eds. *The ovary. Vol.II Physiology*. New York: Academic Press, 1977:316-398.
2. Tyndale-Biscoe CH, Renfree MB. *Reproductive physiology of marsupials*. Cambridge: Cambridge Univ Press, 1987.
3. Rothchild I. The regulation of the mammalian corpus luteum. *Rec Prog Horm Res* 1981; 37:183-298.

4. Berger PJ. Eleven-month 'Embryonic Diapause' in a marsupial. *Nature* 1966; 211:435-436.
5. Sutherland RL, Evans SM, Tyndale-Biscoe CH. Macropodid marsupial luteinizing hormone: validations of assay procedures and changes in concentrations in plasma during the oestrous cycle in the female tammar wallaby (*Macropus eugenii*) *J Endocr* 1980; 86:1-12.
6. Sharman GB, Berger PJ. Embryonic diapause in marsupials. *Adv Reprod Physiol* 1969; 4:211-240.
7. Tyndale-Biscoe CH. Embryonic diapause in a marsupial: roles of the corpus luteum and pituitary in its control. In: Ralph CL, ed. *Comparative endocrinology: developments and directions.* New York: Alan R. Liss Inc. 1986:137-155.
8. Merchant JC. The effect of pregnancy on the interval between one estrus and the next in the tammar wallaby, *Macropus eugenii*. *J Reprod Fert* 1979; 56:459-463.
9. Renfree MB, Green SW, Young IR. Growth of the corpus luteum and its progesterone content during pregnancy in the tammar wallaby, *Macropus eugenii*. *J Reprod Fert* 1979; 57:131-136.
10. Hinds LA, Evans SM, Tyndale-Biscoe CH. In-vitro secretion of progesterone by the corpus luteum of the tammar wallaby, *Macropus eugenii*. *J Reprod Fert* 1983; 67:57-63.
11. Hinds LA, Tyndale-Biscoe CH. Plasma progesterone levels in the pregnant and non-pregnant tammar, *Macropus eugenii*. *J Endocr* 1982a; 93:99-107.
12. Tyndale-Biscoe CH, Hinds LA, Horn CA, Jenkin G. Hormonal changes at oestrus, parturition and post-partum oestrus in the tammar wallaby (*Macropus eugenii*). *J Endocr* 1983; 96:155-161.
13. Hearn JP. Pituitary inhibition of pregnancy. *Nature* 1973; 241:207-208.
14. Hinds LA. Progesterone and prolactin in marsupial reproduction. Ph.D. Thesis, Australian National University, Canberra, 1983.
15. Sernia C, Hinds LA, Tyndale-Biscoe CH. Progesterone metabolism during embryonic diapause in the tammar wallaby, *Macropus eugenii*. *J Reprod Fert* 1980; 60:139-147.
16. Stewart F, Tyndale-Biscoe CH. Prolactin and luteinizing hormone receptors in marsupial corpora lutea: relationship to control of luteal function. *J Endocr* 1982; 92:63-72.
17. Short RV, Flint APF, Renfree MB. Influence of passive immunization against GnRH on pregnancy and parturition in the tammar wallaby, *Macropus eugenii*. *J Reprod Fert* 1985; 75:567-575.
18. Concannon P. Effects of hypophysectomy and of LH administration on luteal phase progesterone levels in the beagle bitch. *J Reprod Fert* 1980; 58:407-410.
19. Heap RB, Perry JS, Rowlands IW. Corpus luteum function in the guinea-pig; arterial and luteal progesterone levels and the effects of hysterectomy and hypophysectomy. *J Reprod Fert* 1967; 13:537-553.
20. Anderson LL, Melampy RM. Hypophysial and uterine influences on pig luteal function. In: Lamming GE, Amoroso EC, eds. *Reproduction in the female mammal.* London: Butterworths, 1967:285-316.
21. Hunter MG. Responsiveness *in vitro* of porcine luteal tissue recovered at two stages of the luteal phase. *J Reprod Fert* 1981; 63:471-476.
22. Tyndale-Biscoe CH, Hawkins J. The corpora lutea of marsupials, aspects of function and control. In: Calaby JC, Tyndale-Biscoe CH, eds. *Reproduction and evolution.* Canberra: Australian Academy of Science, 1977:245-252.
23. Tyndale-Biscoe CH, Hinds LA. Seasonal patterns of circulating progesterone and prolactin and response to bromocriptine in the female tammar, *Macropus eugenii*. *Gen Comp Endocr* 1984; 53:58-68.
24. Tyndale-Biscoe CH, Hinds LA, McConnell SJ. Seasonal breeding in a marsupial: opportunities of a new species for an old problem. *Rec Prog Horm Res* 1986; 42:471-512.
25. Hinds LA, Tyndale-Biscoe CH. Prolactin in the marsupial *Macropus eugenii* during the estrous cycle, pregnancy and lactation. *Biol Reprod* 1982; 26:391-398.
26. Gordon K, Fletcher TP, Renfree MB. Reactivation of the quiescent corpus luteum and diapausing embryo after temporary removal of the sucking stimulus in the tammar wallaby (*Macropus eugenii*). *J Reprod Fert* 1988; 83:401-406.
27. Merchant JC, Calaby JH. Reproductive biology of the red-necked wallaby (*Macropus rufogriseus banksianus*) and Bennett's wallaby (*M.r.rufogriseus*) in captivity. *J Zool Lond* 1981; 194:203-217.
28. Curlewis JD, White AS, Loudon ASI, McNeilly AS. Effects of lactation and season on plasma prolactin concentrations and response to bromocriptine during lactation in the Bennett's wallaby *Macropus rufogriseus rufogriseus*. *J Endocr* 1986; 110:59-66.
29. Hinds LA, Tyndale-Biscoe CH. Seasonal and circadian patterns of circulating plasma prolactin during lactation and seasonal quiescence in the tammar, *Macropus eugenii*. *J Reprod Fert* 1985; 74:551-558.
30. Berger PJ. Reproductive biology of the tammar wallaby, *Macropus eugenii*. Ph.D. Thesis, Tulane University. *Dissert Abst Int* 1970; 31B:3760-3761.
31. Sadleir RMFS, Tyndale-Biscoe CH. Photoperiod and the termination of embryonic diapause in the marsupial *Macropus eugenii*. *Biol Reprod* 1977; 16:605-608.
32. Loudon ASI, Curlewis JD. Refractoriness to melatonin and short daylengths in early seasonal quiescence in the Bennett's wallaby (*Macropus rufogriseus rufogriseus*). *J Reprod Fert* 1987; 81:543-552.

33. Hinds LA, den Ottolander RC. Effect of changing photoperiod on pheripheral plasma prolactin and progesterone concentrations in the tammar wallaby (*Macropus eugenii*). *J Reprod Fert* 1983; 69:631-639.
34. McConnell SJ, Tyndale-Biscoe CH, Hinds LA. Change in duration of elevated concentrations of melatonin is the major factor in photoperiod response of the tammar, *Macropus eugenii*. *J Reprod Fert* 1986; 77:623-632.
35. Author's unpublished observations.

CONTROL OF THE ENDOCRINE FUNCTION OF THE HUMAN PLACENTA BY CYCLIC AMP

Guy E. Ringler, Lee-Chuan Kao, Alfredo Ulloa-Aguirre, and Jerome F. Strauss III

*Departments of Obstetrics and Gynecology
and Pathology and Laboratory Medicine
University of Pennsylvania
School of Medicine
Philadelphia, Pennsylvania 19104 USA*

THE human placenta elaborates a variety of protein and steroidal hormones.[1,2] The major site of synthesis of many of these hormones is the syncytial trophoblast, which arises from fusion of mononuclear cytotrophoblasts.[3-5] Cytotrophoblasts, the replicating trophoblastic elements, initially have a different endocrine repertoire than the syncytial trophoblasts, but eventually undergo a process of differentiation in which they cease dividing, become fusion competent, and acquire the capacity to produce hormones characteristic of the syncytial trophoblast (e.g., chorionic gonadotropin: CG and chorionic somatomammotropin: CS). The biochemical events which underly this process of differentiation have not been elucidated.

A SYSTEM TO STUDY THE MORPHOLOGICAL AND FUNCTIONAL DIFFERENTIATION OF CYTOTROPHOBLASTS

We have developed an *in vitro* system to study the functional and morphological differentiation of cytotrophoblasts at the molecular level.[3] In brief, cytotrophoblasts are prepared by digesting chorionic villus tissue with trypsin and DNase, and separating the dispersed cells on a Percoll gradient. A highly enriched preparation of cytotrophoblastic cells is recovered from the gradient in a density range of 1.048-1.062 g/ml. Freshly isolated cytotrophoblasts do not stain immunocytochemically for CG subunits, CS, or pregnancy specific β_1 glycoprotein (SP1). Thus, they can be distinguished from the syncytial trophoblasts which react positively for these hormones. Cytotrophoblasts prepared from term placenta produce progesterone in short-term incubations when provided with a cholesterol analogue steroid precursor (25-hydroxycholesterol), and possess aromatase activity.

In culture, the cytotrophoblasts differentiate both morphologically and biochemically in a time-dependent manner. During the initial 3-6 hrs, the cells are individual and mononuclear. Over the subsequent 24 to 72 hrs, they aggregate and fuse forming multi-nucleated syncytia. During this same period, the cells acquire the capacity for increased hormone production; between 48 and 72 hrs of culture the cells secrete increasing amounts of CG. In sequence, immunostaining for SP1, CG, and CS appears.[3,6] The fact that freshly isolated cytotrophoblasts possess some steroidogenic activity which is followed later by the production of appreciable amounts of CG and CS suggests that the ontogeny of placental endocrine activities involves expression of steroidogenic activity prior to activation of genes encoding glycoprotein and protein hormones characteristic of the syncytial trophoblast.

While we usually employ term placentae in our preparation of cytotrophoblasts, the method can be used to isolate cytotrophoblasts from first trimester placentae as well, although contamination with non-trophoblastic cell types tends to be greater. A major drawback to the use of term placentae is that the vast majority of cytotrophoblastic cells isolated are not mitotically active under routine culture

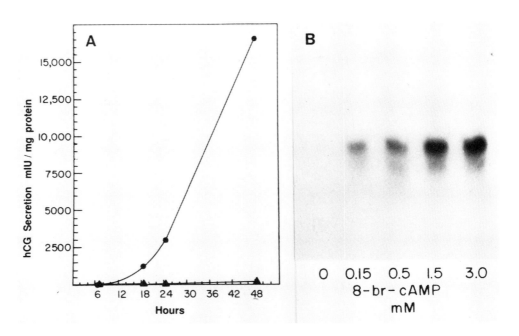

Figure 1. A. *Effects of 8-bromo-cAMP on CG secretion. Cytotrophoblasts were incubated in the absence (▲) or presence (●) of 8-bromo-cAMP (1.5 mM) for 48 hrs. Values presented are for cumulative CG secretion at the indicated times.* B. *Effects of 8-bromo-cAMP on β CG and mRNA levels. Cytotrophoblasts were incubated in the presence of the various amounts of cyclic nucleotide analogue for 48 hrs and RNA was then extracted and analyzed for β CG message. A photograph of a representative autoradiogram is presented.*

conditions. Therefore, it is not possible to explore very early molecular events in the regulation of these cells, including the control of their growth and cessation of replicative activity.

THE RELATIONSHIP BETWEEN TROPHOBLAST MORPHOLOGY AND FUNCTION

The morphological (syncytium formation) and biochemical differentiation of cytotrophoblasts in culture can be dissociated.[6,7] For example, α and β CG subunits and CS can be detected by immunocytochemistry in all morphological forms, including mononuclear cells and syncytia. In addition, when cytotrophoblasts are cultured in serum-free medium, aggregation and fusion do not occur but CG secretion can still be stimulated by agents which increase hormone production (e.g., 8-bromo-cAMP, see below). Thus, the formation of multinucleated cells is not a requirement for expression of CG subunit genes. However, the uninuclear trophoblasts which have been exposed to stimuli provoking expression of CG secretion do undergo a dramatic cytoplasmic differentiation so that they acquire the structural features (e.g., prominent Golgi apparatus and endoplasmic reticulum) characteristic of syncytial trophoblast.

THE ROLE OF CYCLIC AMP IN THE CONTROL OF TROPHOBLAST ENDOCRINE ACTIVITY

Cyclic AMP has been shown to stimulate CG and progesterone secretion by cultured cytotrophoblasts, placental explants, and choriocarcinoma cells lines[6,8-10] (Fig. 1). Moreover, cytotrophoblasts possess adenylate cyclase activity, and factors that activate the endogenous cyclase (e.g., forskolin and cholera toxin) increase both CG and progesterone secretion.[11] Indeed, there is a direct relationship between the production of cyclic AMP by cytotrophoblasts and their secretion of CG.

We have examined the mechanisms by which cyclic AMP increases CG and progesterone secretion. Increased synthesis of α and β CG subunits in response to 8-bromo-cAMP treatment has been demonstrated by pulse labeling trophoblasts with ^{35}S-methionine followed by immunoprecipitation, SDS-PAGE, and fluorography.[8] Northern blot analysis showed that 8-bromo-cyclic AMP causes a striking increase in both α and β CG mRNAs (Fig. 1).[8,9] Thus, cyclic AMP stimulated CG secretion by increasing CG subunit gene expression. As noted above, cyclic AMP analogues also promote cytoplasmic differentiation of the cells consistent with increased secretory activity.

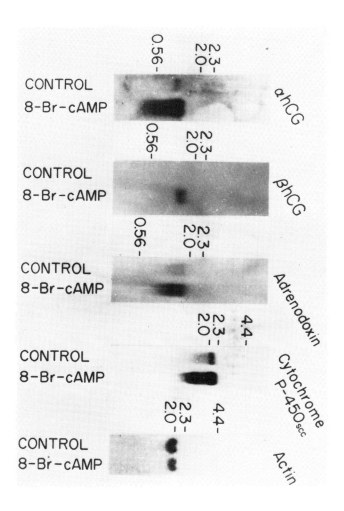

Figure 2. Effect of 8-bromo-cAMP on levels of various mRNAs in cultured cytotrophoblasts. Cytotrophoblasts were cultured for 24 hrs in the absence or presence of 1.5 mM 8-bromo-cAMP. Representative autoradiograms of Northern hybridization analyses are shown. Size markers are in Kb.

To determine if cyclic AMP stimulates steroidogenesis through similar mechanisms, we studied the effects of 8-bromo-cAMP on the abundance of mRNAs encoding two components of the cholesterol side-chain cleavage system, cytochrome P-450scc and adrenodoxin (Fig. 2). Cytochrome P-450scc catalyzes the first and rate-limiting step in the synthesis of all steroid hormones, and adrenodoxin is part of the mitochondrial electron transport system which transfers reducing equivalents to cytochrome P-450scc. Treatment of cytotrophoblasts with 8-bromo-cAMP increased levels of cytochrome P-450scc and adrenodoxin mRNAs 1.8-fold and 5.7-fold, respec-

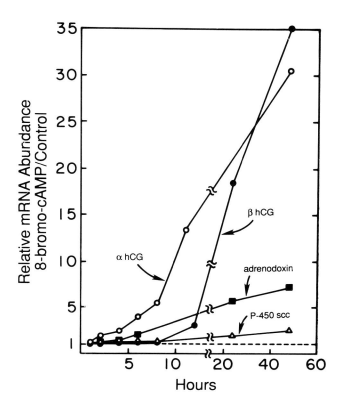

Figure 3. Summary of temporal change of mRNAs in cytotrophoblasts in response to 8-bromo-cAMP. A series of overlapping time-course studies were carried out with cells being exposed to 1.5 mM 8-bromo-cAMP for 1, 2, 4, 6, 8, 12, 24, or 48 hrs. Six studies covered the 1-6 hour time points and 6 studies covered the 8-48 hour time points. The mean values for the relative increments in each mRNA are plotted for each time point.

tively, after 24 hrs, consistent with the increases observed in steroid hormone secretion.[9] The increase in mRNA levels for P-450scc and adrenodoxin is accompanied by increased *de novo* synthesis of these proteins and their accumulation within the cultured trophoblastic cells as demonstrated by pulse labeling with ^{35}S-methionine and immunoprecipitation and immunocytochemical analyses.[12]

MECHANISMS OF CYCLIC AMP CONTROL OF TROPHOBLAST GENE EXPRESSION WITH SPECIAL REFERENCE TO THE GENE ENCODING αCG

Time-course studies revealed a disparity in the temporal pattern in which the CG subunit, cytochrome P-450scc, and adrenodoxin mRNAs accumulate in cultured trophoblasts in response to 8-bromo-cAMP (Fig. 3). α CG mRNA doubled after 4 to 6 hrs of treatment, whereas the first detectable rise in β CG mRNA was at 12 hrs. There was a similar disparity in the effects of 8-bromo-cAMP on accumulation of adrenodoxin and cytochrome P-450scc mRNAs. Adrenodoxin mRNA rose approximately two-fold at 6 hrs of treatment, whereas a two-fold increase in cytochrome P-450scc mRNA appeared consistently only after 24 to 48 hrs of treatment.[9] These observations suggest that separate mechanisms may be involved in the accumulation of the mRNAs that encode the steroidogenic enzymes and CG subunits.

Cyclic AMP activates protein kinases, which then catalyze phosphorylation of various proteins, which produce a change in cellular function. To determine if protein kinases are required for cyclic AMP stimulation of CG production by cytotrophoblasts, cells were treated for 24 hrs with 50 μM H-7, an isoquinolinesulfonamide protein kinase inhibitor, in the presence or absence of 8-bromo-cAMP. H-7 prevented the 8-bromo-cAMP-stimulated rise in CG secretion, without affecting basal CG levels, and it prevented the increase in both α and β CG mRNAs (Fig. 4). H-7 also blocked the 8-bromo-cAMP-stimulated increase in progesterone secretion and the associated rise in cytochrome P-450scc and adrenodoxin mRNAs.[9]

While these findings indicate a requirement for the involvement of a protein kinase in cyclic AMP's mechanism of action, they do not specify the type of kinase involved, since H-7 inhibits a variety of enzymes including protein kinase C, and cyclic GMP and cyclic AMP-dependent protein kinases.[13,14] However, since neither phorbol esters, which activate C kinases, nor 8-bromo-cyclic GMP produce the same striking up-regulation of CG secretion and the CG subunit mRNAs, it is likely that the effects of H-7 are due to inhibition of a cyclic AMP-dependent protein kinase. We postulate therefore that 8-bromo-cyclic AMP activates a protein kinase that phosphorylates a protein(s) which may be involved in regulation of the mRNAs in question.

Protein kinases presumably act on factors that regulate gene transcription. In JEG-3 cells, 8-bromo-cyclic AMP raises α and β CG mRNAs due, at least in part, to increased gene transcription.[15] In bovine adrenal cells, cyclic AMP analogues increase transcription of the cytochrome P-450scc and adrenodoxin genes.[16] The increment in transcription is thought to involve transacting proteins which bind to cis-regulatory elements (enhancers). To examine whether new protein synthesis is required for the stimulatory effects of cyclic AMP analogues on CG and

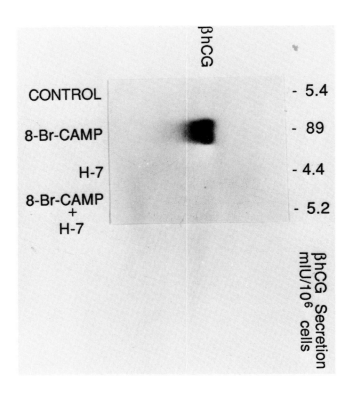

Figure 4. Effects of H-7 on 8-bromo-cyclic AMP action. Cytotrophoblasts were cultured for 24 hrs in the absence or presence of H-7 (50 μM) in the absence or presence of 8-bromo-cyclic AMP (1.5 mM). CG was measured by radioimmunoassay. β CG mRNA was detected by blot hybridization.

adrenodoxin mRNA abundance, we treated trophoblasts with cycloheximide at a dose that inhibits protein synthesis by 95% (as assessed by incorporation of ^{35}S-methionine) and then challenged the cells with 8-bromo-cAMP. Cycloheximide did not prevent the 8-bromo-cAMP stimulated rise in α CG mRNA; however, it reduced basal adrenodoxin mRNA levels and attenuated the effect of 8-bromo-cAMP on adrenodoxin message accumulation.[10] This suggests that if a trans-acting factor is needed for increased α CG gene transcription, it is not short-lived. However, the stimulation of adrenodoxin gene expression was prevented by cycloheximide, consistent with a requirement for synthesis of a protein factor. These observations are consonant with the notion that different mechanisms are involved in the control of the mRNAs encoding hormones and enzymes involved in steroidogenesis.

Considerable information is available regarding the control of the α CG gene, and the cis elements in the 5'-

flanking region of the α CG gene which are required for responsiveness to cyclic AMP have been delineated.[15,17-21] We recently discovered two cytotrophoblast nuclear proteins by gel-shift analysis that bind to regions of the α CG gene 5'-flanking DNA containing the consensus cyclic AMP responsive element (CRE), TGACGTCA, and an adjacent upstream response element (URE) which also appears to be involved in expression of the α CG gene.[22] One protein is present in control and stimulated cells (that binding to the CRE), while the other is only found after 8-bromo-cAMP treatment (that binding to the URE). We suspect that both of these proteins, if they have a role in regulating the α CG gene, are relatively long-lived, based on the fact that concomitant cycloheximide treatment does not prevent the 8-bromo-cAMP-induced increase in α CG mRNA. These proteins may be activated to associate with the CRE and URE as a result of phosphorylation catalyzed by a cyclic AMP-dependent protein kinase and act in concert to increase transcription of the α CG gene. Other transcriptional factors are presumably involved in the control of the β CG genes and those encoding steroidogenic enzymes.

WHAT REGULATES TROPHOBLAST CYCLIC AMP LEVELS?

The factors which might control cyclic AMP levels in trophoblastic cells *in vivo* have not been identified. From our *in vitro* studies we can suggest several candidates including β-adrenergic agents and corticotropin releasing hormone (CRH), each of which activates adenylate cyclase and stimulates secretion of placental hormones.[12,23] Cytotrophoblasts produce CRH, making this polypeptide a viable candidate for an autocrine/paracrine regulator of trophoblast function.[24] CG has been shown to stimulate placental adenylate cyclase and thus could serve as an autocrine agent in a positive feedback loop.[25] High density lipoproteins have also been found to stimulate placental adenylate cyclase and could be an additional factor controlling placental cyclic AMP production.[26] Other factors including prostaglandins and peptide autocrine/paracrine substances (e.g., GnRH and epidermal growth factor) may also have roles in modulating the trophoblast at various times during gestation.[27]

OTHER REGULATORS OF TROPHOBLAST FUNCTION

Cyclic AMP is most certainly not the only intracellular regulator of trophoblast endocrine function. Other second messenger pathways, including the calcium/calmodulin and

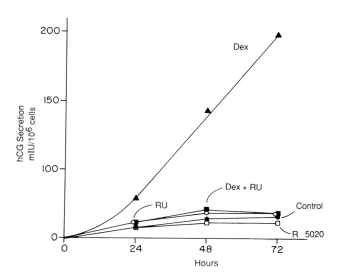

Figure 5. *Effects of dexamethasone on CG secretion. Cytotrophoblasts were cultured in the presence of the various steroidal additions or control medium for 72 hrs and CG secretion was determined at 24 hour intervals. Values are means from triplicate cultures with data normalized to the number of cells plated. Dex is dexamethasone, 1 μM; RU is RU-486, 10 μM; R5020 is 1 μM; control is ethanol vehicle.*

the protein kinase C systems, probably have roles which remain to be elucidated.[27]

We recently found that glucocorticoids stimulate CG secretion by trophoblasts revealing a role for steroid hormones in the expression of placental endocrine activity.[28] Treatment of cytotrophoblasts with 1 μM dexamethasone increased CG secretion by 6-10 fold over a 72-hour period, whereas progesterone and the synthetic progestin, R5020, had no effect (Fig. 5). The stimulatory effects of dexamethasone were completely blocked by the glucocorticoid antagonist, RU-486, indicating action through the glucocorticoid receptor. Northern blot analyses revealed that dexamethasone stimulates CG secretion by increasing the abundance of CG mRNAs, a response which is also blocked by RU-486 (Fig. 6). Dexamethasone augmented the 8-bromo-cAMP-stimulated increase in CG secretion (Table I). This synergism was seen at all concentrations of 8-bromo-cAMP examined, suggesting that glucocorticoids are acting to enhance endocrine activity at a locus after generation of cyclic AMP.

The exact mechanisms by which glucocorticoids increase CG mRNA levels (e.g., transcriptional vs. post-translational control) remain to be elucidated. A direct effect on CG gene expression is possible. The 5'-flanking region of the

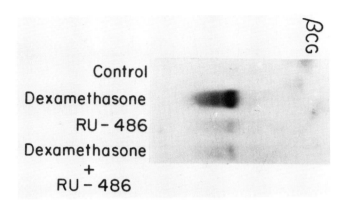

Figure 6. *Effects of RU-486 on dexamethasone induced increments in β CG mRNA. Cells were cultured for 72 hours in the absence or presence of dexamethasone (1 μM), RU-486 (10 μM), or a combination of dexamethasone and RU-486. RNA was processed as described above and β CG mRNA was detected by Northern blot analysis.*

Table I. *Effects of dexamethasone on CG secretion by cultured cytotrophoblasts.*

	CG Secretion mIU/10⁶ cells/24 h
Control	53 ± 17[a]
Dexamethasone (1 μM)	369 ± 84[b]
8-bromo-cyclic AMP (1.5 mM)	1669 ± 421[c]
Dexamethasone plus 8-bromo-cyclic AMP	4873 ± 921[d]

Cytotrophoblasts were cultured for 72 hrs in the presence of the indicated treatments. Media were changed at 24-hr intervals. Values presented are means ± SE from 3 experiments for CG secretion during the last 24 hrs of culture. Values with different superscripts are significantly different from each other ($P < 0.05$).

α CG gene contains DNA sequences with modest homology to the consensus glucocorticoid response element (GRE) sequences.[30] However, the β CG genes do not contain GRE consensus sequences. Therefore, it is not obvious that glucocorticoids regulate the CG genes in a manner similar to that described for well-known glucocorticoid-controlled genes (e.g., tyrosine aminotransferase).[31] Alternatively, glucocorticoid treatment could increase the stability of CG mRNAs, and thus promote accumulation of these messages.

Robinson et al. found that dexamethasone increases CRH gene expression in trophoblasts,[33] and our preliminary studies revealed that dexamethasone increases progesterone secretion (Ringler, Kallen, and Strauss, unpublished data). Thus, the effects of glucocorticoids extend beyond CG secretion.

A MODEL FOR FUNCTIONAL DIFFERENTIATION OF TROPHOBLASTIC CELLS

We envision trophoblast differentiation to be an irreversible progression in which the immature cytotrophoblasts cease mitotic activity and acquire the structural and functional (e.g. cytoplasmic organelles, fusion competence) features of mature trophoblastic elements (i.e., syncytial trophoblasts) including the capacity to produce CG and CS. Thus, as more cytotrophoblasts become terminally differentiated the placenta acquires a greater capacity to elaborate hormones characteristic of the mature trophoblast. Whereas the central event in the control of production of most of these hormones is the turning on of gene expression in association with the differentiation process (e.g., CS), more complex regulation may be involved in the case of other genes (e.g., β CG), accounting for divergent secretory patterns. We suggest that trophoblast differentiation is propelled by sequential actions of autocrine and paracrine agents circulating hormones (e.g., glucocorticoids). The cast of participating autocrine/paracrine and humoral factors, the order in which they act and their mechanisms of action remain to be clarified.

Acknowledgment

We thank Ms. Debbie Coffin for her assistance in the preparation of this manuscript. Work presented in this manuscript was supported by USPHS grant HD-06274, and grants from the Mellon and Rockefeller Foundations.

References

1. Simpson ER, MacDonald PL. Endocrine physiology of the placenta. *Annu Rev Physiol* 1981; 43:163-188.
2. Jaffe RB. The endocrinology of pregnancy. In: Yen SSC, Jaffe RB, eds. *Reproductive endocrinology*. Philadelphia, London, Toronto: W.B. Saunders, 1986.
3. Kliman HJ, Nestler JE, Sermasi E, Sanger JM, Strauss JF III. Purification, characterization and *in vitro* differentiation of cytotrophoblasts from human term placentae. *Endocrinology* 1986; 118:1567-1581.
4. Kliman HJ, Feinman MA, Strauss JF III. Differentiation of human cytotrophoblast into syncytiotrophoblast in culture. *Trophoblast Research* 1987; 2:407-421.

5. Hoshina M, Boothby M, Boime I. Cytological localization of chorionic gonadotropin alpha and placental lactogen mRNAs during development of the human placenta. *J Cell Biol* 1982; 93:190-198.
6. Feinman MA, Kliman HJ, Caltabiano S, Strauss JF III. 8-bromo-3′,5′-adenosine monophosphate stimulates the endocrine activity of human cytotrophoblasts in culture. *J Clin Endocrinol Metab* 1986; 63:1211-1217.
7. Kao L-C, Caltabiano S, Wu S, Strauss JF III, Kliman HJ. The human villous cytotrophoblast: interactions with extracellular matrix proteins, endocrine function and cytoplasmic differentiation in the absence of syncytium formation. *Developmental Biology* 1988; 130:693-702.
8. Ulloa-Aguirre A, August AM, Golos TG et al. 8-bromo-3′,5′-adenosine monophosphate regulates expression of chorionic gonadotropin and fibronectin in human cytotrophoblasts. *J Clin Endocrinol Metab* 1987; 64:1002-1009.
9. Patillo RA, Hussa RO. Early stimulation of human chorionic gonadotropin secretion by dibutyryl cyclic AMP and theophylline in human malignant trophoblast cells *in vitro*; inhibition by actinomycin D, α-amanitin, and cordycepin. *Gynecol Invest* 1975; 6:365-377.
10. Burnside J, Nagelberg SB, Lippman SS, Weintraub BD. Differential regulation of hCG α and β subunit mRNAs in JEG-3 choriocarcinoma cells by 8-bromo-cAMP. *J Biol Chem* 1985; 260:12705-12709.
11. Nulsen JE, Woolkalis MJ, Kopf GS, Strauss JF III. Adenylate cyclase in human cytotrophoblasts: characterization and its role in modulating hCG secretion. *J Clin Endocrinol Metab* 1988; 66:258-265.
12. Nulsen JC, Silavin SL, Kao L-C, Ringler GE, Kliman HJ, Strauss JFIII. Control of the steroidogenic machinery of the human trophoblast by cyclic AMP. *J Reprod Fert* 1989; 37(suppl):147-153.
13. Hidaka H, Inagaki M, Kawamoto S, Sasaki Y. Isoquinolinesulfonamides, novel and potent inhibitors of cyclic nucleotide dependent protein kinase and protein kinase C. *Biochemistry* 1984; 21:5036-5041.
14. Kawamoto S, Hidaka H. 1-(5-Isoquinolinesulfonyl)-2-methylpiperazine (H-7) is a selective inhibitor of protein kinase C in rabbit platelets. *Biochem Biophys Res Commun* 1984; 1:258-264.
15. Jameson JL, Jaffe RC, Gleason SL, Habener JF. Transcriptional regulation of chorionic gonadotropin α and β-subunit gene expression by 8-bromo-adenosine 3′,5′-monophosphate. *Endocrinology* 1986; 119:2560-2567.
16. John ME, John ML, Boggaram V, Simpson ER, Waterman MR. Transcriptional regulation of steroid hydroxylase genes by corticotropin. *Proc Natl Acad Sci USA* 1986; 13:4715-4719.
17. Jameson JL, Deutsch PJ, Gallagher GD, Jaffe RC, Habener JF. Transacting factors interact with a cyclic AMP response element to modulate expression of the human gonadotropin alpha gene. *Mol Cell Biol* 1987; 9:3032-3040.
18. Darnell RB, Boime I. Differential expression of the human gonadotropin alpha gene in ectopic and eutopic cells. *Mol Cell Biol* 1985; 5:3157-3167.
19. Silver BJ, Bokar JA, Virgin JB, Vallen EA, Milsted A, Nilsen JH. Cyclic AMP regulation of the human glycoprotein hormone alpha-subunit gene is mediated by an 18-base-pair element. *Proc Natl Acad Sci USA* 1987; 84:2198-2202.
20. Delegeane AM, Ferland LH, Mellon PL. Tissue-specific enhancer of the human glycoprotein hormone α-subunit gene: dependence on cyclic AMP-inducible elements. *Mol Cell Biol* 1987; 7:3944-4002.
21. Deutsch PJ, Jameson JL, Habener JP. Cyclic AMP responsiveness of human gonadotropin-alpha gene transcription is directed by a repeated 18-base pair enhancer. Alpha-promoter receptivity to the enhancer confers cell-preferential expression. *J Biol Chem* 1987; 25:12169-12174.
22. McNight CE, Strauss JF III, Ulloa-Aguirre A, Solter D. Inducible and constitutively bound trans factors interact with a cyclic AMP responsive element of the human gonadotropin alpha gene. *J Cell Biochem* 1988; UCLA Symposia on Molecular and Cellular Biology. Abstract 197.
23. Petraglia F, Sawchenko PE, Rivier J, Vale W. Evidence for local stimulation of ACTH secretion by corticotropin-releasing factor in human placenta. *Nature* 1987; 328:717-719.
24. Robinson BG, Emanuel RL, Frim DM, Majzoub JA. Glucocorticoid stimulates corticotropin releasing hormone gene expression in human placenta. *Proc Natl Acad Sci* 1988; 85:5244-5248.
25. Menon KMJ, Jaffe RB. Chorionic gonadotropin sensitive adenylate cyclase in human placenta. *J Clin Endocrinol Metab* 1973;36:1104-1109.
26. Wu YO, Jorgensen EV, Handwerger S. High density lipoproteins stimulate placental lactogen and adenosine 3′,5′-monophosphate (cAMP) production in human trophoblast cells, evidence for cAMP as a second messenger in human placental lactogen release. *Endocrinology* 1988; 123:1879-1884.
27. Huot RI, Foidart JM, Nardone RM, Stromberg K. Differential modulation of human chorionic gonadotropin secretion by epidermal growth factor in normal and malignant placental cultures. *J Clinical Endocrinol Metab* 1981; 53:1059-1063.

28. Ritvos O, Butzow R, Jalkanen J, Stenman U, Huhtaniemi, Ranta T. Differential regulation of hCG and progesterone secretion by cholera toxin and phorbol ester in human cytotrophoblasts. *Mol Cell Endocrinol* 1988; 56:165-169.
29. Ringler GE, Kallen CB, Strauss JF III. Regulation of human trophoblast function by glucocorticoids: dexamethasone promotes increased secretion of chorionic gonadotropin. *Endocrinology* 1989; 124:1625-1631.
30. Akerblom IE, Slater EP, Beato M, Baxter JD, Mellon PL. Negative regulation by glucocorticoids through interference with a cAMP responsive enhancer. *Science* 1988; 241:350-353.
31. Lewis EJ, Harrington CA, Chikaraishi DM. Transcriptional regulation of the tyrosine hydroxylase gene by glucocorticoid and cyclic AMP. *Proc Natl Acad Sci USA* 1987; 84:3550-3554.

SECTION VI: IMPLANTATION WINDOW

BIOMOLECULAR MARKERS FOR THE WINDOW OF UTERINE RECEPTIVITY

Ted L. Anderson

The Jones Institute for Reproductive Medicine
Department of Obstetrics and Gynecology
Eastern Virginia Medical School
Norfolk, Virginia 23507 USA

A variety of anatomic, physiologic, molecular, and temporal constraints govern the initial embryo-uterine interactions leading to successful implantation. Appropriate maturation of the blastocyst and the endometrium must be realized, as well as spatial and temporal approximation of these complex tissues.[1] Additionally, heterotypic cell adhesion is required between the apical membranes of two polarized epithelial cell populations that are of disparate genetic (as well as tissue) derivation. Specifically, the trophoblastic epithelium must affix firmly to the uterine luminal epithelium, penetrate this initial barrier, and gain access to the endometrial stroma, wherein lies a plethora of vascular and other components necessary for placentation.[2] As such, the process of implantation, and its regulation, presents a number of cell biological enigmas.

A highly invasive trophoblast allows certain mammalian embryos to implant almost without discretion in a variety of ectopic sites, regardless of host tissue, hormonal milieu, or timing of such an interaction.[3] Conversely, it is overtly conspicuous that the only tissue in which trophoblast invasion does not occur indiscriminately is the natural implantation site, the uterine lining. The endometrium is permissive to blastocyst implantation only during a brief receptive interval, following appropriate hormonal stimulation, as demonstrated by the failure of transferred blastocysts to result in endometrial attachment except at the time of normal uterine receptivity for that species.[4] If there is perturbation of the normal progression of hormonal sequelae, or cellular responses to that stimulation, diminution of reproductive potential often results. On one hand, an insufficient hormonal stimulation can fail to produce the physiological and biochemical components required to support nidation. On the other hand, an excessive hormonal stimulation such as peri-ovulatory administration of progesterone, may lead to implantation failure due to asynchronous embryo-uterine development.[5-7] In human *in vitro* fertilization programs where ovarian hyperstimulation is used to obtain multiple ova for fertilization, excessively high serum levels of estradiol and progesterone often result in advanced endometrial histologic maturation or stromal/epithelial asynchrony,[8] could contribute to embryo-uterine asynchrony, and appear to be partially responsible for the relatively modest rates of successful outcome experienced in these programs. Thus, to achieve nidatory success, coincidence must occur in an embryonic "developmental window," an endometrial "receptive window," and a coordinated "transport window" (which may be achieved *in vivo* or through embryo transfer).

The nature of the embryonic developmental window has been examined by several investigators. Alterations in surface membrane components during the preimplantation differentiation period (surface negativity, lectin binding, and glycoprotein expression) have been described, with particular reference to the development of adhesive properties.[9-12] Examinations in numerous experimental animal systems have clearly defined temporal aspects of normal implantation. Such examination has been extended, through the technology of *in vitro* fertilization and embryo transfer, to describe a similar transport window (not surprisingly) in non-human primates and humans. However, our subjective definitions of uterine receptivity to implantation have been limited to temporal, physiologic, and anatomic observations. Not until recently have we begun to examine more closely the cellular and molecular responses of endometrial cells to hormonal stimulation.

Though differentiation of the trophoblastic epithelium is surely requisite for blastocyst attachment and invasion, a number of reports provide compelling evidence to suggest that differentiation of the endometrium into a receptive state is the primary determinate of successful nidation. The luminal epithelium is the first endometrial surface encountered by implanting embryos and, as such, is the most likely candidate to mediate the seemingly rigid constraints on implantation. Potential roles of the uterine epithelium in various aspects of implantation (including secretion, absorption, and signal transduction) have been described.[13] Cowell[14] provided strong evidence that the implantation barrier manifested by the nonreceptive uterus is mediated by the luminal epithelium with his observation that mouse blastocysts would "implant" in focal areas where the epithelium had been scraped away to expose stroma. Further evidence for a regulatory role of the uterine luminal epithelium in embryo-uterine interactions is provided by a growing number of observations (in a wide variety of species) of endometrial luminal surface modifications related to implantation. In addition to alterations of surface charge and glycocalyx composition, temporal and spatial characteristics of stage-specific protein and glycoprotein expression provide us with markers that permit us to begin to define the parameters of uterine receptivity in molecular terms. Progesterone-stimulated secretory proteins of the endometrium are discussed elsewhere in this volume; thus, this discussion will focus upon stage-specific alterations of the luminal surface and membrane components.

OBSERVATIONS AND DISCUSSION

The Cell Surface

Histological features of luminal and glandular epithelial cells related to physiological states of the endometrium (including uterine receptivity) have been well-described in rodents, rabbits, nonhuman primates, and humans.[15-18] Surface modifications of luminal epithelial cells have also been reported,[19-20] including the stage-specific appearance of "pinopod" protrusions. Accompanying these morphological changes, discrete alterations have been identified in the composition and "morphology" of luminal glycocalyx material in several species.[27-30] Common features include: decreased surface negativity; increased thickness of PAS-positive material; and a more fibrillar glycocalyx structure by electron microscopy. The reduction of luminal surface negativity prior to the time of implantation is consistent with proposed mechanisms of cellular adhesion involving changes in membrane glycoproteins, and with observations that events, such as adhesion and fusion, are enhanced when repulsive charges on the involved cell surfaces are diminished.[31,32]

The significance of increased glycocalyx thickness on the uterine luminal surface at the time of implantation is not clear. Maroudas[33] predicted the exclusion volume of glycocalyx macromolecules on adjacent cells would likely contribute to mutual repulsion. As such, one might predict that a *reduction* of uterine luminal glycocalyx would better facilitate apposition of trophoblastic and endometrial epithelial surfaces. Such a reduction of surface coat material at prospective implantation sites in the rat uterus has been reported,[34] but Enders et al.[35] did not detect direct effects of blastocysts on the uterine epithelial glycocalyx. Reduction of glycocalyx material specifically at sites of embryo-uterine apposition has been demonstrated in the ferret[21] and rabbit.[28] Similar examination of areas of potential trophoblast-endometrial interactions prior to implantation in the primate have not been reported.

Skutelsky et al.[36] proposed that sialic acid plays a "protective role" during differentiation by masking antigenic or recognition sites. Surface negativity of the non-receptive rabbit uterus appears related to the presence of sialic acid;[25] this is likely true in the primate as well. Anderson et al.[28] found that enzymatic removal of sialic acid from the glycocalyx of non-receptive rabbit uteri revealed N-acetyl-glucosamine and galactose residues. Similar removal of sialic acid to reveal D-galactose residues on glycoproteins appears to be a recognition mechanism common to a variety of biological systems. For example, certain serum glycoproteins (e.g., transferrin, fetuin, ceruloplasmin) contain terminal D-galactose-sialic acid dimers;[37] removal of sialic acid from these proteins is necessary for recognition by the liver asialoglycoprotein receptor.[38] Similarities between these carbohydrate recognition systems are attractive in relation to the acquisition of uterine receptivity to implantation.

Lectin Binding

Another hormonally-regulated surface modification is alteration of glycocalyx saccharide composition (lectin binding affinities). Uteri of several species have been examined with respect to binding of numerous lectins; a common feature that has emerged is an increase in WGA and, especially, RCA-I lectin binding during the interval of uterine receptivity. These observations correlate with an increased incorporation of N-acetyl-glucosamine (WGA) and of D-galactose residues (RCA-I) at the luminal surface, or with the unveiling of such moieties already present in the glycocalyx, or both.[26-29] Such observations of uteri from humans and nonhuman primates during the normal menstrual cycle, with particular reference to the window of uterine receptivity, revealed that RCA-I binding appears to be limited to the peri-implantation interval, and disappears prior to the onset of menses.[29-42]

Recognition of galactose-containing glycoproteins by apical membrane endogenous lectins appears to mediate adhesion of chick blastoderm cells,[43] as well as cell-cell or cell-substratum adhesion of some tumor cells in relation to metastatic potential.[44] Considered in this light, observations of increased lectin binding to the uterine luminal surface in temporal relationship to the peri-implantation period suggests the possibility of an embryo recognition and/or adhesion system involving D-galactose. Additional support for this view is derived from reports of stage-specific saccharide-containing and saccharide-recognizing endometrial proteins in the human and nonhuman primate[42] (see discussion below). Further evidence for saccharide involvement during initial embryo-uterine interactions comes from observations that specific inhibitors of galactosyltranferases diminish implantation success when introduced into the uterine lumen during the peri-implantation period in the rabbit (T. Anderson, unpublished observations) and mouse.[45] Similar endogenous lectins (cell surface galactosyltranferases) have been postulated as mediators of fertilization.[46]

Membrane Protein Expression

Investigation of apical membrane protein expression by endometrial epithelial cells in relation to the window of uterine receptivity has been limited. Stage-specific proteins in plasma membrane fractions from rabbit endometrial scrapings, and in extracts of rabbit epithelial membranes isolated by intraluminal incubation of detergent solution, have been described.[28,47] Lectin binding to proteins isolated by the latter method and transferred to nitrocellulose has revealed some are glycoproteins. Of particular interest is a 42 kDa glycoprotein recognized by both WGA and RCA-I that has been purified for antibody production[48] (see below). Other proteins, seemingly present in extracts from nonreceptive and receptive uteri, appeared to be glycosylated differentially depending on the hormonal state, exhibiting lectin binding only in the latter. One prominent example is a 145 kDa glycoprotein exhibiting dramatic increases in lectin binding (particularly Con A) during the receptive interval. Thus, steroid hormones appear to influence epithelial apical membrane protein composition both at the transcription level and by post-translational modification.

Techniques have been developed for isolating luminally exposed membrane components from primate uteri after *in situ* labeling.[40] Cleavable derivatives of biotin, or biotinylated lectins, specifically bind appropriate externally oriented functional groups of proteins or glycoproteins; these are subsequently isolated using avidin affinity chromatography. Similar to observations in the rabbit, both stage-specific expression and stage-specific glycosylation of apical membrane proteins have been described in humans and non-human primates.[39-42] Furthermore, using agarose-immobilized specific sugar residues, stage-specific expression of saccharide-recognizing membrane proteins has been identified in the human endometrium.[42]

The molecular mechanism(s) by which hormones induce stage-specific membrane glycocalyx alterations in luminal epithelial cells is very poorly understood. On one hand, regulation may occur at the level of post-translational modification so that constitutively synthesized proteins are glycosylated differentially depending on the hormonal environment. Support for this notion comes from the demonstration that estradiol stimulation increases cellular levels of mannosylphosphoryldolichol in the mouse uterus, which enhances N-linked glycosylation of proteins.[49] Alternatively, luminal surface alterations may be mediated through differential gene transcription under the influence of a changing hormonal environment, resulting in the synthesis and glycosylation of a variety of stage-specific membrane proteins. Evidence has been provided that both of these mechanisms are operative under the influence of progesterone in the rabbit and primate uterus.[28,39-42]

Antibodies to Stage-Specific Proteins

At least three monoclonal antibodies (Mab) recognizing stage-specific endometrial epithelial membrane markers have been reported. Lampelo et al.[50] reported that Mab EBB2 recognizes apical membranes of luminal (but not glandular) epithelium in rabbits receptive to implantation. Aplin and Seif[51] demonstrated that Mab CC25 recognizes an epitope expressed in the basolateral membrane compartment of human endometrial epithelial cells (luminal and glandular), appearing shortly after ovulation, expressed during the mid and "mid-late" secretory phases, but significantly diminished by the late secretory (pre-menstrual) interval. Similarly, Thor et al.[52] found that Mab B72.3, generated against a metastatic breast carcinoma, recognizes glandular epithelium of the human endometrium specifically during the secretory phase. Unfortunately, specific antigens recognized by EBB2, CC25, and B72.3 have continued to elude characterization. Hoffman et al.[48] recently described the recognition pattern of a monospecific polyclonal antibody raised against a 42 kDa glycoprotein of rabbit luminal epithelial cells. Reactivity of this antibody was localized in the apical cytoplasm of luminal and cryptal epithelial cells as early as day 4. On days 6-7, the time of implantation in rabbits, reactivity was observed primarily at the apical membrane; the presence of this antigen appeared to diminish as early as day 8. No antibody localization was detected in glandular epithelial cells at any stage. Though the specific relationship between apical membrane proteins of the luminal epithelium and implantation remains unknown, temporal and spatial aspects of their expression suggest an integral role in early embryo-uterine interactions.

SUMMARY

Alterations in glycocalyx thickness and morphology toward the time of implantation appear to reflect a "decondensation" due to reduced negativity and increased saccharide complexity of glycoproteins synthesized under specific hormonal stimulation. Increased availability of D-galactose residues in the glycocalyx at this time may be indicative of a carbohydrate-based cell recognition system during the initial phase of embryo-uterine interaction; this hypothesis is supported by the presence of saccharide-recognizing proteins in the luminal membrane at that time. It is impressive that, despite overt differences in mechanisms of implantation and placentation in such a wide variety of species, remarkably similar molecular modifications of the luminal surface occur in relationship to the acquisition of uterine receptivity. As such, it is likely that many of these surface changes represent alterations common to a variety of molecular recognition and adhesion systems, and are not specific for the process of implantation *per se*. Instead, these membrane alterations likely facilitate initial apposition and adhesion of trophoblastic epithelium with the uterine luminal epithelium (regardless of the species) in such a way that other, more implantation-specific and/or species-specific, molecular interactions may be facilitated.

The role of stage-specific apical membrane proteins of uterine luminal epithelial cells remains unclear. However, one might predict that they mediate, among other events, signal transduction between the implanting blastocyst and the endometrium. Sialoglycoproteins on some epithelial cell surfaces appear to serve as "signals" to instigate *Salmonella* adherence and invasion.[53] In light of observations described here, a similar cellular communication can be envisioned with respect to embryo-uterine interactions. Isolation, purification, and characterization of stage-specific membrane proteins will permit continued investigation of unique embryo-uterine interactions at the molecular level. Additionally, it is noteworthy that benefits of this research extend beyond understanding implantation regulation. Knowing the response of endometrial cells to hormonal stimulation at the molecular level should contribute significantly to our understanding of a variety of disease states of the endometrium, including uterine cancers.

References

1. Casimiri V, Psychoyos A. Embryo-endometrial relationships during implantation. In: DeBrux J, Mortel R, Gautray JP, eds. *The endometrium.* New York: Plenum Press, 1981:63-79.
2. Schlafke S, Enders AC. Cellular basis of interaction between trophoblast and uterus at implantation. *Biol Reprod* 1975; 12:41-65.
3. Kirby DRS. The transplantation of mouse eggs and trophoblast to extrauterine sites. In: Daniel JC, ed. *Methods in mammalian embryology.* San Francisco: WH Freeman and Company, 1965:146-156.
4. Finn CA. The implantation reaction. In: Wynn RM, ed. *Biology of the uterus.* New York: Plenum Press, 1977:245-303.
5. Psychoyos A. Hormonal control of uterine receptivity for nidation. *J Reprod Fert* 1976; 25(suppl):17-28.
6. Schacht CJ, Foote RH. Progesterone-induced asynchrony and embryo mortality in rabbits. *Biol Reprod* 1978; 19:534-539.
7. Trounson A, Howlett D, Rogers P, Hoppen H-O. The effect of progesterone supplementation around the time of oocyte recovery in patients superovulated for in vitro fertilization. *Fertil Steril* 1986; 45:532-535.
8. Jones HW. Factors affecting the luteal phase in IVF and ET programs. In: Testart J, Frydman R, eds. *Human in vitro fertilization; INSERM Symposium No. 24.* Amsterdam: Elsevier, 1985:219-235.

9. Nilsson O, Lindkvist I, Ronqvist G. Decreased surface charge of mouse blastocysts at implantation. *Exp Cell Res* 1973; 83:421-423.
10. Johnson LV, Calarco PG. Mammalian preimplantation development: The cell surface. *Anat Rec* 1980; 196:201-219.
11. Magnuson T, Epstein CJ. Characterization of Concanavalin A precipitated proteins from early mouse embryos: A 2-dimensional gel electrophoresis study. *Dev Biol* 1981; 81:193-199.
12. Chavez DJ, Enders AC. Lectin binding of mouse blastocysts: Appearance of *Dolichos bifloris* binding sites on the trophoblast during delayed implantation and their subsequent disappearance during implantation. *Biol Reprod* 1982; 21:545-552.
13. Martin L. What roles are fulfilled by uterine epithelial components in implantation? In: Leroy F, Finn CA, Psychoyos A, Hubinot PO, eds. *Blastocyst-endometrium relationships; Prog Reprod Biol.* Vol. 7, Basel: S Karger, 1980:54-69.
14. Cowell TP. Implantation and development of mouse eggs transferred to the uterus of non-progestational mice. *J Reprod Fert* 1969; 19:239-245.
15. Noyes RW, Dickmann Z. Relation of ovular age to endometrial development. *J Reprod Fert* 1960; 1:186-196.
16. Parr MB. Effects of ovarian hormones on endocytosis at the basal membranes of rat uterine epithelial cells. *Biol Reprod* 1982; 26:909-913.
17. Williams T, Rogers AW. Morphometric studies of the luminal epithelium in the rat uterus to exogenous hormones. *J Anat* 1980; 139:867-881.
18. Hoffman LH, Davies J. Studies on the progestational endometrium of the rabbit. I. Light microscopy, day 0 to day 13 of gonadotrophin-induced pseudopregnancy. *Am J Anat* 1973; 137:423-446.
19. Nilsson BO. Changes of the luminal surface of the rat uterus at blastocyst implantation. *Z Anat Entwickl* 1974; 144:337-342.
20. Martel D, Frydman R, Glissant M, Maggioni C, Roche D, Psychoyos A. Scanning electron microscopy of postovulatory human endometrium in spontaneous and cycles stimulated by hormone treatment. *J Endocr* 1987; 114:319-324.
21. Enders AC, Schlafke S. Implantation in the ferret: Epithelial penetration. *Am J Anat* 1972; 133:291-313.
22. Hewitt K, Beer AE, Grinnell F. Disappearance of anionic sites from the surface of the rat endometrial epithelium at the time of implantation. *Biol Reprod* 1979; 21:691-707.
23. Murphy CR, Rogers AW. Effects of ovarian hormones on cell membranes in the rat uterus. III. The surface carbohydrates at the apex of the luminal epithelium. *Cell Biophys* 1981; 3:305-320.
24. Guillomot M, Fléchon J-E, Wintenberger-Torres S. Cytochemical studies of uterine and trophoblastic surface coats during blastocyst attachment in the ewe. *J Reprod Fert* 1982; 65:1-8.
25. Anderson TL, Hoffman LH. Alterations in the epithelial glycocalyx of rabbit uteri during early pseudopregnancy and pregnancy, and following ovariectomy. *Am J Anat* 1984; 171:321-334.
26. Whyte A, Robson T. Saccharides localized by fluorescent lectins on trophectoderm and endometrium prior to implantation in pigs, sheep, and equids. *Placenta* 1984; 5:533-540.
27. Chavez DJ, Anderson TL. The glycocalyx of the mouse luminal epithelium during estrus, early pregnancy, the peri-implantation period, and delayed implantation. I. Acquisition of *Ricinus communis*-I binding sites during pregnancy. *Biol Reprod* 1985; 32:1135-1142.
28. Anderson TL, Olson GE, Hoffman LH. Stage-specific alterations in the apical membrane glycoproteins of endometrial epithelial cells related to implantation in rabbits. *Biol Reprod* 1986; 36:599-618.
29. Lee M-C, Damjanov I. Pregnancy-related changes in the human endometrium revealed by lectin histochemistry. *Histochemistry* 1985; 82:275-280.
30. Jansen RPS, Turner M, Johannisson E, Landgren B-M, Diczfalusy E. Cyclic changes in human endometrial surface glycoproteins: A quantitative histochemical study. *Fertil Steril* 1985; 44:85-91.
31. Vicker MG, Edwards JG. The effect of neuraminidase on the aggregation of BHK21 cells and BHK21 cells transformed by polyoma virus. *J Cell Sci* 1972; 10:759-768.
32. Weiss L, Nir S, Harlos JP, Subjeck JR. Long-distance interactions between Erlich ascites tumor cells. *J Theor Biol* 1975; 51:439-454.
33. Maroudas NG. Polymer exclusion, cell adhesion, and membrane fusion. *Nature* 1975; 254:695-696.
34. Salizar-Rubio M, Gil-Recansens ME, Hicks JJ, Gonzalez Angulo A. High resolution cytochemical study of the uterine epithelial surface of the rat at identified sites previous to blastocyst-endometrial contact. *Arch Invest Med (Mex).* 1980; 11:117-127.
35. Enders AC, Schlafke S, Welsh AO. Trophoblastic and uterine epithelial surfaces at the time of blastocyst adhesion in the rat. *Am J Anat* 1980; 159:59-72.
36. Skutelsky E, Marikovsky Y, Danon D. Immunoferritin analysis of membrane antigen density: A. Young and old human blood cells. B. Developing erythroid cells and extruded erythroid nuclei. *Eur J Immunol* 1974; 4:512-518.

37. Uhlenbruck G, Baldo BA, Steinhausen G, Schwick HG, Chatterjee BP, Horejsi V, Krajhanzl A, Kocourek J. Additional precipitation reactions of lectins with human serum glycoproteins. *J Clin Chem Clin Biochem* 1978; 16:19-23.
38. Ashwell G, Harford J. Carbohydrate-specific receptors of the liver. *Ann Rev Biochem* 1982; 51:531-554.
39. Anderson TL, Coddington CC, Shen M, Hodgen GD. Defining the window of uterine receptivity: Biochemical evaluation of the endometrium. Fifth World Congress on In Vitro Fertilization and Embryo Transfer. February, 1987, Norfolk, Virginia (abstract).
40. Anderson TL, Sieg SM, Hodgen GD. Membrane composition of the endometrial epithelium: Molecular markers of uterine receptivity to implantation. In: Iizuka R, Semm K, eds. *Human reproduction. Current Status/Future Prospect.* Amsterdam: Elsevier, 1988:513-516.
41. Anderson TL, Simon JA, Hodgen GD. Histochemical characteristics of the endometrial surface related temporally to implantation in the non-human primate *Macaca fascicularis*. *Trophoblast Res* 1989; 4: in press.
42. Anderson TL, Zullo F, Coddington CC, Hodgen GD. Both saccharide-containing and saccharide-binding membrane proteins are expressed in human endometrium during the window of uterine receptivity to implantation. *Soc Gyn Invest* 36th Annual Meeting, San Diego, CA, March 1989.
43. Milos N, Zalik SE. Mechanisms of adhesion among the cells of the early chick blastoderm. Role of the beta-D-galactosamine-binding lectin in the adhesion of extraembryonic endoderm cells. *Differentiation* 1982; 21:175-182.
44. Meromsky L, Lotan R, Raz A. Implications of endogenous tumor cell surface lectins as mediators of cellular interactions and lung colonization. *Cancer Res* 1986; 46:5270-5275.
45. Chavez DJ. Cell surface of mouse blastocysts at the trophectoderm-uterine interface during the adhesive stage of implantation. *Am J Anat* 1986; 176:153-158.
46. Shur BD, Hall NG. A role for mouse sperm surface galactosyltransferase in sperm binding to the egg zona pellucida. *J Cell Biol* 1982; 95:574-579.
47. Lampelo SA, Ricketts AP, Bullock DW. Purification of rabbit endometrial plasma membranes from receptive and nonreceptive uteri. *J Reprod Fert* 1985; 75:475-484.
48. Hoffmann LH, Winfrey VP, Anderson TL, Olson GE. Uterine receptivity to implantation in the rabbit: Evidence for a 42 kDa glycoprotein as a marker of receptivity. *Trophoblast Res* 1989; 4: in press.
49. Carson DD, Tang J-P, Hu G. Estrogen influences dolichol phosphate distribution among glycolipid pools in mouse uteri. *Biochem* 1987; 26:1598-1606.
50. Lampelo SA, Anderson TL, Bullock DW. Monoclonal antibodies recognize a cell surface marker of epithelial differentiation in the rabbit reproductive tract. *J Reprod Fert* 1986; 78:663-672.
51. Aplin J, Seif MW. A monoclonal antibody to a cell surface determinant in human endometrial epithelium: Stage-specific expression in the menstrual cycle. *Am J Obstet Gynecol* 1987; 156:250-253.
52. Thor A, Viglione MJ, Muraro R, Ohuchi N, Schlom F, Gorstein F. Monoclonal antibody B72.3 reactivity with human endometrium: A study of normal and malignant tissue. *Int J Gynecol Pathol* 1987; 6:235-247.
53. Finlay BB, Heffron F, Falkon S. Epithelial cell surfaces induce *Salmonella* proteins required for bacterial adherence and invasion. *Science* 1989; 243:940-943.

SCANNING ELECTRON MICROSCOPY OF THE UTERINE LUMINAL EPITHELIUM AS A MARKER OF THE IMPLANTATION WINDOW

D. Martel, R. Frydman,* L. Sarantis, D. Roche, and A. Psychoyos

Laboratoire de Physiologie de la Reproduction
CNRS UA 549, Hôpital de Bicêtre
Batiment INSERM
78 rue du Général Leclerc,
94270 Le Kremlin Bicêtre, France.

*Service de Gynécologie-Obstétrique
Hopital Antoine Béclère
157 rue de la porte de Trivaux
92140 Clamart, France

IN VITRO fertilization and culture of human ova are now performed with increasing frequency; however, the pregnancy rate which follows replacement of the embryos is far from satisfactory. The crucial point is the likely success of the egg implantation process. Most of the studies concerning the early steps of the implantation process have been performed on small rodents, and in particular, on the rat. It has been established that successful implantation requires the synchronism of embryo development with uterine preparation. The egg must have reached the blastocyst stage and the endometrium must be in a receptive phase. Uterine receptivity, which is by definition the unique situation in which the uterus allows nidation to occur, is a hormone-dependent phenomenon, limited in time.[1] A great deal of information on egg implantation has been accumulated during this last decade. However, evaluation of uterine receptivity in humans and consequently the definition of its chronological limits remains difficult, especially in clinical practice, as histology offers limited information in this respect. In contrast, scanning electron microscopic studies of the uterine luminal surface reveal subtle changes around the expected time of implantation.[2] These changes are similar to those occurring in the rat.[3] The uterine luminal epithelium is composed of two cell types: microvilli-bearing cells and ciliated cells. Only the surface of the microvillous cells evolves depending on specific hormonal effects. Of particular interest are some apical surface protrusions referred to as "pinopods" because they could be considered as a specific marker of the occurrence of uterine receptivity.

ULTRASTRUCTURAL CHANGES OF THE SURFACE OF UTERINE LUMINAL EPITHELIUM AND RECEPTIVITY IN RAT

In this species, uterine receptivity for egg implantation lasts only a few hours. It appears on day 5 of pregnancy and is lost as soon as day 6. The hormonal conditioning responsible for these functional changes is now well defined. In ovariectomized animals, uterine receptivity is induced by a precise temporal sequence of progesterone and estradiol: it is only after a progesterone priming of at least 48 hrs that estradiol will induce 18 hrs later a transient phase of receptivity which is obligatory, followed by a phase of "non receptivity" during which the uterus becomes hostile to non-implanted eggs. Those functional changes are accompanied by striking modifications of the ultrastructure of the surface of the luminal epithelium. These changes are easily observed using scanning electron microscopy.[3,4]

Changes Occurring During Pseudopregnancy and Pregnancy

The apical surface of the uterine luminal epithelium exhibits a continuous evolution throughout day 2 to day 6 of pseudopregnancy. On days 3 and 4 of pseudopregnancy (Fig. 1a), the cell surface is covered with dense long

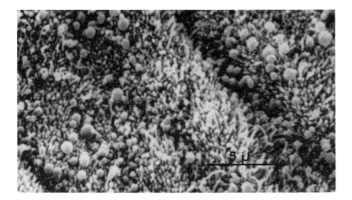

Figure 1a. *Luminal epithelium of the rat uterus on day 3 of pseudopregnancy (pre-receptive period).*

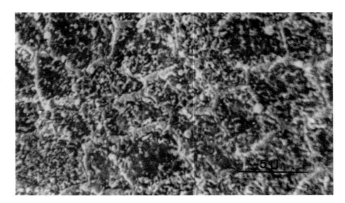

Figure 1c. *Luminal epithelium of the rat uterus on day 7 of pseudopregnancy (non-receptive period).*

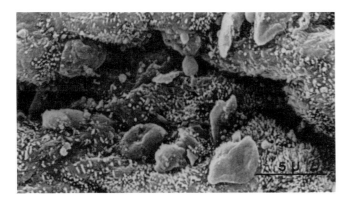

Figure 1b. *Luminal epithelium of the rat uterus on day 5 of pseudopregnancy (receptive period).*

and thick microvilli, and numerous droplets which may be secretory products are present on the cell surface. The appearance changes completely by day 5 (Fig. 1b) (the day of receptive period). The cells appear to swell and their microvilli shorten. From the surface of several cells, large formations protrude towards the uterine lumen; they are referred to as "pinopods." On day 6 of pseudopregnancy and from then on (Fig. 1c), the cell's features change again: the pinopods disappear and those seen occasionally appear to regress, while microvilli are short and the cell shape is polygonal.

Similar ultrastructural modifications have been observed during pregnancy,[3] and the pinopods absent on day 4 are particularly abundant on day 5. Now it seems evident that these structures are actively involved in pinocytosis and endocytosis of uterine fluid or macromolecules.[5,6] Their role at the time of implantation could be the closure of the uterine lumen by removing uterine fluid and/or the uptake of some molecular message released by the embryo. The substitution of microvilli by pinopods on the surface of the epithelial cells, by increasing the surface of embryo-maternal contact, together with the biochemical changes which appear on the epithelial membrane,[7-9] may also facilitate embryonic attachment and are therefore related to uterine receptivity.

Displacement of the Uterine Receptive Period

Administration of progesterone antagonists early in pregnancy or pseudopregnancy had been reported to delay or prolong the occurrence of receptivity in rats[10] and rabbits.[11] Administration of the progesterone antagonist RU-486 (Roussel-Uclaf, Romainville, France) on day 1 of pseudopregnancy (s.c. injection, 5 mg/Kg) resulted in a delay in the evolution of the endometrial luminal surface. Under this treatment the feature of the luminal surface on day 5 (Fig. 2a) was similar to that of control animals on day 4 of pseudopregnancy. Treatment with the antiprogestagen displaced the time of the appearance of fully developed pinopods from day 5 to the following days 6 and 7 of pseudopregnancy (Fig. 2b and c). It is obvious from these observations that there exists a close relationship between the presence of pinopods and the uterine phase of receptivity, both events being postponed by one or more days by the injection of the antiprogesterone.

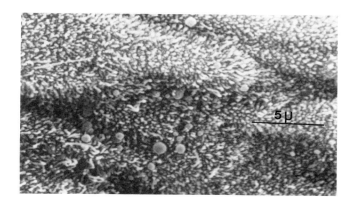

Figure 2a. Luminal epithelium of the rat uterus on day 5 of pseudopregnancy after treatment (s.c. injection) on day 1 of pseudopregnancy with 5 mg/Kg of RU-486.

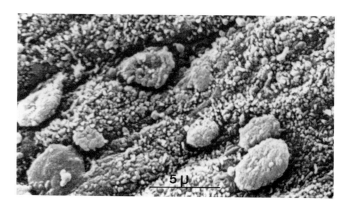

Figure 2b. Luminal epithelium of the rat uterus on day 6 of pseudopregnancy after treatment (s.c. injection) on day 1 of pseudopregnancy with 5 mg/Kg of RU-486.

ULTRASTRUCTURAL CHANGES OF THE SURFACE OF UTERINE LUMINAL EPITHELIUM IN HUMAN

The existence of a limited period of uterine receptivity, an "implantation window," remains to be established in human. The presence of pinopods on the uterine luminal surface in human endometrium[2] is of particular interest, since these structures could be considered as being specific markers of endometrial receptivity, as has been shown in the rat. Therefore, the feature of the luminal surface epithelium was studied during the peri-nidatory period (second part of the cycle) in women during normal, stimulated, and artificial menstrual cycles.

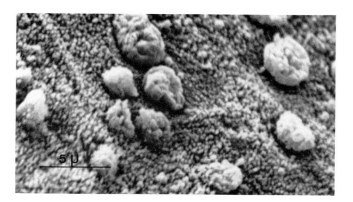

Figure 2c. Luminal epithelium of the rat uterus on day 7 of pseudopregnancy after treatment (s.c. injection) on day 1 of pseudopregnancy with 5mg/Kg of RU-486.

Spontaneous Cycles

Women who volunteered to participate in this study were recruited from a population with normal menstrual cycles. The date of ovulation was calculated from daily determinations of plasma luteinizing hormone[12] for groups among which biopsies were taken on days 2 and 6 after ovulation; or from histological examinations for biopsies taken on day 9 after ovulation.

On day 2 after ovulation, most ($\cong 80\%$) of the observed biopsies (10 specimens) had the same appearance (Fig. 3a). The cells bearing microvilli were slightly ovoid (about 3 μm long) with long and thick microvilli extending towards the uterine lumen. Numerous droplets, approximately 0.3 to 0.6 μm in diameter, covered the cellular surface. The general appearance of these endometrial samples was almost uniform. However, apical protrusions (pinopods) could be seen *occasionally* in cells surrounding a gland orifice.

On Day 6 after ovulation (Fig. 3b), most (78%) of the biopsies observed (13 specimens) were covered with pinopods: the microvilli had completely disappeared and the apical surface of the cells protruded towards the uterine lumen. These pinopods appeared to be at different stages of development in different specimens. They either covered the whole surface of the endometrial sample or occupied large regions between patches of cells bearing microvilli. In all cases the small droplets observed on day 2 after ovulation had disappeared.

On day 9 after ovulation (Fig. 3c), the pinopods had completely regressed and the uterine epithelium regained a regular appearance: the cells had a polygonal shape and were covered with dense short and thin microvilli.

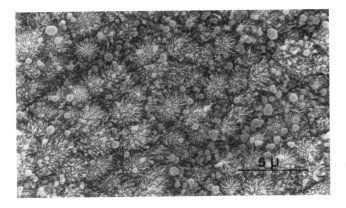

Figure 3a. Luminal epithelium of the human uterus 2 days after ovulation during spontaneous menstrual cycle.

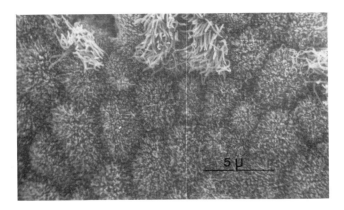

Figure 3c. Luminal epithelium of the human uterus on day 9 after ovulation during spontaneous menstrual cycle.

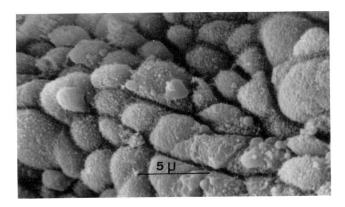

Figure 3b. Luminal epithelium of the human uterus on day 6 after ovulation during spontaneous menstrual cycle.

Our studies using scanning electron microscopy have revealed marked changes in the ultrastructure of the luminal surface epithelium in human endometrium during the secretory phase of the menstrual cycle. The most interesting observation was the transient presence of fully formed pinopods which are, as already described for the rat, limited to the period when the embryo is expected to implant, i.e., day 20 in the case of a fertile cycle. Thus, in spite of the fact that the final steps of the implantation process are quite different in the rat and the human, the first steps appear to follow a similar course in both species.

Stimulated Cycles

Women in this group were recruited from an *in vitro* fertilization program. They received clomiphene citrate (100 mg/day; Merrell, Neuilly sur Seine, France) for 5 consecutive days and beginning on the second day of the menstrual cycle, followed by hMg (two ampules/day; Neopergonal, Serono, Levallois-Perret, France) on days 6, 8, and 10 of the cycle. The hMg treatment was continued until completion of follicular maturation. As soon as a concentration of 1.1-1.5 nmol estradiol/l for each follicle of more than 15 mm was reached, hCG (5000 i.u. Organon, Saint Denis, France) was administered.

On day 2 after ovulation, only $\cong 44\%$ of the biopsies observed (9 specimens) had a luminal surface that was identical in structure to that of the normally cycling group at the same stage (aspect shown in Fig. 3a). Another 44% of the biopsies observed were in advanced stages with pinopods either bulging or well formed.

On day 6 after ovulation, only $\cong 15\%$ of the observed biopsies (13 specimens) had pinopods identical in structure to specimens taken on day 6 after ovulation in the normal cycling group. No formation of pinopods was seen in all the other specimens.

Our results provide evidence that these hormonal treatments modify the appearance of the uterine luminal surface. Ovarian stimulation with clomiphene citrate, hMg, and hCG resulted in altered evolution of the surface of the microvillous cells. The absence of pinopods on day 20 of the menstrual cycle is consistent with an aberrant development of the endometrium which could result from luteal-phase defects occurring after treatment with hMG alone or with clomiphene citrate plus hMG.[13,14] However, it can be suggested from our studies that at least some of the biopsies were out of phase since 44% of them were already in an advanced stage on day 2 after ovulation. It is likely that pinopods had already regressed at the

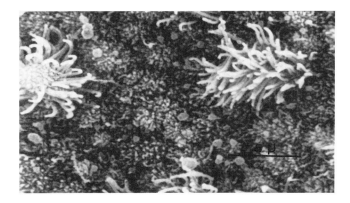

Figure 4a. *Luminal epithelium of the human uterus during artificial cycle, 2 days after the beginning of the progesterone treatment. Appearance of the 28% of the biopsies that exhibited a maturation equivalent to day 16 of a normal menstrual cycle.*

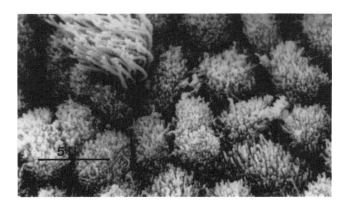

Figure 4b. *Luminal epithelium of the human uterus during artificial cycle, 2 days after the beginning of the progesterone treatment. Appearance of the 43% of the biopsies that were at an advanced stage, equivalent to day 18 of a normal menstrual cycle.*

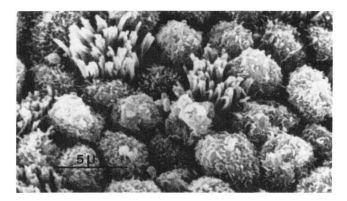

Figure 4c. *Luminal epithelium of the human uterus during artificial cycle, 6 days after the beginning of the progesterone treatment. Well-formed pinopods were seen in the majority of biopsies.*

Replacement Cycles

Women in this group suffered from total or severely reduced ovarian failure and were scheduled for embryo replacement during an artificially induced menstrual cycle. They received estradiol valerate (Progynova, Schering, Lys-Lez-Lannoy, France) 2 mg/day from days 1 to 6 of the artificial cycle; 4 mg/day from days 7 to 9; 6 mg/day from days 10 to 12; 8 mg/day on day 13; and 2 mg/day from day 14 until day 28; Progesterone (Utrogestant, Besins-Iscovesco, Paris, France) was given from days 14 to 28 of the artificial cycle. Endometrial biopsies were taken on days 2 or 6 after the beginning of the progesterone treatment (equivalent days 16 and 20 of the artificial cycle).

On day 2 after the beginning of the progesterone treatment, the appearance of the surface of the luminal epithelium in $\cong 28\%$ (Fig. 4a) of the biopsies observed (7 specimens) was identical to that described for day 16 in a normal cycle. The greater part of the biopsies observed ($\cong 43\%$) were at a more advanced stage (Fig. 4b), with shortened microvilli and bulging pinopods equivalent to day 18 in a normal cycle. One specimen was even more advanced with well-formed pinopods covering the surface.

On day 6 after the beginning of the progesterone treatment, most biopsies ($\cong 71\%$) exhibited well-formed pinopods; however, some of those biopsies had a heterogeneous appearance with large plates of cells corresponding to day 18 of a normal cycle. One biopsy was at a more advanced stage, equivalent to day 21 of a normal cycle.

expected time of initiation of egg implantation (day 6 after ovulation). It is possible that if there exists in the human a limited nidatory period, the endometrium could already be in a non-receptive phase when the embryo reaches the blastocyst stage and is able to implant. In any case, according to our findings, it appears difficult to associate the induction of superovulation with the normal development of the endometrium.

Our results concerning the replacement cycles are encouraging since after 6 days of progesterone treatment following the estradiol priming, pinopods were present on the majority of the biopsies observed. However, in that case, the quality of the endometrial evolution (heterogeneous appearance of the biopsies) could perhaps be ameliorated by a light modification of the progesterone and estradiol protocols. Further studies are therefore necessary to define the precise hormonal requirement for normal endometrial maturation during the pre-nidatory period in the human.

CONCLUSIONS

In the human as in the rat, the presence of completely developed pinopods appears to be restricted to the perinidatory period, and is progesterone dependent. It is, of course, tempting to consider that the time of the appearance and disappearance of these structures indicates in the human as in the rat, the chronological limits of the implantation window. However, further research is needed to clarify this point. These morphological criteria could already be of clinical significance as indicators of the normality of the endometrial evolution under different hormonal conditions, in particular those used for the *in vitro* fertilization programs.

References

1. Psychoyos A. Endocrine control of egg implantation. In: Greep RO, Astwood EB, eds. *Handbook of physiology*. Washington, D.C. 1973:187-215.
2. Martel D, Malet C, Gautray JP, Psychoyos A. Surface changes of the luminal uterine epithelium during human menstrual cycle: a scanning electron microscopic study. In: De Brux J, Mortel R, Gautray JP, eds. *The endometrium: hormonal impacts*. Penum Publishing Corporation 1981:15-29.
3. Psychoyos A, Mandon P. Etude de la surface de l'épithélium uterin au microscope electronique a balayage. Observations chez la rate au 4ème et 5ème jours de la gestation. *C R Acad Sc Paris* 1971; 272:2723-2725.
4. Sarantis L, Roche D, Psychoyos A. Displacement of receptivity for nidation in the rat by progesterone antagonist RU-486: a scanning electron microscopy study. *Human Reprod* 1987; 2:251-255.
5. Enders AC, Nelson DM. Pinocytotic activity in the uterus of the rat. *Am J Anat* 1973; 138:277-299.
6. Parr MB, Parr EL. Uterine luminal epithelium protrusions mediate endocytosis not apocrine secretion in the rat. *Biol Reprod* 1974; 11:220-223.
7. Chavez DJ, Anderson TL. The glycocalyx of the mouse uterine luminal epithelium during estrus, early pregnancy, the peri-implantation period and delayed implantation. I. Acquisition of *Ricinus communis* binding sites during pregnancy. *Biol Reprod* 1985; 32:1135-1142.
8. Murphy CR, Rogers AW. Effects of ovarian hormones on cell membranes in rat uterus. *Cell Biophysics* 1981; 3:305-320.
9. Morris JE, Potter SW. A comparison of developmental changes in surface charge in mouse blastocysts and uterine epithelium using DEAE beads and dextran sulfate in vitro. *Developmental Biology* 1984; 103:190-199.
10. Psychoyos A, Prapas I. Inhibition of egg development and implantation in the rats after post-coital administration of the progesterone antagonist RU 486. *J Reprod Fertil* 1987; 80:487-491.
11. Hegele-Hartung C, Beier HM. Distribution of uteroglobin in the rabbit endometrium after treatment with an antiprogesterone (ZK 98.734): an immunocytochemical study. *Hum Reprod* 1986; 1:497-505.
12. Testart J, Frydman R, Feinstein MC, Thebault A, Roger M, Scoller R. Interpretation of plasma luteinizing hormone assay for the collection of mature oocytes from women: definition of a luteinizing hormone surge initiating rise. *Fertil Steril* 1981; 36:50-60.
13. Jones GS. The role of luteal support for in vitro fertilization. In: Edwards RG, Purdy J, Steptoe PC, eds. *Implantation of the human embryo*. New York: Academic Press 1985:285-302.
14. Edwards RG. Normal and abnormal implantation in the human uterus. In: Edwards RG, Purdy J, Steptoe PC, eds., *Implantation of the human embryo*. New York: Academic Press, 1985:303-333.

UTERINE RECEPTIVITY FOR IMPLANTATION: HUMAN STUDIES

P.A.W. Rogers and C.R. Murphy*

Department of Obstetrics and Gynecology
Monash University
Clayton, Victoria 3168, Australia

*Department of Histology and Embryology
University of Sydney
Sydney, NSW 2006 Australia

RESEARCH projects based on human subjects are governed by a number of serious limitations, in particular ethical considerations and practical restrictions on experimental design. Research in a field like uterine receptivity is further hampered by our lack of understanding of the many and apparently varied mechanisms that exist in the numerous animal models that have been studied to date. The advent in recent years of *in vitro* fertilization (IVF) as a clinical treatment for human infertility has focused much basic and clinical research on the human reproductive process between the latter stages of gametogenesis through to fertilization and implantation. In particular, attention is now being paid to the role of the non-receptive uterus in preventing embryo implantation because it is becoming apparent that this may be one of the major remaining blocks to higher pregnancy rates.[1] In this chapter, a brief review of some animal studies on uterine receptivity will be followed by sections on four different aspects of human receptivity, each of which is based on recent studies made possible by the advent of clinical IVF.

THE ROLE OF THE UTERUS IN CONTROLLING IMPLANTATION: ANIMAL STUDIES

The first stages of interaction and communication between the implanting blastocyst and the maternal endometrium are some of the most important and least well understood during the reproductive process. Current thinking, based primarily on animal models, while not ignoring the role of the blastocyst, favors the view that it is the uterus, appropriately conditioned by ovarian hormones, that predominantly determines the success or otherwise of implantation.[2-5] Further support for this hypothesis comes from numerous studies demonstrating that mammalian embryos can initiate implantation-type vascular reactions in non-uterine tissues with a high degree of success regardless of the sex or hormonal status of the host. Ectopic sites that have been studied in this way include the anterior chamber of the eye,[6-8] the kidney,[9,10] the testis,[11] and the spleen.[12]

Understanding of the uterine mechanisms that control implantation is further complicated by the wide variability that exists from species to species in the method whereby the embryo comes into contact with the endometrium.[13] Among well-studied species such as laboratory rodents, it has been shown that the uterus becomes receptive to the implanting blastocyst for a short period of time a few days after the commencement of continuous progesterone administration.[14,15] Priming estrogen prior to this progesterone is not essential,[15] although a small amount of estrogen must be given at some time after the commencement of progesterone for an implantation receptive uterus to be established. These and other studies have led to the concept of an "implantation window," defined as the period of time when the uterus is receptive to the implanting blastocyst. In addition to the receptive state, it has also been postulated that the uterus goes through "implantation neutral" and "implantation hostile" states.[16] During the neutral phase the embryo can survive in the uterus but will not implant, while during the hostile phase the embryo is actively destroyed. How the uterus effects these receptive, neutral, and hostile states remains largely unclear, although embryo toxic compounds have been demonstrated in uterine flushings from rats and mice taken at times other than when implantation normally occurs.[17,18] Other studies have implicated a major role for the uterine epithelium in preventing implantation unless the correct hormonal priming has occurred.[19] In this work the embryo was only able to implant in the unprimed mouse uterus once the epithelium had been removed.

UTERINE FACTORS CONTRIBUTING TO HUMAN IMPLANTATION FAILURE

Estimates of maximum human fecundability (defined as a percentage of women who will produce a full-term infant per menstrual cycle during which frequent intercourse occurs) range from 14.4% to 31.8% for various populations and age groups of women.[20] Under normal circumstances a number of factors may contribute to this low success rate, including anovulation, intercourse at the wrong time, reduced semen quality, failure of egg or sperm transport, fertilization failure, embryonic mortality, and uterine hostility. Of these potential factors, it is probable that embryonic mortality contributes significantly,[21] as a result of both chromosomal[22] and other developmental abnormalities within the embryo. To date, it has not been possible using information derived from natural conception cycles to determine the role that uterine factors may play in implantation failure.

More recently, the large amount of human implantation data produced following superovulation and multiple embryo transfer by various IVF groups has provided an avenue for exploring the relative contributions of embryonic and uterine factors to implantation failure.[23,24] These studies are based on a hypothetical two parameter model for implantation proposed by Speirs et al.[25] This model assumes that each embryo has a probability (E) of survival, and that in any given patient there is a probability (U) that the uterus will be receptive. Thus, when a single embryo is transferred the probability of pregnancy is represented by the product U x E. This simplistic model makes a number of assumptions: that U and E are independent, that U and E are the only factors influencing implantation, that one embryo successfully implanting does not influence the chance of other embryos implanting, and that the probabilities U and E do not alter significantly within each IVF group with time.

Five large sets of IVF data have been analyzed using this mathematical model for implantation, and values for U and E have been calculated using maximum-likelihood methods (Table I). When these values for U and E were used to construct tables of predicted singleton and multiple implantation rates following embryo transfer for each IVF group, only 2 of the 5 predicted sets of data deviated significantly from the actual observed results (Queen Elizabeth and Norfolk). These results suggest that the U-E model may in fact be a good approximation to the biological events that control implantation. If this is the case, then it is quite evident that low uterine receptivity is playing a significant role in implantation failure in human IVF. It is also of interest to note that Norfolk, the only IVF clinic not to use the anti-estrogen clomiphene citrate as a superovulation drug, has a theoretical uterine receptivity of 0.64. By contrast, the 4 IVF groups that use clomiphene citrate have significantly lower theoretical uterine receptivity values ranging from 0.31 to 0.42.

Table I. *Estimates for uterine receptivity (U) and embryo viability (E) based on implantation data from 5 IVF groups. (± simultaneous 95% confidence limits).*

IVF Group	Uterine Receptivity (U)	Embryo Viability (E)
Monash, Melbourne	0.31 ± 0.07	0.32 ± 0.06
Royal Women's, Melbourne	0.42 ± 0.11	0.23 ± 0.05
Queen Elizabeth, Adelaide	0.42 ± 0.17	0.28 ± 0.10
Norfolk, Virginia	0.64 ± 0.22	0.21 ± 0.08
*Bourne Hall, Cambridge	0.36	0.43

Taken from Rogers et al., 1986[23] and *Walters et al. 1985.[24]

If these theoretical values for uterine receptivity are correct, then two major conclusions may be drawn. First, as has been shown in a number of other species, the human uterus has selective mechanisms by which the implanting embryo can be accepted or rejected. Second, if IVF pregnancy rates are going to be improved significantly, then it will be necessary to address the problem of low uterine receptivity. This is particularly important since problems with low embryo viability can be overcome to some extent by replacing more embryos, whereas uterine receptivity is always fixed for each patient and rapidly becomes the dominant negative factor controlling the overall pregnancy rate once 3 or more good embryos are transferred to the uterus.

ENDOCRINOLOGICAL REQUIREMENTS FOR UTERINE RECEPTIVITY IN THE HUMAN

Prior to IVF and embryo transfer becoming routine clinical treatments for human infertility, very little data were available concerning the sequence and amounts of estrogen and progesterone necessary to prepare the endometrium for implantation. Studies of circulating estrogen and progesterone levels during the normal menstrual cycle show wide variability from woman to woman.[26] However, there is little understanding of how these varying levels of estrogen and progesterone within the wide normal range may influence receptivity. Although it is known that excessive estrogen administered post-ovulation can prevent implantation,[27] not much is known about the pre- and peri-implantation levels of estrogen and progesterone required for successful implantation. In one study which examined 527 cycles in 67 subfertile patients it was found that significantly more viable pregnancies occurred among patients with an estrogen-to-progesterone ratio in the range of 7.63 to 12.22 (calculated as estrogen in pmol/l divided by progesterone in nmol/l).[28] Steroid levels were measured in circulating blood taken at the presumed time of implantation.

IVF has generated large amounts of accurate endocrine data on the circulating levels of estrogen and progesterone during stimulated cycles. In addition, receptive cycles are clearly identified by pregnancy following embryo transfer. Unfortunately, this major increase in previously difficult to obtain data has tended to confuse rather than clarify the situation. As with the variability seen in the natural cycle, pregnancies have been achieved by numerous IVF groups using a wide range of stimulation-protocols that have resulted in an even wider range of circulating estrogen and progesterone levels. Some groups have identified follicular phase estrogen profiles that indicate a higher prospect of pregnancy,[29] although it is possible that these profiles just reflect better follicle development and oocyte quality, and are not acting preferentially on uterine receptivity.

The reporting of the world's first donor oocyte pregnancy in a woman with premature ovarian failure[30] opened a valuable experimental avenue for further exploring the estrogen and progesterone levels required for implantation. In these patients, exogenous estrogen and progesterone is given solely to create a receptive uterine environment, since there is no need to manipulate the follicular phase of the cycle to produce an oocyte. The first steroid replacement regimens developed were based very closely on the standardized 28-day menstrual cycle, with increasing levels of estrogen during the first half of the cycle and progesterone commencing mid-cycle.[30,31] More recently, successful replacement regimens have been developed that use a constant dose of estrogen over a variable period up to the time that the donor oocyte is obtained.[32,33] Progesterone is then given to the patient from either the day before or the day of oocyte collection from the donor. This new approach has the advantage of permitting a much wider window of time in which the donor and the recipient can be synchronized. Examples of cyclical and variable length steroid replacement schedules used at Monash are given in Figure 1. Using the variable length schedule we have achieved pregnancies with follicular phases ranging from 14 to 21 days. Histological and ultrastructural studies of endometrial morphology that are currently under way suggest that these limits may well be extended considerably further. Indeed, it is not inconceivable that, as with some animal species,[15] follicular phase estrogen might be completely unnecessary for the development of uterine receptivity in the human.

Undoubtedly the endocrinological parameters necessary for uterine receptivity will become more clearly defined as studies such as those described above continue. Unfortunately, interpretation of results will always be plagued by the wide natural variation in uterine response to estrogen and progesterone that occurs in the human.[43]

THE IMPLANTATION WINDOW IN HUMANS

The search for morphological or biochemical markers of uterine receptivity that permit quantification of the human implantation window have been unsuccessful to date. The relationship of various morphological criteria to the receptive period are discussed in the final section of this chapter. In one of the few other studies in search of a mechanism whereby the uterus may reject the embryo,[35] it was found that human uterine flushings from different stages of the menstrual cycle had no significant effect on the *in vitro* development of mouse blastocysts. This is despite the apparent presence of uterine derived embryotoxic factors in some animal species.[17,18]

Until morphological or biochemical markers of receptivity are discovered, definition of the implantation window

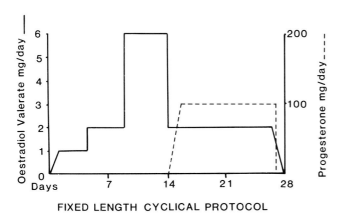
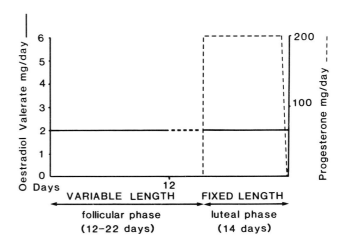

Figure 1. Cyclical and variable length protocols for donor oocyte recipients requiring steroid replacement therapy for premature ovarian failure.

in the human will rely on data generated by asynchronous embryo transfers in human donor oocyte or embryo programs. In a review of 30 published pregnancies in patients receiving donated oocytes for premature ovarian failure,[35] it was estimated that successful implantation occurred when the embryo was anywhere from 36 hrs in front to 48 hrs behind the uterus. These calculations give an implantation window of at least 3½ days. A summary of this and some additional new data, representing a total of 52 pregnancies, is given in Table II. The calculations in Table II are based on the assumption that, as in animals,[14,15] the commencement of progesterone in the human will initiate a "clock" that results in the uterus passing through a receptive phase or window. Uterine age is thus calculated as the time from when the uterus first received progesterone, and embryonic age is taken from the time of ovulation. The synchrony calculations in this table are based on the 2 assumptions that in the natural cycle: (a) significant progesterone secretion starts 12 hrs before ovulation and (b) fertilization occurs 6 hrs after ovulation. Where it has not been possible from the published information to accurately estimate the timing of embryonic development relative to the point in time that the uterus first received progesterone, a question mark (?) has been placed next to the calculated synchrony.

Of particular interest in Table II is the work of Formigli et al.[37] These workers used embryos lavaged from the uteri of donors 5 days post-ovulation, and report pregnancies in cases where the recipient was anywhere from 4 days in front to 3 days behind the donor at the time of ovulation. However, there may be possible sources of error in the calculations of timing in this study. For example, ovulation was only assessed by daily ultrasound of the ovaries monitoring for disappearance of the follicle, and could therefore be up to 24 hrs out. More importantly, it was not possible to exclude the possibility of spontaneous pregnancy in 5 out of 6 patients with ovarian function. Accepting these limitations, this study suggests that the human implantation window may be up to 7 days, twice that previously demonstrated by donor oocyte and embryo results.

MORPHOLOGICAL STUDIES IN SEARCH OF MARKERS FOR HUMAN UTERINE RECEPTIVITY

It has long been recognized that the human endometrium typically undergoes cyclical changes in histological appearance in response to changing levels of estrogen and progesterone during the menstrual cycle. This has been reported both at the light microscope level[41] and using scanning (SEM) and transmission (TEM) electron microscopy.[42,43] However, despite numerous studies it has not yet been possible to link any given morphological criterion unequivocally with the physiological status of uterine receptivity. There are two major reasons for this lack of success. First, it is not ethically permissible to plan experiments where endometrial biopsies are taken from a uterus that contains an implanting embryo and can thus be proven receptive for embryo implantation. The second problem lies in the variability seen between biopsies taken at the same stage of the cycle from different patients, and

Table II. Summary of data on embryonic uterine synchrony based on human donor oocyte and embryo transfers.

Source	Pregnancies reported	Uterus ahead of embryo (hours)	Uterus behind embryo (hours)
(1) Monash donor oocyte Standard cyclical protocol	11		18-39
(2) Monash donor oocyte Variable length protocol	5		24-36
(3) Feichtinger and Kemeter (1985)[38]	1		18
(4) Navot et al. (1986)[31]	2	4-28	
(5) Rosenwaks (1987)[39]	8	0-40	0-24
(6) Serhal and Craft (1987)[32]	7	12	
(7) Asche et al. (1988)[33]	6		18
(8) Formigli et al. (1987)[37]	8	0-96	0-72
(9) Junca et al. (1988)[40]	4	0(?)	

between biopsies taken from the same patient on subsequent cycles.[44]

Studies on endometrial morphology in our group at Monash have concentrated on SEM of the epithelial surface in patients on steroid replacement therapy for premature ovarian failure.[34,45] The advantages of this group for such studies include the fact that each patient receives an accurately determined steroid replacement schedule and that uterine receptivity is tested by embryo transfer in one or more cycles. However, it should be realized that patients suffering premature ovarian failure may possibly have other reproductive deficiencies that could contribute to reduced fecundity, although pregnancy results from IVF donor oocyte programs reported to date do not support this latter contention.[36]

In a SEM study of 26 biopsies taken from 23 patients each receiving a standard 28-day steroid replacement regimen,[34] 7 epithelial morphological characteristics were given relative scores of 1 to 4. The scoring criteria were based on previously published human and animal results[46,47] and gave a high score for appearances that are believed to be receptive, and a low score for appearances that are supposedly non-receptive. (Examples of low and high scoring biopsies are shown in Fig. 2.) Morphological criteria and scoring were as follows:

(1) Bulging cell apices, score 4. Flat or sunken apices, score 1.
(2) Irregular microvilli, score 4. Long, uniform microvilli, score 1.
(3) Few and sparse microvilli, score 4. Dense microvilli, score 1.
(4) Gland openings slit-like, score 4. Gland openings round, score 1.
(5) Surface contours smooth, score 4. Surface contours rough, score 1.
(6) Many blebs and apical protrusions, score 4. Few or none, score 1.
(7) Few ciliated cells, score 4. Many ciliated cells, score 1.

Two interesting conclusions resulted from this work. It was clear that there was no correlation between endocrine profiles as measured by daily radioimmunoassay (RIA) of circulating blood and the morphological criteria measured in the study. In other words, patients with similar endocrine profiles had widely different endometrial scores. The second more tentative conclusion was that the morphological features being measured probably did not relate to receptivity, at least in any direct sense. This conclusion was based on the observation that 3 patients who became pregnant in subsequent transfer cycles had scores of 1.33, 2.14, and 2.29, compared with an average score for the whole group of 2.44, while 3 patients with average scores of 3.43, 3.33, and 3.20 who received transfers failed to become pregnant. Further evidence to support the hypothesis that these morphological criteria do not in themselves define receptivity comes from observations made on a biopsy taken unknowingly from a conception cycle.[48] This patient, with a diagnosis of primary ovarian

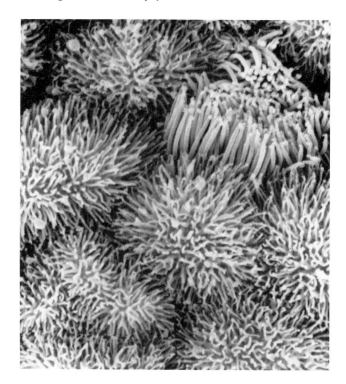 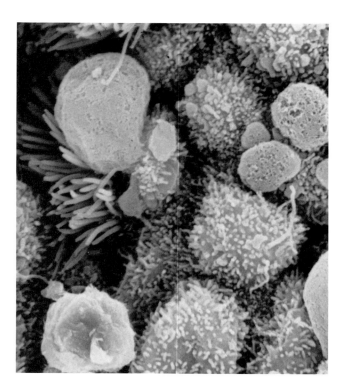

Figure 2. *Scanning electron micrographs showing widely different uterine epithelial surface morphology. It has been suggested that the long dense microvilli seen in the left photograph were consistent with a nonreceptive state, while the morphological features seen in the right photograph were more indicative of a receptive uterus. Recent studies have now questioned these conclusions.*[34,38] *(X5000).*

failure, spontaneously ovulated on day 10 of steroid replacement therapy (as judged by her spontaneous LH surge) and was biopsied on day 18 of the cycle, 8 days post ovulation. Retrospective analysis of daily bloods detected the first appearance of βhCG on day 19, the day following the biopsy. The average morphological score for this biopsy was 2.43 (see Fig. 3). Although it is possible that this relatively low score is because the biopsy was taken 1-2 days after implantation, we believe that a more probable interpretation is that the embryo implanted despite the presence of a number of morphological characteristics previously thought to be unfavorable for implantation.

We are presently continuing these morphological studies[49] comparing endometria from natural cycles with biopsies collected both during standard cyclical steroid replacement therapy and also during the new variable length follicular phase therapy (Fig. 1). This latter protocol has been remarkably successful at achieving pregnancies (5 from 14 transfers, 36%; versus 10 from 50 transfers with the old standard protocol, 20%).

A further study presently under way in our group is freeze-fracture electron microscope analysis of tight junctions between uterine epithelial cells. It is known that these

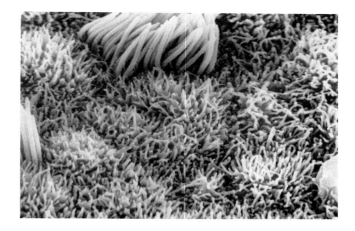

Figure 3. *Uterine epithelial surface ultrastructure one to two days post implantation (day 22 of a standardized 28 day cycle). Note the long microvilli and general similar appearance of the "unreceptive" biopsy shown in Figure 2. (X5400).*

tight junctions alter markedly during the estrous cycle in the rat[50] and also during the menstrual cycle in the human.[51] Intercellular tight junctions play an important role in regulating the passage of substances across the epithelium, and as such may play a significant role in regulating the movement of embryonic messengers, or even the embryo itself, around the time of implantation. Preliminary studies have shown a considerable reduction in the depth of the tight junctions down the lateral wall of the epithelial cells approximately 5-6 days after the commencement of progesterone. Whether or not this observation is general, and if it is, whether it correlates to a reduction in epithelial strength or permeability prior to embryo invasion, is currently under investigation.

References

1. Short RV. When a conception fails to become a pregnancy. In: *Maternal recognition of pregnancy. Ciba Foundation: Excerpta Medica*, 1979; 377-394.
2. Sherman MI, Wudl LR. The implanting mouse blastocyst. *Cell Surface Rev* 1976; 1:81-125.
3. Murphy CR, Rogers AW. Effects of ovarian hormones on cell membranes in the rat uterus. III. The surface carbohydrates at the apex of the luminal epithelium. *Cell Biophysics* 1981; 3:305-320.
4. Murphy CR, Swift JF, Mukherjee TM, Rogers AW. Changes in the fine structure of the apical plasma membrane of endometrial epithelial cells during implantation in the rat. *J Cell Sci* 1982; 55:1-12.
5. Anderson TL, Hoffmann LH. Alterations in epithelial glycocalyx of rabbit uteri during early pseudopregnancy and pregnancy, and following ovariectomy. *Am J Anat* 1984; 171:321-324.
6. Runner MN. Development of mouse eggs in the anterior chamber of the eye. *Anat Rec* 1947; 98:1-17.
7. Fawcett DW, Wislocki GB, Waldo CM. The development of mouse ova in the anterior chamber of the eye and in the abdominal cavity. *Am J Anat* 1947; 81:413-443.
8. Rogers PAW, Macpherson AM, Beaton LA. Vascular response in a non-uterine site to implantation-stage embryos in the rat and guinea-pig: in vivo and ultrastructural studies. *Cell Tissue Res* 1988; 254:217-224.
9. Fawcett DW. The development of mouse ova under the capsule of the kidney. *Anat Rec* 1950; 108:71-91.
10. Kirby DRS. Development of mouse eggs beneath the kidney capsule. *Nature* 1960; 187:707-708.
11. Kirby DRS. The development of mouse blastocysts transplanted to the scrotal and cryptorchid testis. *J Anat* 1963; 97:119-130.
12. Kirby DRS. Development of the mouse blastocyst transplanted to the spleen. *J Reprod Fertil* 1963; 5:1-12.
13. Finn CA, Porter DG. Implantation of ova. In: Finn CA, ed. *The uterus. Handbooks in reproductive biology*, Vol. 1, London: *Elek Science* 1975; 57-73.
14. De Feo VJ. Determination of the sensitive period for the induction of deciduomata in the rat by different inducing procedures. *Endocrinology* 1963; 73:488-497.
15. Humphrey KW. Induction of implantation of blastocysts transferred to ovariectomized mice. *J Endocr* 1969; 44:299-303.
16. Psychoyos A. Hormonal control of ovoimplantation. *Vitams Horm* 1973; 31:201-256.
17. Psychoyos A, Casimiri V. Factors involved in uterine receptivity and refractoriness. *Prog Reprod Biol* 1980; 7:143-157.
18. Weitlauf HM. Factors in mouse uterine fluid that inhibit the incorporation of ³H-uridine by blastocysts in vitro. *J Reprod Fertil* 1978; 52:321-325.
19. Cowell TP. Implantation and development of mouse eggs transferred to the uteri of non-progestational mice. *J Reprod Fert* 1969; 19:239-245.
20. Leridon H. *Human fertility*. Chicago: University of Chicago Press, 1977.
21. Hertig AT, Rock J, Adams EC. A description of 34 human ova within the first 17 days of development. *Am J Anat* 1956; 98:435-493.
22. Boué J, Boué A, Lazar P. Retrospective and prospective epidemiological studies of 1500 karyotyped spontaneous human abortions. *Teratology* 1975; 12:11-26.
23. Rogers PAW, Milne BJ, Trounson AO. A model to show human uterine receptivity and embryo viability following ovarian stimulation for in vitro fertilization. *J Vitro Fert Emb Trans* 1986; 3:93-98.
24. Walters DE, Edwards DG, Meistrich ML. A statistical evaluation of implantation after replacing one or more human embryos. *J Reprod Fert* 1985; 74:557-563.
25. Speirs AL, Lopata A, Gronow MJ, Kellow GN, Johnston WIH. Analysis of the benefits and risks of multiple embryo transfer. *Fertil Steril* 1983; 39:468-471.
26. Landgren BM, Undén AL, Diczfalusy E. Hormonal profile of the cycle in 68 normally menstruating women. *Acta Endocr* 1980; 94:89-98.
27. Morris JM, Van Wagenen G. Interception: The use of postovulatory oestrogens to prevent implantation. *J Am Obstet Gynecol* 1973; 115:101-106.
28. Sharp NC, Anthony F, Williams J, Masson GM, Miller JF. Oestradiol and progesterone levels at the time of implanta-

28. tion and their effect upon its success in a subfertile population. [Abstract] In: *Proceedings of the Sixth Scientific Meeting of the Fertility Society of Australia.* Sydney, Australia, 1987:43.
29. Jones HW, Acosta A, Andrews MC, et al. The importance of the follicular phase to success and failure in in vitro fertilization. *Fertil Steril* 1983; 40:317-321.
30. Lutjen P, Trounson A, Leeton J, Findlay J, Wood C, Renou P. The establishment and maintenance of pregnancy using in vitro fertilization and embryo donation in a patient with primary ovarian failure. *Nature* 1984; 307:174-175.
31. Navot D, Laufer N, Kopolovic J, et al. Artificially induced endometrial cycles and establishment of pregnancies in the absence of ovaries. *N Engl J Med* 1986; 314:806-811.
32. Serhal P, Craft I. Simplified treatment for ovum donation. *Lancet* 1987; I:687-688.
33. Asche RH, Balmoceda JP, Ord T, et al. Oocyte donation and gamete intrafallopian transfer in premature ovarian failure. *Fertil Steril* 1988; 49:263-267.
34. Rogers PAW, Murphy CR, Cameron I, et al. Uterine receptivity in women receiving steroid replacement therapy for premature ovarian failure: ultrastructural and endocrinological parameters. *Human Reprod* 1988; submitted.
35. Aitken RJ, Maathuis JB. Effect of human uterine flushings collected at various states of the menstrual cycle on mouse blastocysts in vitro. *J Reprod Fertil* 1978; 53:137-140.
36. Rogers P, Leeton J, Cameron IT, Murphy C, Healy DL, Lutjen P. Oocyte Donation. In: Wood C, Trounson A, eds. *Clinical in vitro fertilization and embryo transfer.* 2nd Edition. Berlin: Springer-Verlag, 1988:143-154.
37. Formigli L, Formigli G, Roccio C. Donation of fertilized uterine ova to infertile women. *Fertil Steril* 1987; 47:162-165.
38. Feichtinger W, Kemeter P. Pregnancy after total ovariectomy achieved by ovum donation. *Lancet* 1985; II:722-723.
39. Rosenwaks Z. Donor eggs: their application in modern reproductive technologies. *Fertil Steril* 1987; 47:895-909.
40. Junca A-M, Cohen J, Mandelbaum J, et al. Anonymous and non-anonymous oocyte donation preliminary results. *Human Reprod* 1988; 3:121-123.
41. Noyes RW, Hertig AT, Rock J. Dating the endometrial biopsy. *Fertil Steril* 1950; 1:3-25.
42. Lawn AM. The ultrastructure of the endometrium during the sexual cycle. In: Bishop MWH, ed. *Advances in reproductive biology.* Vol. 6. London: Elek, 1973:61-97.
43. Martel D, Malet C, Gautray JP, Psychoyos A. Surface changes of the luminal uterine epithelium during the human menstrual cycle: a scanning electron microscopic study. In: de Brus J, Martel J, Gautray JP, eds. *The endometrium: hormonal impacts.* New York: Plenum Publishing Corporation, 1981:15-29.
44. Balasch J, Vanrell JA, Montserrat C, Márquez M, González-Merlo J. The endometrial biopsy for diagnosis of luteal phase deficiency. *Fertil Steril* 1985; 44:699-701.
45. Murphy CR, Rogers PAW, Leeton J, Hosie M, Beaton L, Macpherson A. Surface ultrastructure of uterine epithelial cells in women with premature ovarian failure following steroid hormone replacement. *Acta Anat* 1987; 130:348-350.
46. Ljungkvist I. Attachment reaction of rat uterine luminal epithelium IV. The cellular changes in the attachment reaction and its hormonal regulation. *Fertil Steril* 1972; 23:847-865.
47. Ferenczy A. Surface ultrastructural response of the human uterine lining epithelium to hormonal environment. A scanning electron microscopic study. *Acta Cytol* 1977; 21:566-572.
48. Rogers PAW, Murphy CR, Leeton J, Hosie M, Beaton L, Macpherson A. An ultrastructural study of human uterine epithelium from a patient with a confirmed pregnancy. *Acta Anat* 1988; in press.
49. Hosie M, Murphy CR, Rogers PAW, Leeton J, Healy DL. A morphometric scoring system for scanning electron microscopic data of the human endometrium. [Abstract] In: *Proceedings of the seventh scientific meeting of the Fertility Society of Australia.* Newcastle, 1988:P12.
50. Murphy CR, Swift JG, Mukherjee TM, Rogers AW. The structure of tight junctions between uterine luminal epithelial cells at different stages of pregnancy in the rat. *Cell Tissue Res* 1982; 223:281-286.
51. Murphy CR, Swift JG, Need JA, Mukherjee TM, Rogers AW. A freeze-fracture electron microscopic study of tight junctions of epithelial cells in the human uterus. *Anat Embryol* 1982; 163:367-370.

THE LUTEAL PHASE AND NIDATION IN RELATION TO *IN VITRO* FERTILIZATION TREATMENT

Bernard Lejeune and Fernand Leroy

Human Reproduction Research Unit and IVF Clinic
St. Pierre Hospital
Free University Brussels
Brussels, Belgium

THE implantation process is under strict hormonal control. In most species, progesterone (P) is mandatory for normal nidation.[1] However, while in guinea pigs and hamsters implantation only requires P, in rats and mice it is induced by a rise of estradiol (E2) occurring on day 4 of gestation.[2] This E2 rise entails a biphasic effect on the endometrium involving a receptive phase followed by a refractory state during which implantation remains no longer possible.[3]

In the human, an important secretion of P occurs during the luteal phase together with a moderate hump in the profile of E2 levels. However, no direct argument in favor of an obligatory role of this E2 rise in implantation is available so far. Gorillas[4] and chimpanzees[5] disclose similar endocrine profiles after ovulation but most other monkeys studied hitherto show low and stable levels of E2 during the luteal phase.[6-8]

By contrast, P is necessary for maintaining pregnancy in our species as indicated by the detrimental effect of corpus luteum ablation in early pregnancy[9] and by the abortive action of the antiprogesterone mifepristone (RU-486).[10,11]

THE LUTEAL PHASE IN *IN VITRO* FERTILIZATION CYCLES

Inadequacy of the luteal phase has been identified as a causal factor in infertility and preclinical abortion since the late 1940's.[12] However, the prevalence and clinical significance as well as diagnostic methods and treatment of luteal phase defects have remained controverted issues (for a review see ref. 13).

The diagnosis of this condition still rests on endometrial morphology[14] but this method is hardly applicable to cycles involving embryo replacement. On the other hand, low P levels have been correlated with endometrial criteria of luteal inadequacy and with unexplained infertility.[15-18] Luteal phase duration appears to be equally important since the tendency to have short luteal phases has been found associated with high rates of preclinical abortion.[19]

These different criteria for luteal defects, however, are difficult to apply to *in vitro* fertilization (IVF) cycles. P and E2 levels are far greater in stimulated than in spontaneous cycles, i.e., at least 4 to 5 and 8 to 10 times higher, respectively, in the early luteal phase. Therefore, the E2 to P ratio is elevated and luteal phase defects cannot be defined in terms of absolute E2 and P levels.

This situation might be related to asynchronic development of follicles within the recruited cohort. Small follicles would seem to be weakly sensitive to LH because of their reduced numbers of LH receptors[20] and to go on secreting an excess of E2 after the LH surge or hCG injection. Under stimulation, cases of polycistic ovarian disease are characterized by the growth of numerous small follicles and the occurrence of a premature LH surge. In such cases, an elevated E2 to P ratio is also observed in the preimplantation period. These endocrine anomalies are found to entail a decreased rate of ongoing IVF

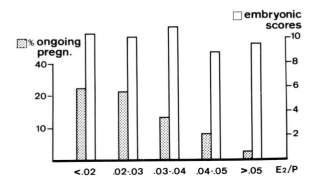

Figure 1. Embryonic scores and pregnancy rates in relation to E2 to P ratio on luteal day 3.

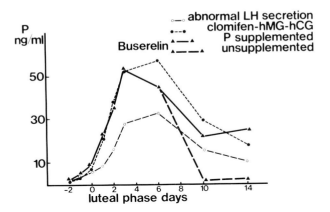

Figure 3. P levels during luteal phases of IVF cycles according to different protocols of stimulation and luteal supplementation.

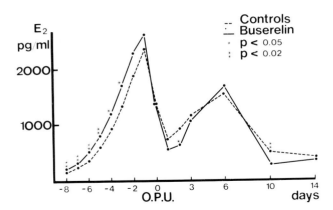

Figure 2. E2 levels during IVF trials under classical Clomiphen-hMG stimulation (controls) or Buserelin inhibition with hMG stimulation. Day 0 = oocyte pickup.

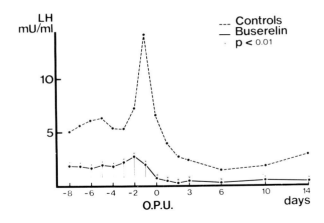

Figure 4. LH levels during IVF cycles effected under Clomiphen-hMG-hCG (controls) of Buserelin-hMG-hCG treatment.

pregnancies[21,22] whereas embryonic vitality scores[23] remain similar along the whole range of the E2 to P ratio (Fig. 1).

In keeping with these data, are the well-known efficacy of an excess of postovulatory estrogen for pregnancy interception[24] and the unfavorable influence of a high E2 to P ratio on the implantation rate in laboratory rodents.[25]

A relative excess of E2 in the early luteal phase appears morphologically correlated with underdevelopment of the "nuclear channel system" and of giant mitochondria in epithelial and glandular cells of the endometrium.[26]

The use of a GnRH analogue (Buserelin) in IVF cycles entails values of the E2 to P ratio in the early luteal days that are lower than those observed after classical clomid-hMG stimulation (Fig. 2).

This difference might explain the better results that are allegedly obtained after pituitary inhibition with this type of drug.[27] Buserelin, however, often induces a drastic shortening of luteal phase duration, more than one third of patients becoming menstruated between days 8 and 10 after oocyte pick-up (OPU) (Fig. 3.).

This shortening is probably related to the downfall of LH levels which occurs after using the analogue and persists during the luteal phase (Fig. 4). Permissive levels of

Table I. *Effects of luteal supplementation with P after IVF in cases with antecedents of luteal defects.*

	Supplemented n=23	Non-supplemented n=25	P
Preovulatory E2 peak (pg/ml)	1850±609	1741±815	N.S.
Nb oocytes retrieved	7.1±2.7	5.7±3.3	N.S.
Vitality score of transferred embryos	12.7±4.6	11.3±4.7	N.S.
E2/P×10³ (luteal day 3)	22.9±18.9	41.0±30.6	<0.02
Ongoing pregnancies	8 (38%)	3 (11%)	
Chemical and aborted pregnancies	2 ⎫ 15	6 ⎫ 22	<0.05
Implantation failures	13 ⎭	16 ⎭	

Table II. *P supplementation in IVF pregnancies associated with low E2 (<200 pg/ml) on luteal day 10. (percent in parentheses.)*

Pregnancies	Supplemented	Not Supplemented	P
Ongoing	9 (43)	3 (13)	
Aborted	5 (24)	6 (25)	<0.05
Biochemical	7 (33)	15 (63)	

Table III. *P supplementation in IVF pregnancies associated with low E2 (<200 pg/ml) on luteal day 14. (percent in parentheses.)*

Pregnancies	Supplemented	Not Supplemented	P
Ongoing	5 (18)	3 (7)	
Aborted	7 (25)	20 (46)	0.05 - 0.1
Biochemical	16 (57)	120 (46)	

Table IV. *P supplementation in IVF pregnancies with low E2 (<200 pg/ml) on luteal day 17. (percent in parentheses.)*

Pregnancies	Supplemented	Not Supplemented	P
Ongoing	3 (14)	0 (0)	
Aborted	4 (19)	2 (9)	0.05 - 0.1
Biochemical	14 (67)	20 (91)	

LH have indeed been shown to be necessary to maintain corpus luteum function in primates.[28,29]

USEFULNESS OF LUTEAL SUPPORT IN IVF CYCLES

In many IVF programs the luteal phase is sytematically supported by repeatedly injecting either hCG or P. However, only a few studies have been published so far on this topic and none has been able to show any significant increase of success rates attributable to such policy. Most studies were conducted on small series, showing only a nonsignificant general trend to better results under suppletive treatment.[30-35] A meta-analysis of these different investigations has been performed but no benefit of luteal supplementation could be demonstrated.[36]

However, according to our own data there would be a place for P treatment in IVF patients burdened with luteal phase defects. This would be especially true for cases showing an imbalance of E2 to P ratio in the preimplantation period and also for the group tending to have shortened luteal phases. These anomalies are observed in about 20% of IVF cycles carried out under classical Clomiphen-hMG stimulation.

We were able to conduct a prospective randomized study on luteal supplementation with high doses of P (100 mg/day) in a group of patients having shown either a short luteal phase, low P levels, or an E2 to P ratio over 0.04 in a previous IVF cycle. The overall percentage of pregnancies remained similar but ongoing pregnancies were significantly more numerous in the supplemented group despite the smallness of the sample (Table I).

From a retrospective study on 449 embryo replacements without any luteal supportive treatment it appeared that low P levels (i.e., below 5 ng/ml) on day 10 after OPU were almost always associated with E2 values below 200 pg/ml. These trials also entailed a normal overall pregnancy rate (22%) but yielded only a very low proportion of ongoing pregnancies (4%). It is impossible from these data to determine whether the low steroid levels are involved in the cause, or are the consequence, of pregnancy demise. However, when comparing the fate of pregnancies obtained from cycles with low E2 (below 200 pg/ml) on day 10 of the luteal phase, in relation to the random application (21 cases) or abstention (24 cases) of P treatment, it was observed that the ongoing pregnancy rate was significantly better among P-supplemented cases (Table II).

The effect of P support is no longer significant among cases with low E2 levels (below 200 pg/ml) observed on days 14 and 17 (Tables III and IV).

On the whole these observations suggest that luteal defects evidenced before or around day 10 are probably primary ones and can be corrected by luteal support. Failed corpus luteum rescue occurring after day 10 is probably secondary to the existence of an abnormal conceptus. However, two cases were observed out of 200 ongoing IVF pregnancies in which E2 levels remained below 200 pg/ml until 8 weeks of gestation. P support was maintained in these cases until 10 weeks of amenorrhea allowing further normal evolution of pregnancy.

CONCLUSIONS

As in almost all species, human implantation requires vast amounts of P to be secreted after ovulation. By contrast, the necessity of a simultaneous elevation of E2 levels is far from demonstrated and excessive estrogen secretion in the early luteal phase appears even detrimental to implantation.

In IVF, different stimulation protocols may induce various disturbances of the luteal phase such as relative hyperestrogenism and drastic shortening in duration. Relative hyperestrogenism of the early luteal phase induces morphological anomalies of the endometrium and reduces the ongoing pregnancy rate in IVF in association with an increase of biochemical pregnancies and implantation failures. Shortening of the luteal phase observed after treatment with GnRH analogues seems to have a similar effect and is probably due to the drop of LH secretion. This latter persists after OPU and is even more marked during the luteal phase.

Luteal supplementation by daily intramuscular injections appears useful when applied after treatment with a GnRH analogue (Fig. 3) or to a sub-population with antecedents of luteal phase defects. These latter cases, however, are diluted in the general population. Therefore, indiscriminate application of suppletive treatment to every IVF patient tends to blur any beneficial effect obtained in selected cases.

Acknowledgment

The data presented in this review were collected thanks to financial support from the Belgian Fund for Medical Research.

References

1. Marcus GJ, Shelesnyak MC. Steroids in nidation. In: Briggs MH, ed. *Advances in steroid biochemistry and pharmacology.* New York: Academic Press, 1970; 2:373-440.
2. Finn CA, Martin L. Endocrine control of implantation. *J Reprod Fertil* 1973; 39:195-206.
3. Psychoyos A. Hormonal control of ovo-implantation. *Vitams Horm*, 1973; 31:201-256.
4. Hodges JK, Hearn JP. The prediction and detection of ovulation: applications to comparative medicine and conservation. In: Jeffcoate SL, ed. *Ovulation: Methods for its prediction and detection.* New York: John Willy & Sons Ltd., 1983:103-122.
5. Lasley BL, Hodges JK, Czekala NM. Monitoring the female reproductive cycle of great apes and other primate species by determination of estrogen and LH in small volumes of urine. *J Reprod Fert* 1980; Suppl. 28:121-129.
6. Knobil E. On the control of gonadotropin secretion in the rhesus monkey. *Rec Progr Horm Res* 1974; 30:1-46.
7. Martel D. Récepteurs de l'oestradiol et de la progestérone et préparation utérine à l'implantation de l'oeuf. *Thèse de doctorat.* Paris, 1981.
8. Aidara D, Badawi M, Tahiri-Zagret C, Robyn C. Changes in concentrations of serum prolactin, FSH, oestradiol and progesterone and the sex skin during the menstrual cycle in the mangabey monkey. *J Reprod Fert* 1981; 62:475-481.
9. Csapo AI, Pulkinen M. Indispensability of the human corpus luteum in the maintenance of early pregnancy. Luteectomy evidence. *Obstet Gynecol Survey* 1978; 33:69-81.
10. Herman W, Wyss R, Riondel A, Philibert D, Teutsch G, Sakiz E, Baulieu EE. Effet d'un stéroïde antiprogesterone chez la femme: interruption du cycle menstruel et de la grossesse au début. *Contracept Fert Sex* 1982; 10, 6:389-393.
11. Lahteenmaki P, Rapeli T, Kaariainen M, Alfthan H, Ylikorlala O. Late postcoital treatment against pregnancy with antiprogesterone RU-486. *Fertil Steril* 1988; 6-8.
12. Jones GS. Some newer aspects of management of infertility. *J Am Med Assoc* 1949; 141:1123-1129.
13. McNeely MJ, Soules MR. The diagnosis of luteal phase deficiency: a critical review. *Fertil Steril* 1988; 50:1-15.
14. Balash J, Van Rell JA, Creus M, Marquez M, Gonzalez-Merlo J. The endometrial biopsy for diagnosis of luteal phase deficiency. *Fertil Steril* 1985; 44:699-701.
15. Radvanska E, Swyer GIM. Plasma progesterone estimations in infertile women and in women under treatment with clomiphene and chorionic gonadotropin. *J Obstet Gynaecol Br Comm* 1974; 81:107-112.
16. Jones GS, Aksell S, Wentz AC. Serum progesterone values in the luteal phase defects: effect of chorionic gonadotropin. *Obstet Gynecol* 1974; 44:26-31.
17. Gautray JP, De Brux J, Tajchner G, Robel P, Mouren M. Clinical investigation of the menstrual cycle. III Clinical, endometrial and endocrine aspects of luteal defect. *Fertil Steril* 1981; 35:296-303.
18. Smith SK, Lenton EA, Cooke ID. Plasma gonadotropin and ovarian steroid concentrations in women with a short luteal phase. *J Reprod Fert* 1985; 75:363-365.
19. Cline DL. Unsuspected subclinical pregnancies in patients with luteal phase defects. *Am J Obstet Gynecol* 1979; 134:438-444.
20. Hillier SG, Ross GT. Independence of steroidogenic capacity and luteinizing hormone receptor induction in developing granulosa cells. *Endocrinology* 1978; 102:937-946.
21. Gidley-Baird A, O'Neill C, Sinosich MJ, Porter RN, Pike IL, Saunders DM. Failure of implantation in human in vitro fertilization and embryo transfer patients: the effects of altered progesterone/estrogen ratios in human and mice. *Fertil Steril* 1985; 45:69-74.
22. Lejeune B, Camus M, Deschacht J, Leroy F. Differences in the luteal phases after failed or successful in vitro fertilization and embryo replacement. *J In Vitro Fertilization* 1986; 3:358-363.
23. Puissant F, Van Rysselberge M, Barlow P, Deweze J, Leroy F. Embryo scoring as a prognostic tool in IVF treatment. *Human Reprod* 1987; 2:705-708.
24. Morris JM, Van Wagenen G. Interception: the use of post-ovulatory estrogens to prevent implantation. *Am J Obstet Gynecol* 1973; 115:101-105.
25. Walton EA, Huntley S, Kennedy TG, Armstrong DT. Possible causes of implantation failure in superovulated immature rats. *Biol Reprod* 1982; 27:847-852.
26. Dehou MF, Lejeune B, Arijs C, Leroy F. Endometrial morphology in stimulated in vitro fertilization cycles and after steroid replacement therapy in cases of primary ovarian failure. *Fertil Steril* 1987; 48:995-1000.
27. Neveu S, Hédon B, Maris P, Bringer J, Arnal F, Deschamps F, Cristol P, Humeau C. Expérience en fécondation in vitro d'un agoniste de GnRH: la Busereline. *Contracept Fert Sex* 1987; 15:774-777.
28. Knobil E. On the regulation of the primate corpus luteum. *Biol Reprod* 1973; 8:246-256.
29. Hutchinson JS, Zelesnik AJ. The rhesus monkey corpus luteum is dependent on pituitary gonadotropin secretion throughout the luteal phase of the menstrual cycle. *Endocrinology* 1984; 115:1780-1784.
30. Mahadevan M, Leader A, Taylor O. Effects of low dose human chorionic gonadotropin on corpus luteum function

after embryo transfer. *J In Vitro Fertil* 1985; 2:190-194.
31. Leeton J, Trounson A, Jessup D. Support of the luteal phase in *in vitro* fertilization program: results of controlled trial with intramuscular proluton. *J In Vitro Fertil* 1985; 2:166-169.
32. Yovich JL, McColm SC, Yovich JM, Matson PL. Early luteal serum progesterone concentrations are higher in pregnancy cycles. *Fertil Steril*, 1985; 44:185-189.
33. Trounson A, Howlet D, Rogers P, Hoppen MO. The effect of progesterone supplementation around the time of oocyte recovery in patients superovulated for *in vitro* fertilization. *Fertil Steril* 1986; 45:532-535.
34. Belaisch-Allart J, Testart J, Fries N, Forman RG, Frydman R. The effect of dihydrogesterone supplementation in an IVF programme. *Human Reprod* 1987; 2:183-186.
35. McBain JC, Clarke GA, Molloy D, Yeates J, Johnston WIH, McKenna M. A randomized trial of progesterone support following ovarian stimulation with clomiphene-hMG for IVF and GIFT. *Fifth World Congress on In Vitro Fertilization and Embryo Transfer.* Norfolk, Virginia, 1987; abstract 126.
36. Daya S. Efficacy of progesterone support in the luteal phase following *in vitro* fertilization and embryo transfer: meta-analysis of clinical trials. *Human Reprod* 1988; 3:731-735.

Index

A
Abembryonic pole, 14
Adherens junctions, 13
Adrenodoxin, 209
Alprazolam, 20
Amnion matrix, 57, 59, 60, 62-72
Antibodies, 72, 154, 156, 173, 191, 198, 221
Antiluteolysins, 17, 28, 75, 78
Antiluteolytic factor, 75
Antimesometrium 127, 145, 146, 191
Apoptosis, 105-115
Arachidonic acid, 80
Attachment, 47, 51
Autocrine, 159, 213

B
β-lactoglobulin-related secretory proteins, 153, 159
bTP-1, 25-28
Baboon, 152-160, 196
Badgers, 191
Big bang, 2-4, 7
Binucleate cells (BNC), 117
Blastocoel, 11, 13, 14
Blastocyst, 11, 13, 55, 75
    attachment, 17, 31
    energy metabolism 39-43
    expansion, 13, 14
    formation, 13
    implantation, 117, 191, 196
    orientation, 51
    positioning, 50
    spacing, 49-50, 191
Blastomere, 12
Bonnet monkey, 196

C
CAMs, 83
Caruncles, 75, 117
Catechol estrogen, 135
Cell asynchrony, 11
Cell culture
    ovine endometrial cells, 75
Cell surface, 220
Chimpanzee, 48, 196
Chorionic gonadotropin, 196
Conceptus, 14, 173
    derived proteins, 25
Corneal matrix, 61-72

Corpus luteum, 189, 191, 192, 201
    autonomy, 203
    endocrine control of, 202
    prolactin inhibition of, 203
    rescue, 25, 195, 196
Cotyledons, 117
Cow, 25, 48, 52, 117-123, 191
Cultural evolution, 1
Cyclic AMP, 210-211, 213
Cycloheximide, 32, 156
Cynomolgus monkey, 195
Cytochrome P-450scc, 209
Cytocortex, 11
Ctyokeratin, 14, 77
Cytoskeleton, 11
Cytotrophoblast, 209-216

D
Decidua, 12, 127-133, 145, 151-161, 173
Decidual
    cells, 31, 41, 55, 127, 145
    cell response, 17, 48, 50
    cell morphology, 127-133
    crypt, 127
    function, 151
    luteotropin, 145
    protein, 145
    tissue, 49
Decidualization, 36, 47, 135-139, 145, 151, 191, 195
Deer, 122, 190
Desmosome, 11, 13, 77
Donor oocyte, 231

E
Early pregnancy factor (EPF), 19, 20
Electron microscopy, 51, 57-58, 60-62, 70-77, 99-100, 225-230
Embryo, 25, 31, 47, 219
    growth factors, 175
    metabolism, 40
    mouse, 39-43
    peri-implantation, 171
    post-implantation, 171
    pre-implantation, 17, 18
Embryonic
    axis, 14
    knob, 51
    mediators, 25-30
Endocrine
    pre-requisites for implantation, 231

Endometrial
    cells, 75-80
    function, 151
    protein secretion, 152-162
    ultrastructure, 231
    vascular permeability, 135
Endometrium, 12, 17, 18, 31, 39, 75-80, 135, 152, 195
Epithelial cells, 75, 31-36, 39, 47-48, 61, 75-80, 105-115
Epithelium, 31-37, 64, 65
    trophoblast interaction with, 96
Estrus, 20
Estradiol, 17, 31-36, 154, 156, 180
Estrogen, 31-37, 78, 136, 195, 196
Expanding universe, 2-3
Extracellular matrix (ECM), 55-72, 83

F
Ferrets, 191, 192
Fetomaternal cell fusion, 117-123
Fetomaternal interface, 171, 173
Fetoplacental unit, 191
Fibroblast, 57, 71, 154
Fibronectin, 19, 57, 77, 83

G
Giant cells, 102, 173
Glucose metabolism, 40-41
Glycocalyx, 52, 77, 98
Glycoproteins, 18
Goat, 48, 117-123
Golgi, 110
Growth factors, 175
Guinea pig, 48, 51

H
Histamine, 18, 135, 195
Horse, 48
Human, 48, 52, 55, 60, 75, 152, 154, 191, 195, 227, 231
    chorionic gonadotropin (hCG), 56, 209
    evolution, 5-6
    secretory proteins, endometrium, 152
Hydroxysteroid dehydrogenase, 18

I
Iloprost, 19
Immune response, 48, 49, 173
Immune system, 172
Immunohistochemical studies, 77, 85, 154, 156
Immunohistocompatibility, 185
Immunosuppression, 190
Implantation, 17, 31-37, 42, 47, 55, 117, 135, 219, 231
    adhesion, 48, 49
    apposition, 48, 49
    central, 48
    chamber, 71, 105
    delayed, 51, 191
    displacement, 83
    eccentric, 48
    fusion, 83
    invasive, 48, 51, 83
    interstitial, 48
    models for establishing hormonal requirements of, 197-198
    site in mouse uterus, 106
    window, 17, 231, 238
Indomethacin, 173
Inflammation, 48
Inflammatory response, 105
Insulin-like growth factor binding protein, 154-160
Interferons (IFNs), 26-28, 78
In vitro models
    cell cultures
        human tissue, 83-89
        isolated endometrial cells, 75-81
        stromal cells, 75
    of implantation, 84
        rodents, 55
        sheep, 75
        humans, 83
IVF, 231

L
Lactogens, 122
Laminin, 85
Lectins, 220
Leukotrienes, 138
Light microscopy, 97
Luteal implantation factor, 191
Luteal phase, 239-244
Luteolysins, 28

M
Mammals, 47, 55
Marmosets, 196
Marsupials, 207
Matrix
    human amnion, 62
    Matrigel, 57, 59, 60-72, 77
    rat corneal, 59

vascular smooth muscle cell, 59
Membrane proteins, 221
Menstrual cycle, 152, 154, 196, 227-229
Menstruation, 47
Mesometrium, 127, 146
Metrial gland, 179
Microcarrier beads, 77
Microvilli, 59, 61, 65, 117
Mink, 191
Morphology, 12, 68, 127, 209-210
Morula, 11
Mouse, 48-52, 55, 56, 58, 59, 60-62, 105, 127
mRNA, 27, 28, 34, 36, 37
Mustelid carnivores, 191

N
Necrosis, 105, 114
Nidation, 47, 83, 191, 239
Nidatory
    estradiol, 31-37
    estrogen, 52

O
Orientation, 47, 49, 51
Origin of life, 4-5
Oviduct, 189-190
oTP-1, 25-28, 78-80, 185-186
Ovine trophoblast, 75-80
Ovum, 47

P
Paracrine action, 75, 157, 159, 213
Peri-implantation, 152, 171-178, 195
Post-implantation, 171-178, 196
Pre-implantation, 75, 173
Phospholipid, 19
Pig, 47, 48, 49, 52, 191
Placenta, 47, 48, 50, 85, 86, 117, 151
Placentation
    chorio-allantoic, 55
    epitheliochorial, 55, 151
    hemochorial, 55, 151
    yolk sac, 55
Plasminogen activators, 85, 89
Plasminogen activator inhibitors, 89
Platelet-activating factor, 139
Polarity, 11-12, 59, 61, 68, 77
Pregnancy, 225
    -associated proteins, 156
    establishment of, 19, 75-80, 192, 195

    maintenance of, 189, 192, 195, 197
    maternal recognition of, 19, 25, 185
Primary decidual zone (PDZ), 106, 112, 163-169
Primates, 151, 195
Prolactin, 154, 201
Prolactin-like hormone, 145, 179
Progesterone, 17, 18, 31-36, 49, 51, 78, 154, 180, 195, 196, 209
    action, 219
    effect on
        blocking further ovulations, 190
        decidual formation, 191
        oviductal functions, 189
        proteins regulated by, 152
        uterine contractility, 190
        uterine physiology, 190
Programmed cell death, 48, 113
Prostaglandins, 75, 135-139, 195
    PGF, 27, 75
    PGE, 18, 27, 28, 75, 77-78, 191
    synthesis, 78
Proteins, 18, 25, 32-36, 83
    decidual, 146, 151-162
    oTP-1, 75
    kinase, 209
    membrane, 221
    secretory, 75, 151-162
    stage-specific, 18
    synthesis, 78
Proteoglycans, 83

R
Rabbit, 48, 50, 52, 105
Rat, 31-36, 48, 52, 56, 59, 60-72, 105, 127, 145, 149, 191, 225
Receptivity (see under Uterine)
Relaxin, 50, 191
Rhesus macaque, 152, 197
RNA, 32
Rodents, 49, 51, 191
Ruminants, 117-123 (see also sheep, cow, goat, horse, ewe)

S
Science and Theology, 7
Secretory proteins (see under proteins)
Sheep, 25, 50, 75, 117-123
Species variation, 47, 49
Spotted skunks, 191, 192
Steroids, 18, 75, 156, 179, 191-192, 195, 197
Stroma, 31-37, 155, 156

Stromal cells, 17, 31-37, 62-72, 77
Syncytium, 48

T
Tammar, 201
Tight junction, 11, 12-13
TIMP, 89
Trinucleate cells (TNC), 119, 120
Trophectoderm, 13, 75
Trophoblast, 47-52, 55, 58, 62-72, 83, 210-316
    cAMP, 213
    cells, 105, 185
    hemotropic invasion, 95
    knob structure, 96, 101
    morphology, 210-211
    mouse, 58, 60
Trophoblastin (see oTP-1)
Tumor metastasis, 185

U
Ultrastructure, 12
Urokinase, 89
Uterine
    epithelial cells, 55, 105-115
    fluid, 39
    lumen, 39, 225, 227
    metabolism, 39
    microvasculature, 39
    prereceptive, 31-32
    receptivity, 31-32, 195, 219-224, 226, 231
    stromal cells, 56, 67-72
Uteroglobulin, 190
Uterus, 47, 219
    surface properties, 97

V
Vascular permeability, 50

W
Weasels, 191
Window (see implantation)

XYZ
Zona pellucida, 51, 56, 117
Zonular occludens (see tight junction)
ZO-1, 12-13